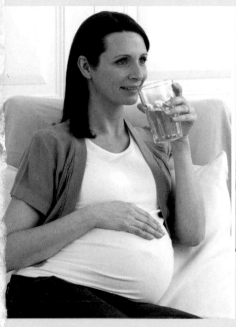
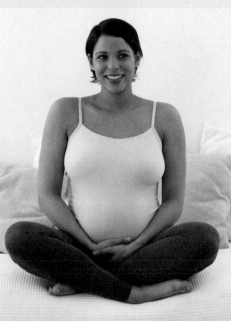
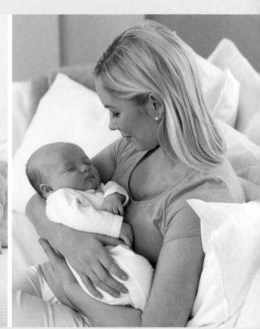

my
Pregnancy

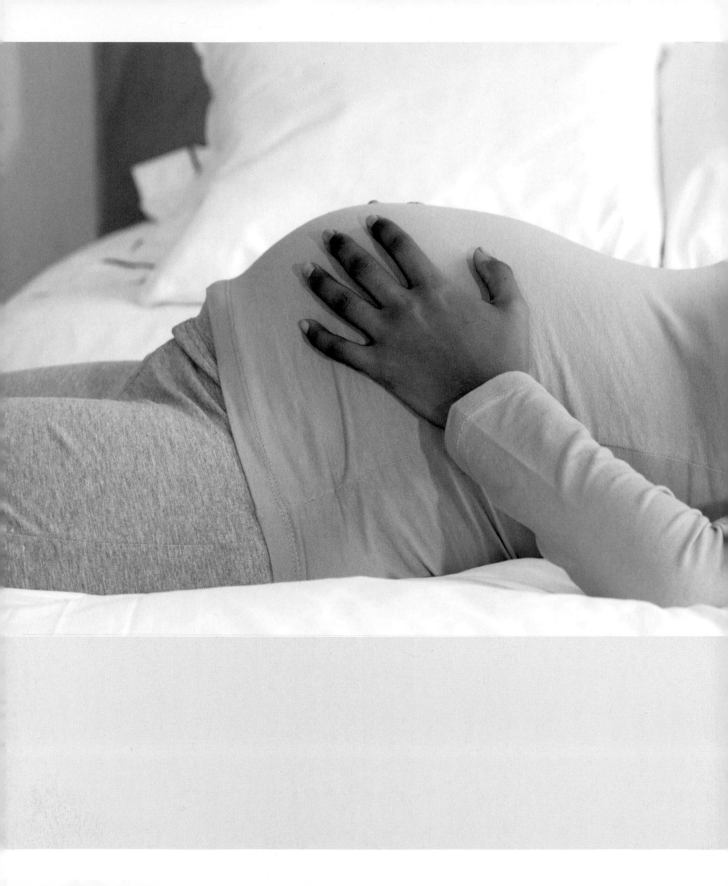

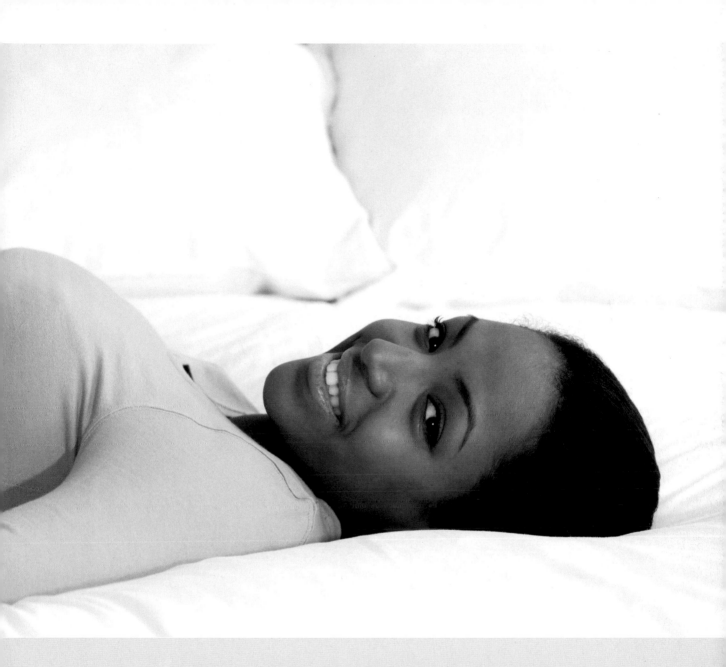

my
Pregnancy
Canadian Edition

Project Editors Claire Cross, Emma Maule
Canadian Editor Barbara Campbell
Editor Beth Landis Hester
Designers Hannah Moore, Wendy Bartlet
Senior Editor Amanda Lebentz
Senior Art Editors Sara Kimmins, Anne Fisher
Editorial Consultant Karen Sullivan
Consultant Editor Lisa Fields
Managing Editor Penny Warren
Managing Art Editors Glenda Fisher, Marianne Markham
Publisher Peggy Vance
Art Directors Peter Luff, Lisa Lanzarini
Production Editor Ben Marcus
Creative Technical Support Sonia Charbonnier
Senior Production Controller Man Fai Lau
Photography Vanessa Davies

First Canadian Edition, 2012

Dorling Kindersley is represented in Canada by
Tourmaline Editions Inc.
662 King Street West, Suite 304
Toronto, Ontario M5V 1M7

12 13 14 15   10 9 8 7 6 5 4 3 2 1

001–183441–Mar/2012

Published in Great Britain by Dorling Kindersley Limited.

Library and Archives Canada Cataloguing in Publication
My pregnancy / general editor, Virginia
Beckett. -- 1st Canadian ed.
Includes index.
ISBN 978-1-55363-176-7
1. Pregnancy--Popular works. 2. Childbirth--Popular
works. 3. Infants--Care--Popular works. I. Beckett, Virginia
RG525.M9 2012   618.2   C2011-904864-7

DK books are available at special discounts when purchased in bulk for corporate
sales, sales promotions, premiums, fund-raising, or educational use. For details, please
contact specialmarkets@tourmaline.ca.

Printed and bound in Singapore by Tien Wah Press

Discover more at
www.dk.com

Contents

Ready for pregnancy?

My health and lifestyle

My prenatal care

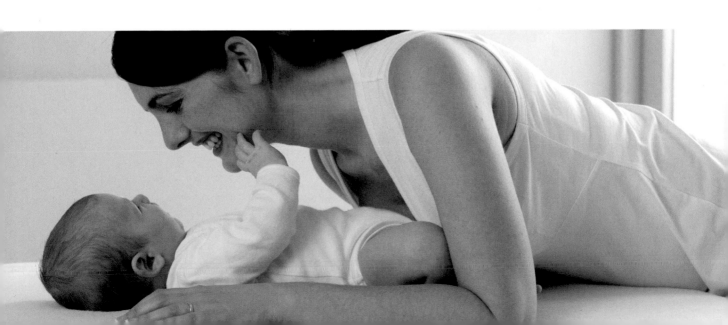

My pregnancy calendar

Preparing for motherhood

My labor and birth

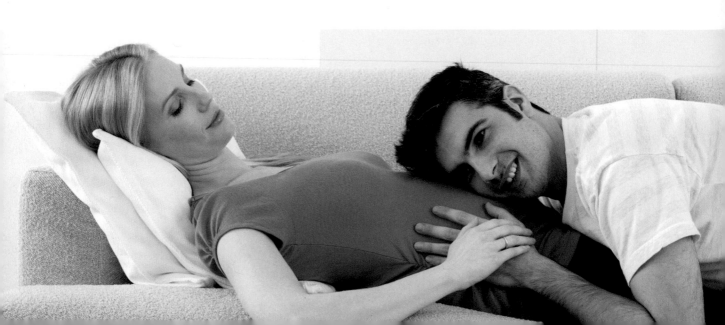

My new baby and me

My first weeks as a mom

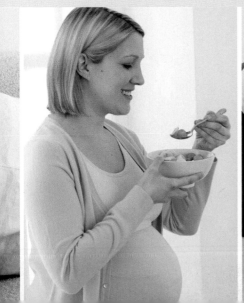
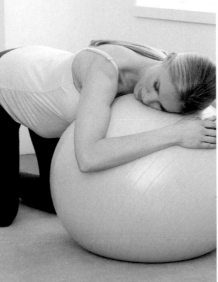
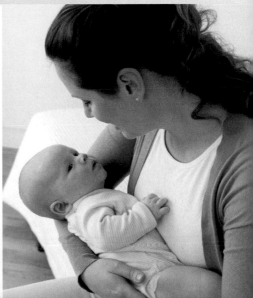

Foreword

Our book offers a different perspective on pregnancy. Not only is each contributor an expert in their field, we are all moms. We have experienced the excitement and uncertainty of pregnancy and the need for reliable information. We hope that by sharing with you the stories of our pregnancies and the early days with our babies, as well as our professional knowledge, you will gain the confidence that you will need over the coming months.

We firmly believe that you are the expert on your pregnancy. Perhaps it doesn't feel like that right now. Even though I had planned to conceive, when I first found out that I was pregnant, I was overwhelmed with the enormity of what was about to happen to me. I'd been a practicing obstetrician for a few years by then, which gave me some insight, but actually living through the ups and downs of pregnancy myself was different! So, you can know quite a lot about pregnancy, and still feel a bit shaky about the coming months—and that's before you even think about parenthood!

When I see moms-to-be in my day-to-day practice, it concerns me that so many of them don't really understand much of what is happening to them. Pregnancy and childbirth often seem shrouded in mystery, partly because of the terminology that health professionals use. A century ago, women would have grown up having witnessed women in labor at home. Modern obstetrics and midwifery have made

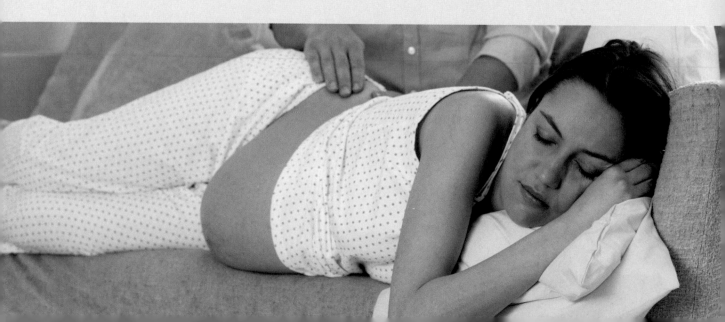

pregnancy much safer but perhaps have moved this life event "behind closed doors." Let us—two obstetricians, a midwife, a dietician, a fitness expert, a psychologist, and a pediatrician—enlighten you on the realities of pregnancy, and share with you our combined experience.

We hope to be your companions for your pregnancy, pointing you in the right direction but giving you the confidence to make your own choices. We aim to explain the changes that will happen to your body, to guide you through the care you will receive and all the different health professionals you may meet, to help you stay in the best of health throughout your pregnancy, and to achieve the delivery that is right for you. We'll take you through your pregnancy, step-by-step, so that when you have to make decisions for you and your baby, you have all the information you need to do so right at hand.

You are embarking on the amazing adventure that is parenthood. We're with you every step of the way.

Virginia Beckett

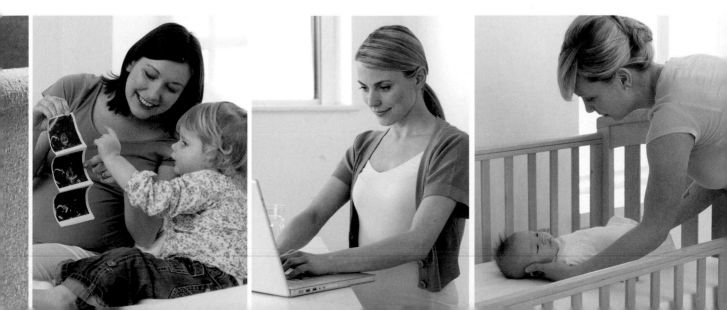

Meet your experts

Introducing our seven moms, all professionals in their own fields, who have pooled their expertise and experience to help you through every step of your pregnancy, from conception right up to your baby's birth—and beyond.

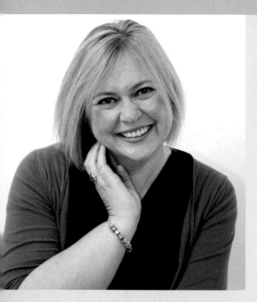

Dr. Virginia Beckett

Dr. Virginia Beckett has worked as an obstetrician and gynecologist for 19 years. She is now a consultant in one of the busiest maternity units in the UK, in Bradford, Yorkshire. She specializes in caring for women with high-risk pregnancies, and runs a satellite IVF unit.

Being particularly interested in fertility, she helps many couples at the pre-conception stage, improving their chances of a successful and healthy pregnancy.

Virginia strongly believes in a team approach to patient care, with a well-informed patient at the center of the team. It was partly as a result of this firmly held principle that Virginia began to work with the UK's Health Education Authority on its pregnancy publications.

MEDIA WORK
Virginia was medical editor for HEA's *The Pregnancy Book,* and contributed to *Birth to Five,* both of which were given free to women in England in their first pregnancy. She was also medical advisor for *The Rough Guide to Pregnancy* (Rough Guides, 2010). She is a spokesperson for the UK's Royal College of Obstetricians and Gynaecologists (RCOG) and regularly comments on reproductive health in newspapers and magazines, as well as on the radio and television.

Virginia has a son, Rowan, and a daughter, Lydia. Virginia worked through both her pregnancies, then took extended maternity leave. She has experienced full-time and part-time working as a parent. These experiences help her enormously as she guides the women she cares for through their pregnancies. Her aim is to help women achieve the best pregnancy and labor possible for them and their babies.

Talking about her involvement with this book, Virginia says, "I am passionate about empowering women by providing them with all the information that they need to make the right choices for them and their babies. Producing this book with other like-minded women has been a real pleasure."

"Producing this book with other like-minded women has been a real pleasure"

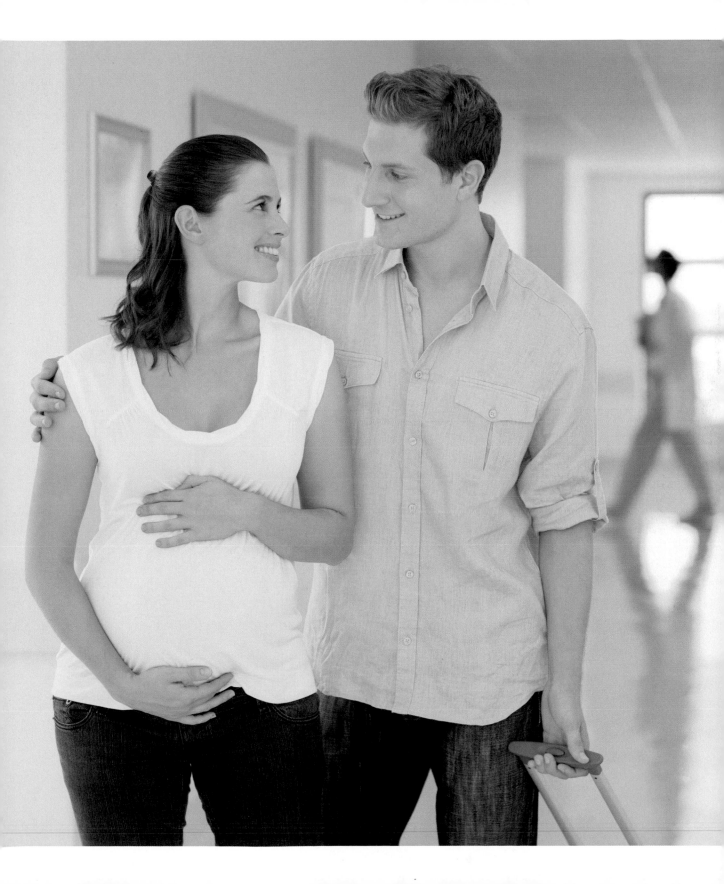

Dr. Moneli Golara

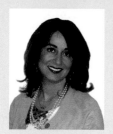

Dr. Moneli Golara is an obstetrician and gynecologist. She has practiced in this field for 20 years, specializing in high-risk and complicated pregnancies. She also undertook two years in clinical research, mainly in conditions such as preeclampsia and prematurity. She now provides care for a large population of pregnant women in north London. She is the mother of two children.

Moneli says, "Pregnancy and childbirth is an overwhelming experience, one that I have been through twice. As well as being the happiest time, it can also bring confusing choices and anxieties.

Pregnant women can feel very vulnerable and need information from reliable sources. By contributing to this book, I hope to help women understand the changes their bodies go through and be able to make informed choices without compromising their safety or that of their babies."

Dr. Laura Jana

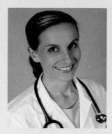

Dr. Laura Jana is an Omaha-based pediatrician and award-winning co-author of *Heading Home with Your Newborn* and *Food Fights*. Laura runs her own company, Practical Parenting Consulting, and is known for her efforts to promote healthy lifestyles for children and offer credible advice to new and expectant parents. She is also a media spokesperson for the American Academy of Pediatrics (AAP) and an expert consultant for various academic organizations and major corporations. Laura is the mother of three children. She is a published children's book author, and an early-literacy advocate. For more about Laura go to www.drlaurajana.com.

Laura says, "Although my own pregnancies were quite a while ago and I had the benefit of medical training, I have always made it a point to remember what it is like for women as they prepare themselves for the miracle of birth and all that follows."

Nikki Khan

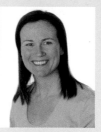

Nikki Khan is a registered and practicing midwife who qualified in 1989. She is the resident expert midwife for *Prima Baby & Pregnancy* magazine, a position she has held since 2001. She is also the expert midwife for popular UK baby products Infacol and Sudocrem, and has worked at Chelsea and Westminster Hospital in London since 1998. She writes a childbirthing blog on her website (www.nikkikhan.co.uk), and she also runs an email and telephone advice hotline.

Nikki had been delivering babies for 17 years before she herself gave birth to her daughter, Nadia.

"Being a midwife and a first-time mother at 40 has given me a wide range of knowledge, which has made me more aware of women's anxieties during pregnancy and childbirth. I hope I can give some pragmatic insight into pregnancy and childbirth, and empower women to make informed decisions about their care."

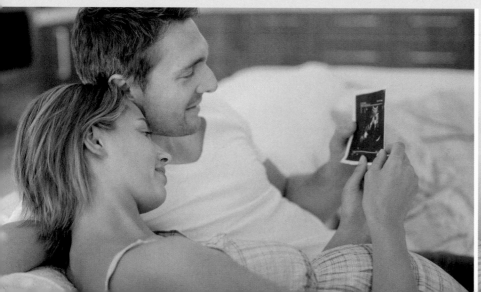

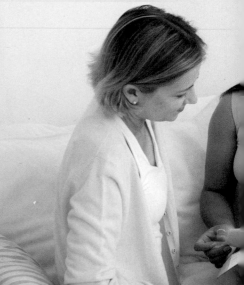

Dr. Claire Halsey

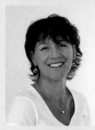

Dr. Claire Halsey is a clinical psychologist of 30 years' standing, working mainly with children and families.

She is also a journalist and author focusing on the areas of child psychology, parenting, and child development. Claire wrote Dorling Kindersley's *Baby Development: Everything You Need to Know* (2012). She has been featured on television as a child-development expert and appears on parentchannel.tv. She is mother to three boys. Her eldest son has had cerebral palsy since birth, so Claire and her family have navigated a range of services to support his health and education.

Claire says, "Having a baby is exciting, moving, and probably involves the steepest learning curve you'll ever experience. I was delighted to contribute to this book, which offers a valuable single resource where parents-to-be can easily find answers to many of their questions."

Tara Lee

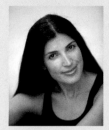

Tara Lee has been practicing yoga for 20 years and teaching yoga for 10 years. She became interested in prenatal yoga while pregnant with her first child. Tara has released three yoga DVDs guiding women through their pregnancies, births, and the transition into motherhood. She has designed a range of yoga clothing for pregnant women, for Blossom.

Tara runs training courses for yoga teachers and birth preparation workshops for couples, as well as teaching privately. She is also a trained doula. Tara has a daughter, Lola, and a son, Jago.

"During my pregnancies I wanted as much information as possible, and read every book I could lay my hands on. Having a baby is the most wonderful experience but it is also exhausting and can seem incredibly overwhelming, which is why I was delighted to contribute to this book so that I can pass on some of my knowledge from my own experiences."

Fiona Ford

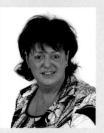

Fiona Ford has worked as a dietitian in the field of maternal and infant nutrition for over 20 years. She was co-director of the Centre for Pregnancy Nutrition (CPN) in the UK, where a national "Eating for Pregnancy" helpline and website were based. The CPN's model is now firmly established within the UK, and used in websites for the Food Standards Agency, BabyCenter, Gurgle, and Wellbeing (RCOG).

Fiona is media spokesperson for maternal and infant nutrition for the British Dietetic Association. She has two grown children, Geraldine and William.

Fiona says, "I feel it's very important to provide pregnant women with sensible, up-to-date information on safe and healthy nutrition, because it is one of the most important factors they can control to ensure the health of their babies. In this book, I wanted to help guide women through pregnancy and prepare them for motherhood."

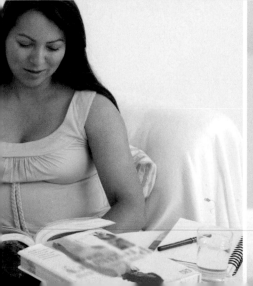

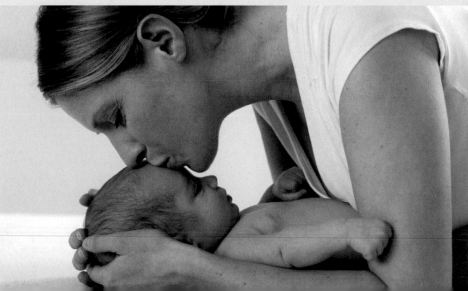

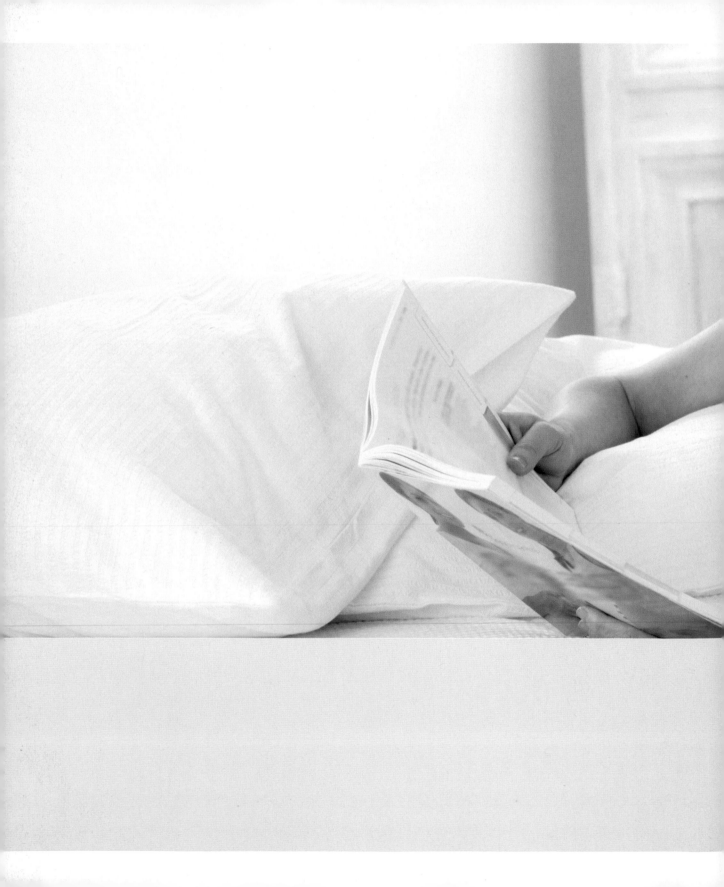

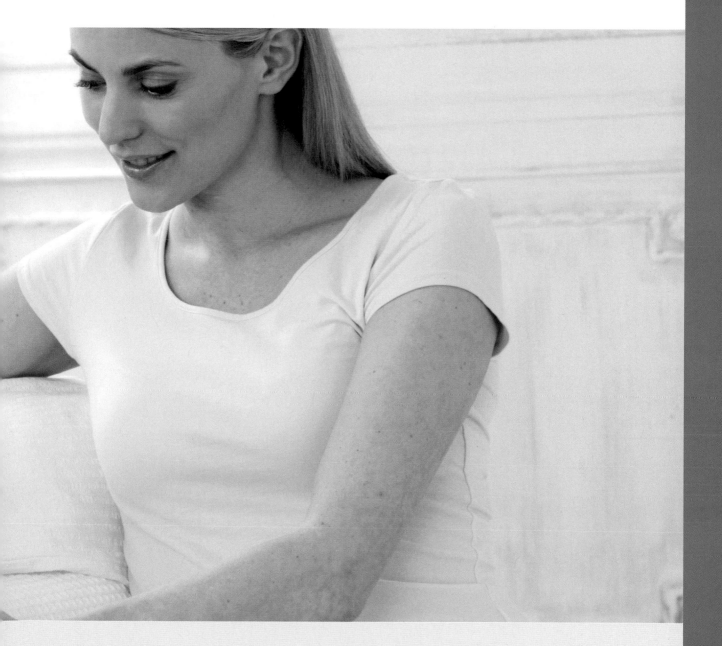

Ready for pregnancy?

You can't plan for everything, but by preparing emotionally, physically, and practically to start a family, you're taking the best approach.

I want to be a mom

The decision to have a baby is probably one of the most exciting and emotionally charged of your life. However, bringing up a baby is a lifelong commitment, and there are important issues to consider before you try to become pregnant.

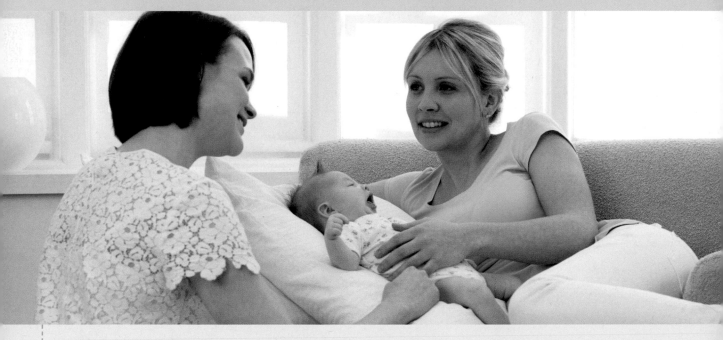

IS MOTHERHOOD FOR ME?
Talking to friends or family who have recently had a baby about the emotional and financial implications can help you to make the right choices.

Having a baby doesn't just mean making a few adjustments here and there; it changes your life forever in the most profound ways. Caring for a child brings huge responsibilities and, of course, incredible rewards. The best way to prepare for pregnancy and beyond is to think through every aspect of your decision with your partner to make sure you are both equally committed to raising a family. You might want to consider whether the timing is right for you both, and whether your relationship is strong enough to cope with the demands that will be placed upon it. There may be implications for your careers, and there will certainly be practical and financial issues to discuss and plan for. The better you can sort your lives out beforehand,

the more relaxed and enjoyable your pregnancy is likely to be. That said, it's also true that if you delay having a child until the timing is exactly right, the "perfect" moment may never come. So for some couples, it's a case of just "jumping in." And, while you may have some control over when you have a baby, there are biological factors involved. After about 35, female fertility decreases, so it may be more difficult to become pregnant (see pp.28–29).

Your relationship

In trying to reach your decision about whether to have a baby, ask yourself questions about your relationship. Is now the right time for you both? Are you and your partner prepared for an inevitable change in lifestyle? If either partner feels coerced or not quite ready to commit, is it better to postpone having a baby for a while? Also consider your motivation. Is this baby an expression of your love or is there an element of hope that this might mend a relationship that is struggling? If your partner does not share your desire for a baby, then becoming pregnant is likely to lead to distrust and resentment.

Even if you are both in agreement that you want a baby, there are still many issues that need to be sorted out ahead of time. Do you agree about how you want to bring up your baby? How do you feel about discipline? What are your views on nutrition? How might you share the workload of caring for a baby—for example, will your partner get up to give bottles at night?

PRACTICAL ISSUES

Before starting a family, it's a good idea to consider practicalities, such as your finances, work, and housing. Having a child is expensive and an ongoing commitment that is not going to diminish as your child grows older. Talk to other couples who already have a family to try to find out what having a baby actually costs. You'll need all sorts of equipment: a crib, car seats, stair gates, clothing, diapers, toys. How will you manage if one of you decides to stay at home as a full-time caregiver?

If you plan to return to work after having a baby, then you should have a plan for childcare. Whether it is your parents, your partner's parents, a combination of the two, day care, nannies, or au pairs, you need to think about the various options and the costs.

Think about whether your house is suitable for a baby. For example, is it near a busy road? If so, you may need to take safety measures such as installing a fence or gate. Where will your baby sleep? Although it is recommended that she sleeps in your room at first (to protect against sudden infant death syndrome, see p.357), she'll soon need her own room.

HOW WILL YOU COPE?

Finally, spend some time thinking about your own well-being. Are you ready for another person to be completely dependent on you and are you willing to give up some of your own independence? Many women swear that having a baby won't change their lifestyle. But inevitably it does: Even the simplest trip to the supermarket may require major organizational skills!

It is also worth considering what help and support from friends and relatives you may need, and whether it is available to you.

> "It's a good idea to consider practicalities, such as your finances, work, and housing"

Is there ever a perfect time?

One of the most common questions I get asked by my friends is when the best time is to have a baby. Well, there never is a perfect time. Women often wait for the "right" time, whether it is because of their careers, relationships, or other factors. Don't put it off for too long. Our bodies are at their optimal reproductive stage until our mid 30s. Once you pass this stage and approach the late 30s to early 40s, not only does your fertility decrease, complications in pregnancy increase. If having a baby is in the cards, then I would say it should be a priority. Your career can always wait. I see so many women who seek advice for fertility because they left it too late. MG

I think this very much depends on one's circumstances, since there's no question that having a baby represents a major life change and overhaul of one's daily routines. My husband and I met in medical school and got married during our residency (first year out of medical school). While no one I know thinks that getting pregnant during residency is a great idea, neither is it going to be easy after you finish your medical training and move, or start a new job. Unless my husband and I had decided to wait an additional eight-plus years to finish all of our training (and associated moves), and settle into a new city and a new job, there simply wasn't a good time (much less the perfect time). So we decided we'd just figure things out when the time came. That time came only two months after we started trying, when I became pregnant for the first time. Yes, it was a juggle when we had my daughter six months before I finished my residency in pediatrics (complete with every third or fourth night spent at the hospital). And it was even more of a juggle when we had our second less than 16 months after the first, and our third a total of three-and-a-half years after our first. Having made it through the blur of the first few years of parenthood (sleep deprivation and all), I can still say that we wouldn't have wanted it any other way. LJ

Is my body ready?

An important part of planning a pregnancy is to recognize that your own health affects your baby from the day you are pregnant (and then through childhood). Improving your health also boosts your chances of becoming pregnant.

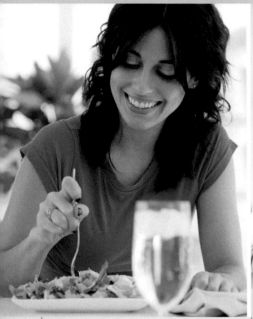

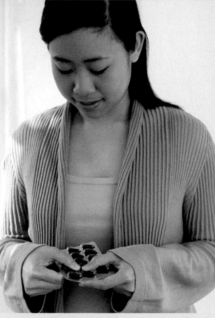

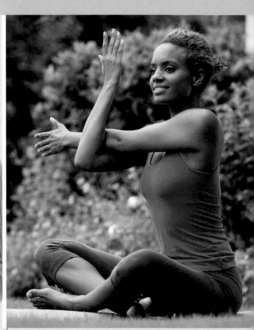

THINK ABOUT YOUR DIET
Maintaining your health by eating a nutritious and varied diet will increase your chances of becoming pregnant.

TAKE FOLIC ACID
The B vitamin folic acid is essential for your baby's healthy development. Start taking it before you try to conceive.

KEEP EXERCISING
Exercise will help you to get fit and stay fit for the rigors of pregnancy and labor. Being in shape will make giving birth easier.

To give your baby the best start in life and to optimize your own health, you should get your body into peak condition before you try to conceive. You should be eating a healthy, balanced diet. If you are overweight, aim to begin a sensible weight-loss program. Look at your lifestyle. Smoking, alcohol, and drugs (including some prescription drugs) can be very dangerous to a developing fetus, and can also interfere with fertility. It's a sensible precaution to limit your exposure to chemicals in the home, and if you have concerns about workplace hazards, you should discuss them with your employer. Pre-pregnancy blood and urine tests can tell you whether you need to be immunized or have an infection that requires treatment.

Diet and activity

The best diet for optimal health is a varied one that supplies you with the nutrients you need. About 40–50 percent of your diet should come from unrefined carbohydrates (such as whole-grain breads, cereals and pastas, and colored rices) and fruits and vegetables. This will not only supply you with the slowly released energy that you need, but also good levels of fiber to promote healthy digestion. Aim for two portions of good-quality whole grains with each meal, and at least seven different fruits and vegetables every day. The other important elements of your diet are proteins (lean meat, legumes, nuts, and seeds) and dairy produce (milk, cheese and yogurt). Fat is also important, but the types you choose are crucial. Avoid all trans fats, and focus on the healthy fats found in nuts, avocados, olives, and oily fish. Many of these are excellent sources of essential fatty acids (see p.51), which promote optimal health. Avoiding junk food, such as cookies and soda, will help stabilize your blood sugar levels. There are some foods that should be avoided altogether (see pp.54–55).

WEIGHT CONTROL

Being a healthy weight is important before conception. To find out whether you are in a healthy range you need to know your body mass index (BMI). If your BMI is over 25, you are overweight; a BMI of 30 or more means that you are obese. If you are overweight, it may be more difficult to get pregnant. Obesity puts you at greater risk of complications during pregnancy, labor, and delivery, and there is a greater risk of wound infection after a caesarean. Stillbirths and premature births are higher in women who are obese.

If you are overweight, and especially if you are obese, you should try to lose weight before becoming pregnant. Consult your doctor for advice or ask to be referred to a weight-loss program.

FITNESS

Exercising regularly and maintaining fitness are important for everyone, but especially if you are planning to become pregnant. The more active you are now, the easier it will be to stay active during pregnancy. In addition, regular exercise can help you to achieve or stay at a healthy weight, can help reduce stress (which may help fertility), and can make childbirth easier. Experts recommend that you exercise moderately for 30 minutes a day, 4 days a week. You can break down activity into 10-minute slots. If you haven't been very active before, start slowly. You'll find it easier to exercise if you choose activities that you enjoy. Building activity into your daily life is a great way to increase exercise levels: For example, get off the bus one stop early and walk, use the stairs instead of the elevator, and walk or bike for short trips.

Remember that you don't necessarily need to join a gym and follow a strict routine. In fact, now is not the time to enter into an intensive program. There is evidence that overly vigorous exercise can reduce fertility, especially in women with low body fat.

Your emotional well-being

When you consider your health in preparation for pregnancy, don't forget that your emotional well-being can play a part in how soon you conceive. Studies have shown that depression, stress, and anxiety can make it more difficult to become pregnant. Review your mood and stress levels, and, just as you are working to be in top physical form, take steps to improve your frame of mind and reduce stress in your life. You could use self-help strategies such as relaxation methods, yoga, and meditation. Setting aside regular time to de-stress, spending some time outdoors in the fresh air, and engaging in exercise can all help give you a mental boost.

If you have experienced difficulties with depression or anxiety in the past, you may be more vulnerable to problems associated with childbirth, such as postpartum depression. Begin to build up a supportive network of friends. If you feel down for more than a few weeks and this is getting in the way of your everyday life, ask your doctor for help.

Folic acid supplements

Start taking folic acid before you get pregnant and throughout your pregnancy.

WHY SHOULD I TAKE FOLIC ACID?
Folic acid is a vitamin that occurs naturally in certain foods. You need a good supply of folic acid when you are pregnant to help with the development of your baby. If you take folic acid pills in early pregnancy, you reduce the risk of having a baby born with a neural tube defect, such as spina bifida. There is also evidence that folic acid reduces the risk of having a baby born with a cleft lip and palate or a heart defect, and that it also makes pre-term labor and miscarriage less likely. You can buy folic acid at your local pharmacy, either as a stand-alone dietary supplement or as a component of multivitamins.

The usual dose is 0.4 to 1 milligram a day. If you have an increased risk of having a child with a neural tube defect, then the dose is 5 milligrams a day, for which you need a prescription. You are at higher risk if: you are obese; a previous pregnancy was affected by a neural tube defect; you or your partner has a neural tube defect; you are taking medication for epilepsy; or you have celiac disease, diabetes, sickle cell anemia, or thalassemia. Only ever take more than the usual dose if told to do so by your doctor.

Start from the time you plan to become pregnant and stop using birth control. If the pregnancy was unplanned, start taking folic acid supplements as soon as you find out. A recent study looked at the effect of taking folic acid for a year before becoming pregnant and found a significant decrease in the rate of pre-term delivery.

Environmental hazards

If you think your job may pose a risk to your pregnancy, you should discuss this with your employer. You may be worried about the effect of chemicals, or about exposure to germs if you work with cats, sheep, or other animals. If you are not yet ready to discuss your plans but you have a health and safety concern at work, go to motherisk.org to find out more information on chemicals and other substances that may harm your developing baby. You'll learn about chemicals that may lead to miscarriage, birth defects, or low birth weight, such as lead and exposure to x-rays, plus ways to protect yourself.

At home, we use many different chemicals, both for household tasks and personal use. In most cases, there is no hard evidence that these chemicals have harmful effects on fertility or pregnancy. However, it is best to minimize exposure: Wear rubber gloves for household tasks and avoid breathing in fumes. Choose products that are recommended for their low environmental impact, since they also contain fewer chemicals (see pp.58–59).

MEDICATIONS

Some medications can be harmful to a developing baby, especially if taken in the early weeks of pregnancy. Therefore, always tell a doctor or dentist who prescribes you medication that you are pregnant or intend to become pregnant. Many medications prescribed to treat long-term problems such as asthma are safe in pregnancy, but some others are not. If you are taking medication, you should always check with your doctor before you try to conceive. In some cases, medication may need to be changed (see pp.24–25).

Ideally, it's best not to take over-the-counter (OTC) medicines, including herbal remedies, while you are trying to conceive or are pregnant. That's not to say you can't use medicine if you're feeling really unwell. But to be on the safe side, check with your doctor, midwife, or pharmacist before taking any medicine. If your doctor thinks you need medicine, she'll be able to recommend a safe prescription drug or the name of a safe OTC medication.

Social habits

Before you start trying for a baby, you should review your social habits and, if necessary, take steps to change them.

QUITTING SMOKING

If you smoke, you are strongly advised to stop smoking before getting pregnant. Tobacco smoke contains poisonous chemicals that pass into your baby's blood and can slow her growth. The risks of miscarriage, premature birth, or stillbirth are higher if you smoke. Babies born to mothers who smoked when pregnant also have an increased risk of developing attention deficit hyperactivity disorder (ADHD) when they are older. Children of smoking parents are at increased risk of sudden

SAFE CLEANING
It's advisable to wear rubber gloves when using cleaning products. Try switching to eco-friendly products, which are likely to contain fewer harmful chemicals.

GIVING UP SMOKING
Nicotine patches may help you quit. Nicotine replacement is still not ideal, but it's better for your baby than cigarettes.

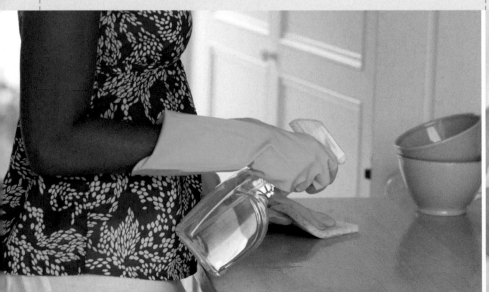

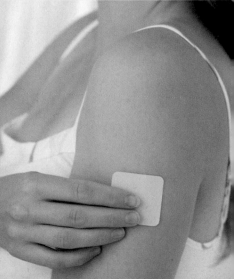

infant death syndrome (SIDS) and are more likely to develop chest infections, asthma, and glue ear. For many women who smoke, planning to become pregnant is a good incentive to stop smoking. It is also often a good time to persuade partners to give up. If you find it difficult to quit smoking, seek advice and help from your doctor or pharmacist.

AVOIDING ALCOHOL

Advice from Health Canada is that you should not drink if you are pregnant or trying to become pregnant. Heavy drinking increases your risk of miscarriage and can cause serious harm to your baby's growth and brain development. A condition called fetal alcohol spectrum disorder (FASD) develops in some babies born to mothers who drink heavily. A baby with this disorder can have severe physical and mental problems. The exact amount of alcohol that is safe during pregnancy is not known. This is why the advice is not to drink at all. If you do choose to drink when pregnant, limit yourself to one

ALCOHOL ADVICE
You may wish to stick to non-alcoholic drinks such as fruit juices during pregnancy, to make sure your baby stays safe.

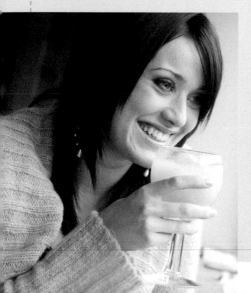

drink on infrequent occasions and try to avoid it entirely for the first 12 weeks, when your baby is most vulnerable. Never binge drink or get drunk. If you find it difficult to cut down or stop drinking, seek help from your doctor.

RECREATIONAL DRUGS

If you use recreational drugs, you are strongly advised to stop before getting pregnant. There is an increasing amount of evidence to suggest that they pose a risk of damage to the baby. Marijuana, for example, has been linked with premature birth and low birth weight. If you cannot stop using drugs, see your doctor for help. A blood test for hepatitis C, hepatitis B, and HIV is advised if you take certain recreational drugs and plan to become pregnant, or are pregnant.

Pre-pregnancy medical checkups

If you have an existing medical problem, such as epilepsy, diabetes, or asthma, it is important that you see your doctor at least three months before you plan to conceive. You may need your medication adjusted or extra monitoring during pregnancy (see pp.24–25).

Even if you are healthy, you may wish to have medical tests before you become pregnant to check your immunity to certain diseases that can harm the developing baby. You can also be screened for infections that could be passed on to the baby or for genetic disorders that could affect your baby.

RUBELLA (GERMAN MEASLES)

Before trying to become pregnant for the first time, you should make sure that you are immune to rubella. The rubella virus causes a mild illness, but can result in

miscarriage or seriously harm your unborn baby, especially in the early stages of growth. Most women are immune to rubella, having been immunized as children or having suffered from the virus. However, childhood immunization does not always work. A blood test can show if you are immune; if not, you can be vaccinated. You should not become pregnant for three months after the injection, and ideally not until your immunity has been confirmed by a further blood test, since the live vaccine can cause abnormalities in the baby.

CHICKEN POX

Contracting chicken pox during pregnancy can cause complications for the mother and for the unborn baby. If you have already had chicken pox (most people have it during childhood), you are immune, and there is nothing to worry about. However, if you're not sure, you can have a blood test to check. If the tests show you are not immune, you can be vaccinated. You will need to wait for three months after the vaccination before trying to conceive.

HEPATITIS B

A mother who is infected with the hepatitis B virus, which causes a liver disease, can easily pass it on to her newborn baby, so babies at high risk are immunized. If you are at high risk of catching hepatitis B you should be immunized before becoming pregnant. This applies if you:
• Have a job in which you may be exposed to people with hepatitis B, such as healthcare worker or employee at a daycare or residential center.
• Inject drugs or share bills or straws for snorting recreational drugs.
• Change sexual partners frequently.
• Live in close contact with someone infected with hepatitis B.

Healthy fatherhood

It's common to overlook how important a man's health is in the process of conception. Men's semen is renewed every three months, so fathers-to-be should make sure they are as healthy as possible before conception.

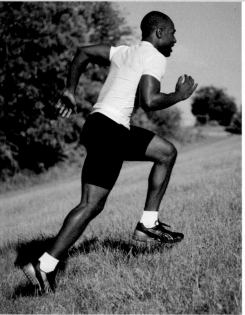

KEEPING FIT
A cardio workout, such as a jog or run, a couple of times a week will keep your partner's heart in good working order.

PEDAL POWER
Cycling is a good form of exercise in moderation—limit it to less than three hours a week to protect against impotence.

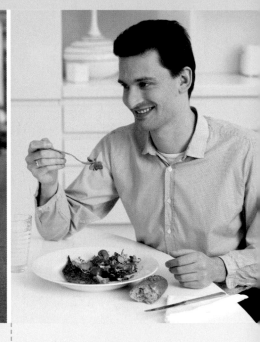

EATING HEALTHILY
Encourage your partner to eat a balanced diet, including proteins and leafy greens, to ensure he is in the best shape to make a baby.

There are many steps a man can take to improve his fertility. Eating a healthy diet with enough vitamins and minerals is vital to ensure that his reproductive system is in tip-top condition. Getting plenty of exercise, not smoking, and avoiding excessive alcohol consumption are also important for his reproductive health. Research suggests that estrogen-like chemicals in many of our foods (such as soy products and beer) and products (such as paints and synthetic cleaners) can damage sperm production. By making careful choices, your partner may boost his fertility. Some nutritional supplements can also be beneficial in improving fertility. Of course, if you and your partner have been trying to conceive for a long period without success, a doctor should check you both to rule out treatable medical conditions.

Diet and exercise

Your partner should eat plenty of fresh fruits, vegetables, whole grains, and legumes to boost his fertility. He also needs to maintain a healthy weight. Obese men can have a reduced sperm count and lowered testosterone levels. Encourage your partner to exercise; doing so enhances fertility by keeping weight at a healthy level and relieves stress and anxiety. However, excessive amounts of exercise (marathon running and associated training) can lead to a lowered sperm count. If your partner is unsure of the type of exercise that's best for him, a trainer can recommend an exercise program to help improve his weight and fitness levels.

Smoking can have an impact on male sperm count, so if you are trying for a baby you both should encourage each other to stop smoking. Binge drinking, heavy alcohol consumption, anabolic steroids, and using recreational drugs can also reduce male fertility.

To produce a large amount of sperm, the testes need to be kept at a lower temperature than the rest of the body. For this reason, men who are trying to start a family are advised to avoid hot baths and Jacuzzis and use showers instead. Boxer shorts are better than briefs, and men should avoid sitting or driving for long periods of time.

BOOSTING FERTILITY

The average man today has half the sperm of his counterpart 50 years ago, and it is of poorer quality. This is believed to be caused by exposure to chemicals that mimic the effects of estrogen. Your partner can prevent or minimize the impact of these chemicals by avoiding plastic containers for storing food or water; using non-bleached paper products; eating organic food and using organic toiletries; and avoiding hormone-containing animal or dairy products. Eating lots of foods high in antioxidants, such as green leafy vegetables, kale, carrots, citrus fruits, broccoli, and cauliflower, may help to counteract the damaging effects of these chemicals.

Nutritional supplements can help boost fertility. The most important of these are vitamin C and zinc.

The male reproductive system

A man's testes—two oval-shaped glands—produce sperm that fertilize a woman's egg during conception. The testes also make testosterone, the male sex hormone. Only at puberty do these glands become active. The testes lie outside the body in a pouch called the scrotum, where they can stay at the best temperature for producing sperm—about 5.5°F (3°C) lower than body temperature. Inside each testis are many folded vessels called "seminiferous tubules," where sperm are made. Thousands of sperm are produced every second, each one maturing as it travels through the tubules. The sperm then pass into the epididymis, a coiled tube that lies on top of each testis, where they finish maturing and are stored. The whole maturation process takes two and a half to three months.

A man's penis is made up of columns of spongy tissue. During sexual arousal, these fill with blood and the penis becomes hard so that it can enter the woman's vagina. Just before ejaculation, sperm are squeezed out of the epididymis and travel along a long, looped tube called the vas deferens, and then into the urethra, the tube that leads to the outside.

Along the way, several glands, including the prostate, add secretions to the sperm, providing them with energy and nutrients. At the moment of ejaculation, the sperm and secretions (together known as seminal fluid) are ejected from the man's body.

MALE ORGANS
The testes are housed outside of the main part of the male's body, in a sac called the scrotum, which sits behind the penis.

SPERM UP CLOSE
Healthy sperm have oval heads and long tails, which work together to propel them forward.

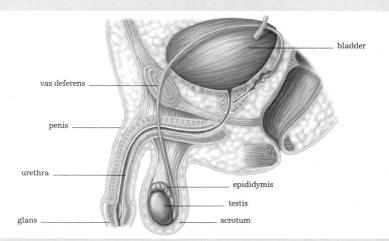

- bladder
- vas deferens
- penis
- urethra
- glans
- epididymis
- testis
- scrotum

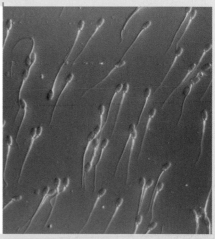

My health concerns

Having a health problem such as asthma or high blood pressure does not mean that you cannot have a healthy pregnancy and a normal, healthy baby. However, you may need careful management to minimize possible risks to you or your baby.

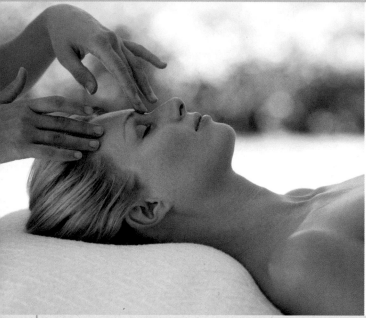

MASSAGE AWAY MIGRAINES
You may find that a soothing head massage can help with migraines. Having a massage may also help to generally relieve stress, which can be a migraine trigger.

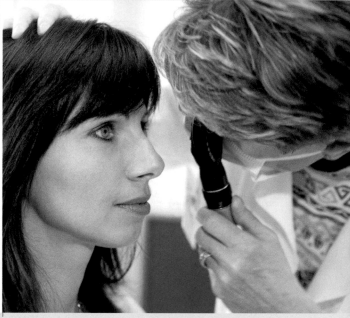

GET YOUR EYES TESTED
If you have diabetes, it is recommended that you have regular eye exams throughout your pregnancy, because diabetic eye problems can develop or increase at this time.

If you have an existing health problem and are planning to have a baby, you should make an appointment with your doctor, ideally before conceiving.

Planning ahead

Your treatment may need to be tailored so that your condition is well controlled, making complications less likely. If you are taking medication, you may need to change to a different one and you may require extra tests or ultrasounds during

pregnancy. Before you conceive, make sure that all your routine screenings, such as Pap smears or blood pressure checks, are up to date.

ASTHMA
It's important for a healthy pregnancy that your asthma symptoms stay under control. Uncontrolled asthma poses a risk to your health and increases the chance of your baby having a low birth weight. As soon as you know you are pregnant, see your doctor for advice. You should keep on taking your prescribed

asthma treatments through pregnancy. Unless symptoms become worse, you don't need to make any changes. Symptoms of worsening asthma include: a cough that's worse at night, early in the morning, or during exercise; wheezing; breathlessness; and tightness in the chest. Symptoms can be made worse by acid reflux—leakage of stomach acid back up into the gullet (esophagus). If you have any of the symptoms listed above or you have reflux, speak to your doctor. Your self-management should mean that you can adjust your asthma treatment as necessary, for example by increasing your "controller" (inhaled steroids) medication if you have a cough or cold. This is safe during pregnancy. To minimize asthma attacks, don't smoke and try to avoid triggers, such as pet dander, pollen, or dust mites.

DIABETES

If you have diabetes, whether it's type 1 or type 2, get advice from your doctor or specialist before trying to conceive.

Like all women planning to have a baby, you'll be advised to take folic acid supplements to prevent your baby from being born with a neural tube defect such as spina bifida, in which the spinal column fails to close. Because the risk of such defects is higher for babies born to diabetic women, you'll need to take a much higher dose than usual—your doctor will prescribe the right amount.

Having diabetes increases your risk of miscarriage, and means that your baby is at greater risk of a high delivery weight (which can make labor and birth more difficult), respiratory problems at birth, heart and other birth defects, jaundice, and low blood-sugar levels.

Diabetes also increases your risk of pregnancy complications and complications associated with diabetes, including problems with vision, called diabetic retinopathy. However, by controlling your blood sugar levels you greatly reduce the likelihood of these problems occurring. This means taking care with your diet and monitoring your blood sugar levels accurately and often. Remember that the most harm to a baby happens in the early weeks of pregnancy, so it is vitally important that you maintain normal blood sugar levels if you are planning to get pregnant.

During pregnancy you will have more frequent prenatal visits, additional ultrasounds, and extra blood tests to monitor your blood sugar.

EPILEPSY

If you have epilepsy and are planning to get pregnant, it is extremely important that you talk to your doctor before you conceive. Some of the drugs used to control seizures carry a small risk of causing physical defects in your developing baby. These include neural tube defects such as spina bifida, heart defects, and cleft lip and palate. However, by planning ahead, these risks can be minimized. The majority of pregnant women with epilepsy have healthy pregnancies and give birth to healthy babies.

Your doctor's aim will be to minimize the risks to your baby while making sure your epilepsy is well controlled. This may involve changing your medication or lowering the dose. If you take drugs to control your epilepsy, you'll be advised to take a high daily dose of folic acid (your doctor will prescribe the right dose) as soon as you start trying for a baby. This may help prevent neural tube defects, such as spina bifida. Anti-epileptic drugs interfere with the absorption of folic acid by the body, which is why you need a high dose.

When you're pregnant, the anatomy scan at 18 to 20 weeks will check for any problems with your baby's development such as a cleft lip and palate. You may need extra blood tests to check the levels of anti-epileptic drugs in your blood.

MIGRAINES

The best way to treat migraines while you are trying to conceive and during pregnancy is to avoid them. Many women find that they can reduce the number of attacks simply by getting an adequate amount of sleep, eating regularly, and avoiding known triggers, such as chocolate and smoke. Stress can also be a trigger, so you may want to consider self-help measures such as yoga or massage. If these measures are not

sufficient and you feel you need some pain relief, talk to your doctor first. If you are given your doctor's go-ahead, it should be okay to take acetaminophen during pregnancy for occasional headaches. If acetaminophen doesn't work, your doctor may prescribe a different medication.

HIGH BLOOD PRESSURE

If you are taking medication for high blood pressure, talk to your doctor before you get pregnant. Some drug treatments are not recommended during pregnancy, and you may need to switch to different medication. It is important to keep your blood pressure under control during pregnancy, because high blood pressure can be dangerous for you and your baby. During pregnancy, you'll have frequent tests to check your blood pressure. Taking drugs to lower blood pressure can reduce blood flow to the placenta and affect your baby's growth, so you may have additional ultrasounds during your pregnancy to make sure she is growing normally.

DEPRESSION

Research suggests that some drugs used for treating depression are not safe to use during pregnancy. However, untreated depression during pregnancy may be harmful to you or your baby, increasing the risk of pre-term labor and low-birthweight babies. Therefore, if you suffer from depression and are planning to get pregnant, you need to get advice about the best way to control this during your pregnancy. If you are already taking anti-depressant drugs, you should never change your dose or stop them unless you have discussed the change with your doctor. Make an appointment to discuss your medication with your doctor at the earliest opportunity, and preferably before you start trying to conceive.

My menstrual cycle

A woman's monthly cycle, from the first day of her period to the day before her next period, is known as the menstrual cycle. A period, or menstruation, is the shedding of the lining of the uterus (endometrium) accompanied by bleeding.

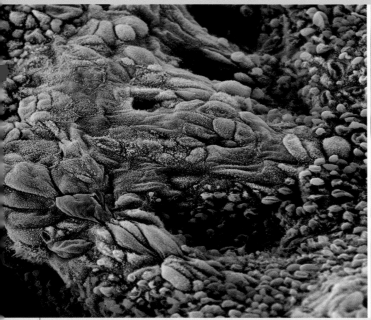

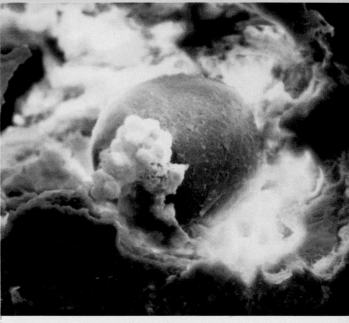

LINING OF THE UTERUS
The tissues of the lining of your womb (known as the endometrium) are shed monthly in response to the hormonal changes of your menstrual cycle. These then grow back until your next period.

EGG BEING RELEASED
Roughly once a month, an egg (or sometimes two) will be released from your ovaries into the fallopian tube. If fertilization does not occur, it will be expelled from your body during your next period.

During the menstrual cycle, an egg in one of the ovaries ripens and is released into a fallopian tube, while the lining of the uterus thickens in preparation for pregnancy. If the egg is fertilized, it will implant into the uterine lining and begin to grow. If it is not fertilized, the egg will be expelled when the uterine lining is shed.

The average length of the menstrual cycle is 28 days. However, only 10–15 percent of women have cycles that are exactly this length, with cycles normally ranging from about 25 to 35 days.

Menstrual cycles tend to be more irregular during the teenage years and after the age of 40.

Hormonal phases

The menstrual cycle is regulated by hormones. Luteinizing hormone (LH) and follicle-stimulating hormone (FSH), which are produced by the pituitary gland in the brain, promote ovulation and stimulate the ovaries to produce estrogen and progesterone. The cycle

can be divided roughly into two halves, which are called the follicular phase and the luteal phase.

FOLLICULAR PHASE
This phase begins on the first day of menstrual bleeding (day 1). However, the main event in this phase is the development of follicles in the ovaries. At the beginning of the follicular phase, the lining of the uterus (endometrium) is thick with fluids and nutrients designed to nourish an embryo. If no egg has been fertilized, estrogen and progesterone

levels are low. As a result, the top layers of the endometrium are shed, and menstrual bleeding occurs. While the lining is being sloughed off, the blood vessels in the uterus constrict, which can cause cramp-like pains.

Meanwhile, invisible changes are happening inside one of your ovaries. Under the influence of FSH, follicles (containing immature eggs) begin to develop. As they grow, they secrete estrogen. When levels of estrogen are high enough, a surge of LH completes maturation of an egg and prompts its release from the ovary (ovulation). Although between three and thirty follicles start to develop, usually only one egg matures completely and is released. Ovulation occurs, in an average 28-day cycle, at day 13 or 14. An egg can be fertilized for only about 12–24 hours after its release.

Around ovulation, some women feel a dull pain on one side of the lower abdomen. The pain, called middle pain or "mittelschmerz" as it occurs midway through a cycle, lasts a couple of minutes up to a few hours. The pain is felt on the same side as the ovary that released the egg, but its precise cause is unknown.

LUTEAL PHASE
The luteal phase begins after ovulation. It lasts about 14 days (unless fertilization occurs) and ends just before a menstrual period. In this phase, the ruptured follicle closes after releasing the egg and forms a structure called the corpus luteum, which produces progesterone. This hormone stimulates the uterine lining to thicken further, ready to receive an egg if it is fertilized.

If an egg is not fertilized, levels of estrogen and progesterone fall and the uterine lining starts to break down. The menstrual cycle starts again with bleeding, as tissue and blood from the broken-down lining leave the body.

The female reproductive system

A woman's reproductive organs include: two ovaries where eggs develop, are stored, and are then released; the womb (uterus), where a fertilized egg implants into the endometrium and a pregnancy develops; two thin tubes called fallopian tubes, which connect the ovaries to the womb; the cervix, the lower part of the womb that connects to the vagina; and the vagina, a tube of muscle connecting the cervix to the outside of the body.

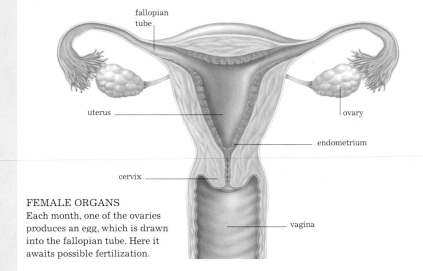

FEMALE ORGANS
Each month, one of the ovaries produces an egg, which is drawn into the fallopian tube. Here it awaits possible fertilization.

An egg's monthly cycle to maturity inside an ovary is shown along the top of the chart (below). It is released from its follicle around day 14, midway through the most fertile phase of your cycle. The bottom of the chart shows the corresponding development of the lining of the uterus—shedding at the start of a period, then rebuilding in preparation for a fertilized egg. If the egg isn't fertilized, it sheds the next time you have a period.

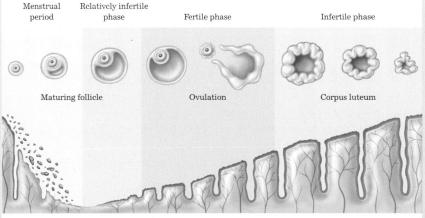

| Menstrual period | Relatively infertile phase | Fertile phase | Infertile phase |

Maturing follicle   Ovulation   Corpus luteum

1 2 3 4 5 6 7 8 9 10 11 12 13 14 15 16 17 18 19 20 21 22 23 24 25 26 27 28
DAYS OF CYCLE

Age and fertility

Greater awareness of the impact of age on a woman's fertility has emerged as more women opt to start their families later. Less well known is the effect of age on male fertility.

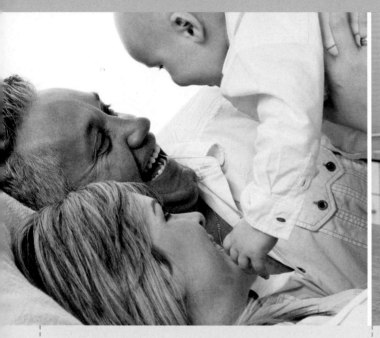

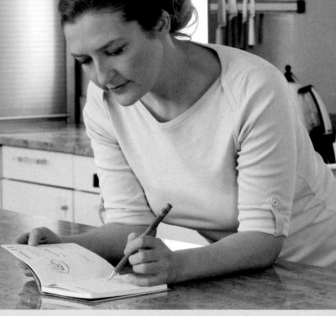

DIFFERENCES BETWEEN MEN AND WOMEN
While female fertility declines beyond the age of 35, men remain able to father a child past 60. However, there is evidence that the offspring of older fathers run an increased risk of health problems.

KEEP AN EYE ON YOUR PERIODS
You may want to record your periods to make sure they are occurring regularly and so you can predict when you ovulate, in order to know when you are at your most fertile.

Fertility in women is at its peak between age 16 and 24. It gradually declines up to the age of 35, then drops dramatically. When you're 40, you are half as fertile as you were at 35. It may take much longer to get pregnant when you reach your late 30s or early 40s, and you may have problems conceiving at all. However, it is important to consider that biological age and physical age are very different in some people. Some women at 30 have a biological age similar to a 25-year-old, and others have a biological age similar to a 40-year-old. This depends on factors such as past and present health, lifestyle, and constitution. Some women conceive naturally at 44 because they are so healthy. As in women, there is much individual variation in men. A man who follows a healthy lifestyle is more likely to maintain his fertility for longer.

Women's fertility

In women, the main reason that fertility decreases with age is a decline in the quantity and quality of her eggs.

A female baby is born with about 1 to 2 million egg follicles (containing immature eggs), but by puberty these will have degenerated to about 300,000. The eggs will also have aged by 12–13 years. During each monthly cycle, an egg (sometimes two) reaches maturity and is released from a follicle, ready to be fertilized. The older a woman is, the fewer eggs she has. The quality of eggs—how prepared the eggs are to develop into embryos—also declines with age. This means there will be fewer good-quality eggs available for fertilization.

WHY EGG QUALITY DECREASES

Egg quality is largely determined by two factors: the number of chromosomes present within a given egg, and the energy available to the egg.

An egg needs to have the right number of chromosomes and should be capable of combining these chromosomes with sperm. Some of your eggs just do not have the right number of chromosomes—this is a natural occurrence—making it impossible to have a successful pregnancy. Eggs require energy to split after fertilization. This is provided by tiny cell components called mitochondria that convert fuel to energy. Mitochondria tend to become less efficient with age. As a result, any egg that is fertilized may run out of energy, which means that it may not be able to divide.

Egg quality determines a woman's ability to get pregnant, as well as to stay pregnant and avoid complications.

An egg that is of poor quality may not properly implant in the uterus even though it has been fertilized. However, eggs that are successfully implanted may not be healthy enough to sustain themselves and will result in miscarriage.

Men's fertility

Men continue to produce sperm throughout life, and it has been assumed that fertility remains the same from puberty until the end of a man's life. However, it seems that, like women, men have a biological clock ticking away their reproductive years. The decline in fertility in men is slower than in women, but the quality and quantity of sperm both decrease with age.

After age 40, a man is likely to take longer to make his partner pregnant, and the risk that she'll have a

miscarriage is also greater. With age, the quantity and motility (ability to move) of a man's sperm decline. As a result, it becomes more difficult for the sperm to fertilize an egg.

One study showed that if the man is under 25, there is about an 8 percent chance that a couple will take longer than a year to conceive; if the man is over 35, this doubles to 15 percent. In addition, women whose partners are over 35 experience more miscarriages regardless of their own age.

This may be due to the build-up of genetic damage in the sperm of older men, leading to rejection of the faulty embryo. These changes aren't as sudden or noticeable as female menopause, but happen gradually over time. Older men are also more likely to develop medical conditions, such as diabetes, that interfere with their libido or ability to get an erection.

Male and female fertility throughout life

As women grow older the likelihood of getting pregnant falls steeply while the likelihood of infertility rises sharply. Male fertility, partially determined by testosterone levels, is also affected by age. Testosterone is always present in men, and rises until the age of 39 (with a small rise then fall during puberty) when it decreases by about a third. In theory, men in their 70s and 80s can father children, but illness and impotence can affect their ability to do so.

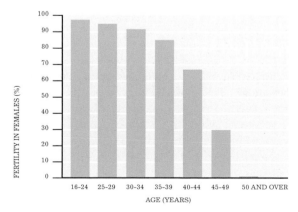

FEMALE FERTILITY
As this chart shows, fertility decreases as a woman gets older. By the age of 50, most women will be unable to have a baby naturally.

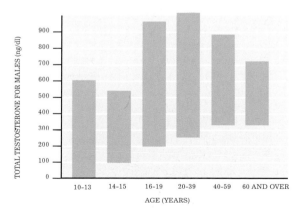

MALE FERTILITY
Testosterone is always present in men and peaks between the ages of 20 and 39, when they are at their most fertile.

When sperm meets egg

Your pregnancy begins when a sperm successfully fertilizes an egg, forming a new cell. For this to happen, the sperm must reach the fallopian tube around the time of ovulation, when one or more eggs are released from a woman's ovary.

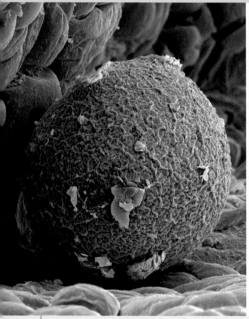

EGG TRAVELING
Once an egg has been released, the sides of the fallopian tube periodically contract, helping the egg to travel toward the uterus.

SPERM TRAVELING
Sperm need to navigate a considerable distance to get to the egg, and they use their long tails to propel themselves.

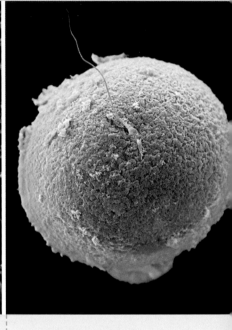

SPERM FERTILIZES EGG
Fewer than 100,000 sperm get into the cervix, only 200 reach the fallopian tubes, and just one can fertilize the egg.

What happens?

Ovulation occurs about midway through a woman's menstrual cycle, and if intercourse has occurred recently, then one of the 100–300 million sperm that have been released may successfully penetrate the outside zone of the egg and fertilize it. Once this occurs, the fertilized egg starts dividing rapidly as it moves down the fallopian tube into the uterus. After about nine days, it implants itself in the uterus and starts developing into an embryo.

OVULATION
Each month, in one of a woman's two ovaries, a group of immature eggs start to develop in small fluid-filled sacs called follicles. Normally, one of the follicles is selected to complete development (maturation). The mature follicle ruptures and releases the egg from the ovary (in the process called ovulation) into the fallopian tube. The egg remains in the fallopian tube and can be fertilized for about 12–24 hours after ovulation. The ruptured follicle develops into a structure called the corpus luteum, which secretes progesterone. This hormone helps thicken the lining of the uterus (endometrium) in preparation for implantation if an egg is fertilized. If an egg is not fertilized, hormone levels fall and the thickened lining of the uterus starts to break down. The lining tissue is shed during your menstrual period.

THE JOURNEY OF SPERM
During sex, a man ejaculates about a teaspoonful (5ml) of semen, containing 100–300 million sperm, into a woman's vagina. The environment is fairly hostile

"At the moment of fertilization, your baby's genetic makeup is complete, including its gender—this is decided by the sperm"

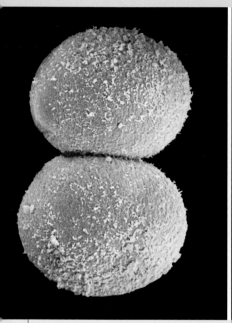

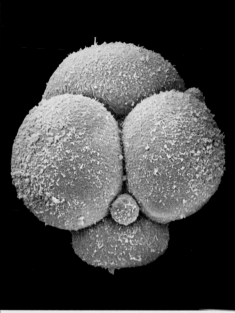

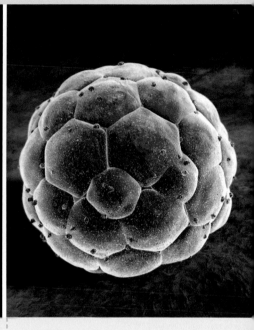

EGG SPLITS INTO TWO
As soon as an egg is fertilized, its cells begin to multiply, dividing first into two cells. The egg is now known as a "zygote."

EGG SPLITS AGAIN
The cells of the zygote split again as it travels down the fallopian tube on its way to the uterus. The trip takes about three to five days.

ATTACHING TO THE UTERUS
When cell division is complete, the zygote becomes a ball of cells known as a blastocyst, which imbeds itself in the wall of the uterus.

to sperm; vaginal secretions are acidic so as to combat bacteria and prevent infections. Cervical mucus also forms a barrier to sperm. During ovulation the mucus becomes more fluid and elastic, making it easier for sperm to get through. Sperm can live up to a week in utero, waiting for the release of an egg.

FERTILIZATION
The first sperm to reach the egg in the fallopian tube binds to its surface, releasing chemicals to help it break through the egg's protective coating.

Once the sperm has penetrated the egg, changes occur in the egg's protein coating to prevent other sperm from entering. The head of the sperm, containing its genetic material, fuses with the nucleus of the egg, forming a single cell.

IMPLANTATION
Within 24 hours after fertilization, the egg (now called a zygote) begins dividing rapidly into many cells as it travels along the fallopian tube. After about three days, it becomes a compact cluster of cells and enters the uterus. Cell division

continues until there is a mass of about 100 cells, known as a blastocyst, which breaks out of its protective covering and embeds itself in the uterine lining. Implantation starts about five days after fertilization and is complete by about day nine. Some women notice spotting (or slight bleeding) for one or two days around the time of implantation. Once the blastocyst is implanted, it starts to produce the hormone human chorionic gonadotrophin (hCG), which stimulates the ovaries to produce hormones that help maintain the pregnancy.

Am I pregnant?

Some women are particularly sensitive to changes in their body and spot signs of pregnancy within a week of conception. Many others do not notice any early signs, and their first clue may be a missed period.

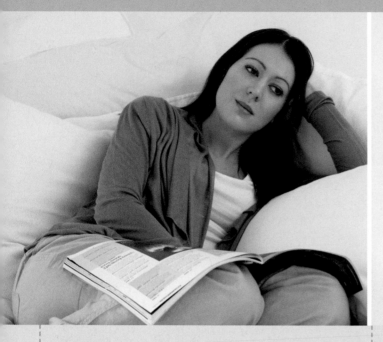

FEELING TIRED
One of the first signs of pregnancy may be utter exhaustion, along with tearfulness and feeling overemotional.

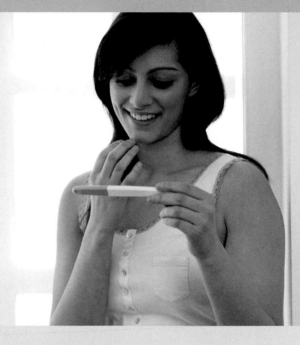

I'M PREGNANT!
A sense of excitement, anticipation, and "mission accomplished" may accompany the confirmation of your pregnancy.

Whenever you first suspect that you might be pregnant, you'll want to find out for sure as soon as possible. You can take a pregnancy test at home quickly and easily from the first day of your missed period.

Early signs

About a week after conception, the embryo pushes itself into the wall of the uterus. This can cause some light bleeding or spots of blood. Some women interpret this as a light period and do not suspect they might be pregnant. You may even get mild stomach cramps while the embryo is moving. Severe stomach cramps may indicate an ectopic pregnancy (see pp.44–45).

As early as one to two weeks after conception, you might notice a difference in your breasts. They might be sensitive to the touch, they may be sore, tingle, or they may change shape and become swollen, so that your bra may not fit as well as normal. These signs are similar to what some women experience just before their period is due, but they are usually much more pronounced.

A missed period is for many women the first indication they might be pregnant. As the embryo embeds into the lining of the uterus, it produces hormones that prevent the lining from breaking down (causing a period). However, women who have irregular periods may not suspect they are pregnant for weeks or even months.

Feeling tired, overemotional, and tearful are common in early pregnancy. Other symptoms you may experience include having to urinate frequently, nausea and vomiting, shortness of breath, constipation, and backache.

PREGNANCY TESTS

If you suspect you might be pregnant, you can take a home test using one of the many pregnancy tests available over the counter. The tests use chemicals that can detect the hormone human chorionic gonadotrophin (hCG) in your urine. This hormone is produced by the implanting embryo and appears in your urine if you are pregnant. You can take a pregnancy test on the first day of a missed period. Some tests claim they can produce results up to five days before your period is due, but these may not be as accurate.

If your test result is positive, you're almost certainly pregnant. However, it is possible to have a positive test result if you've had an early miscarriage, since hCG stays in your body for a few weeks afterwards. If you're worried, seek medical advice. A negative test is less reliable. For example, if you do a pregnancy test too early, you could be pregnant, but there may not be enough hCG in your body to give a positive test result. If you still think you're pregnant after a negative result, wait a week and try again, or see your doctor.

YOUR DUE DATE

Once your pregnancy has been confirmed, you can calculate your due date. Pregnancy is measured as 40 weeks from the first day of your last menstrual period. Although it may seem odd that the time when you had not even ovulated is included, this is done to standardize the duration of pregnancy. The timing of ovulation is different in women, and most women will remember the first day of their last period. Your due date may be changed after your first ultrasound, when the baby is measured accurately.

In a few circumstances, you may be offered a blood test to detect and measure the amount of hCG in your body. For example, if you are having fertility treatment, you may want to check whether it has been successful even before a missed period. This will be discussed with your healthcare experts.

Figuring out your expected date of delivery

To figure out your expected date of delivery (EDD)—also known as the due date—you need to know when you started your last menstrual period (LMP). Look up your LMP date (in **bold** type) on the chart below to discover when your baby is expected. For example, if your LMP was January 13, then your baby will be due on October 20.

January	**1**	**2**	**3**	**4**	**5**	**6**	**7**	**8**	**9**	**10**	**11**	**12**	**13**	**14**	**15**	**16**	**17**	**18**	**19**	**20**	**21**	**22**	**23**	**24**	**25**	**26**	**27**	**28**	**29**	**30**	**31**
Oct/Nov	8	9	10	11	12	13	14	15	16	17	18	19	20	21	22	23	24	25	26	27	28	29	30	31	1	2	3	4	5	6	7
February	**1**	**2**	**3**	**4**	**5**	**6**	**7**	**8**	**9**	**10**	**11**	**12**	**13**	**14**	**15**	**16**	**17**	**18**	**19**	**20**	**21**	**22**	**23**	**24**	**25**	**26**	**27**	**28**			
Nov/Dec	8	9	10	11	12	13	14	15	16	17	18	19	20	21	22	23	24	25	26	27	28	29	30	1	2	3	4	5			
March	**1**	**2**	**3**	**4**	**5**	**6**	**7**	**8**	**9**	**10**	**11**	**12**	**13**	**14**	**15**	**16**	**17**	**18**	**19**	**20**	**21**	**22**	**23**	**24**	**25**	**26**	**27**	**28**	**29**	**30**	**31**
Dec/Jan	6	7	8	9	10	11	12	13	14	15	16	17	18	19	20	21	22	23	24	25	26	27	28	29	30	31	1	2	3	4	5
April	**1**	**2**	**3**	**4**	**5**	**6**	**7**	**8**	**9**	**10**	**11**	**12**	**13**	**14**	**15**	**16**	**17**	**18**	**19**	**20**	**21**	**22**	**23**	**24**	**25**	**26**	**27**	**28**	**29**	**30**	
Jan/Feb	6	7	8	9	10	11	12	13	14	15	16	17	18	19	20	21	22	23	24	25	26	27	28	29	30	31	1	2	3	4	
May	**1**	**2**	**3**	**4**	**5**	**6**	**7**	**8**	**9**	**10**	**11**	**12**	**13**	**14**	**15**	**16**	**17**	**18**	**19**	**20**	**21**	**22**	**23**	**24**	**25**	**26**	**27**	**28**	**29**	**30**	**31**
Feb/Mar	5	6	7	8	9	10	11	12	13	14	15	16	17	18	19	20	21	22	23	24	25	26	27	28	1	2	3	4	5	6	7
June	**1**	**2**	**3**	**4**	**5**	**6**	**7**	**8**	**9**	**10**	**11**	**12**	**13**	**14**	**15**	**16**	**17**	**18**	**19**	**20**	**21**	**22**	**23**	**24**	**25**	**26**	**27**	**28**	**29**	**30**	
Mar/Apr	8	9	10	11	12	13	14	15	16	17	18	19	20	21	22	23	24	25	26	27	28	29	30	31	1	2	3	4	5	6	
July	**1**	**2**	**3**	**4**	**5**	**6**	**7**	**8**	**9**	**10**	**11**	**12**	**13**	**14**	**15**	**16**	**17**	**18**	**19**	**20**	**21**	**22**	**23**	**24**	**25**	**26**	**27**	**28**	**29**	**30**	**31**
Apr/May	7	8	9	10	11	12	13	14	15	16	17	18	19	20	21	22	23	24	25	26	27	28	29	30	1	2	3	4	5	6	7
August	**1**	**2**	**3**	**4**	**5**	**6**	**7**	**8**	**9**	**10**	**11**	**12**	**13**	**14**	**15**	**16**	**17**	**18**	**19**	**20**	**21**	**22**	**23**	**24**	**25**	**26**	**27**	**28**	**29**	**30**	**31**
May/June	8	9	10	11	12	13	14	15	16	17	18	19	20	21	22	23	24	25	26	27	28	29	30	31	1	2	3	4	5	6	7
September	**1**	**2**	**3**	**4**	**5**	**6**	**7**	**8**	**9**	**10**	**11**	**12**	**13**	**14**	**15**	**16**	**17**	**18**	**19**	**20**	**21**	**22**	**23**	**24**	**25**	**26**	**27**	**28**	**29**	**30**	
June/July	8	9	10	11	12	13	14	15	16	17	18	19	20	21	22	23	24	25	26	27	28	29	30	1	2	3	4	5	6	7	
October	**1**	**2**	**3**	**4**	**5**	**6**	**7**	**8**	**9**	**10**	**11**	**12**	**13**	**14**	**15**	**16**	**17**	**18**	**19**	**20**	**21**	**22**	**23**	**24**	**25**	**26**	**27**	**28**	**29**	**30**	**31**
July/Aug	8	9	10	11	12	13	14	15	16	17	18	19	20	21	22	23	24	25	26	27	28	29	30	31	1	2	3	4	5	6	7
November	**1**	**2**	**3**	**4**	**5**	**6**	**7**	**8**	**9**	**10**	**11**	**12**	**13**	**14**	**15**	**16**	**17**	**18**	**19**	**20**	**21**	**22**	**23**	**24**	**25**	**26**	**27**	**28**	**29**	**30**	
Aug/Sep	8	9	10	11	12	13	14	15	16	17	18	19	20	21	22	23	24	25	26	27	28	29	30	31	1	2	3	4	5	6	
December	**1**	**2**	**3**	**4**	**5**	**6**	**7**	**8**	**9**	**10**	**11**	**12**	**13**	**14**	**15**	**16**	**17**	**18**	**19**	**20**	**21**	**22**	**23**	**24**	**25**	**26**	**27**	**28**	**29**	**30**	**31**
Sep/Oct	7	8	9	10	11	12	13	14	15	16	17	18	19	20	21	22	23	24	25	26	27	28	29	30	1	2	3	4	5	6	7

I'm still not pregnant

Pregnancy is easily achieved for some, but requires a bit more effort for others. If you have not conceived as soon as you had hoped, try not to worry. There are positive steps you can take to improve your chances.

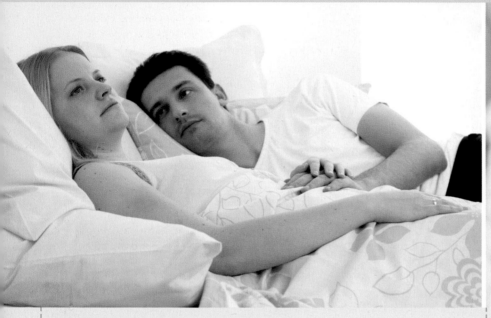

DON'T GIVE UP HOPE
It can take many months to become pregnant, and regular intimacy offers a wonderful opportunity to cement your relationship in advance of becoming parents.

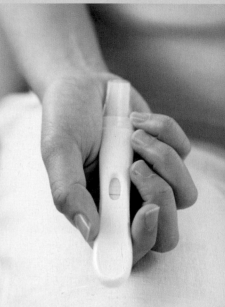

PREDICTING OVULATION
Ovulation predictor kits measure a hormone in your urine that tells you when you are likely to ovulate.

Fertility experts agree that having regular unprotected sex (several times a week) throughout your menstrual cycle is the best way to make a baby. You should ideally be having sex every few days so that there will always be a supply of sperm in the right place whenever you ovulate. For some couples, work commitments and lifestyle can make regular sex difficult. It can be helpful to identify when you ovulate, so you can then try to ensure that you have sex at least once or twice around this time. However, having sex according to a timetable can be stressful. Being relaxed and enjoying your sex life is probably the best way of boosting your chances of conception.

How long will it take?

Most couples who are trying for a baby will conceive within six months. By about one year, 85 percent of couples who have been having regular unprotected intercourse will conceive. It's generally recommended that if you are under 35, you should seek advice after one year of trying; however, if you are over 35, it's probably better to do this after six months.

ENJOYING SEX
Frequent sex is the best way to increase your chances of conceiving. However, when sex becomes merely a means of getting pregnant, your enjoyment—and feelings of intimacy—can suffer. If sex starts feeling like a chore, it's hard to keep up the babymaking pace for long.

You do have the choice to make your lovemaking more passionate, with time spent on foreplay and communicating your needs to each other. Tune in to each other sexually by discussing what you each enjoy, fantasies you may have, or positions you like, and guide each other during sex to make it more enjoyable. Use rooms other than the bedroom or have sex at a different time of day.

Much of the pleasure of sex is in the intimacy of the act; it is created by your thoughts and emotions as well as the physical sensations you experience. Spend time on intimacy for its own sake, which may not lead to sex. Try massage, simply holding hands, romantic meals together, or sharing stories from the beginning of your relationship. These remind you that you have a loving bond and that sex is the expression of that—as well as a way to create your baby.

POSITIONS FOR CONCEPTION

It has been claimed that the man-on-top (missionary) position increases the chance of conception, since it will deposit sperm closer to the cervix. However, there is no evidence to support this idea. Similarly, there is no evidence that a woman is more likely to conceive if she climaxes just after the man ejaculates.

Knowing when you ovulate

Your most fertile time is from about four to five days before ovulation until 24 to 48 hours afterward. If you can pinpoint when you ovulate, you can increase your chance of conception by having sex during your most fertile period. Some women know when they are about to ovulate because they have period-type lower abdominal cramps or breast tenderness just before ovulation, while others experience an increased sex drive during their most fertile phase. However, many women do not experience any signs.

On average, ovulation takes place about midcycle, so knowing the length of your menstrual cycle can guide you as to when it will occur. In practice, most women do not have average cycles. For greater accuracy, you'll need to use other ways to identify the timing of ovulation, as described below.

BASAL BODY TEMPERATURE

Your basal body temperature (BBT) is the lowest temperature of your body during rest. After you ovulate, increased hormone levels in your body cause a very slight (approximately 0.4 degree) rise in temperature, which lasts until your next period. If you record your temperature every day throughout your menstrual cycle, you'll be able to see where a rise in temperature has occurred, pinpointing ovulation. You need to take your temperature first thing in the morning, before even getting out of bed, using a basal thermometer. This thermometer, available from pharmacies, measures very tiny changes in temperature. Monitoring BBT only tells you when you have ovulated and does not predict ovulation. However, by charting your temperature for several cycles, you should be able to identify a pattern that provides a guide to when ovulation is likely. Not everyone finds this helpful—indeed, many couples find this method laborious and difficult.

MONITORING CERVICAL MUCUS

Monitoring the appearance and texture of mucus secreted by your cervix during your menstrual cycle can enable you to predict when ovulation will occur. The secretions alter in response to changing levels of estrogen throughout your cycle. Just after your period, mucus is scant. As estrogen levels rise, the amount of mucus increases, and it will probably seem sticky and appear cloudy or creamy. At ovulation, the mucus becomes clear and stretchy, often described as resembling egg white. After ovulation, your estrogen levels drop (unless fertilization has occurred), and the amount of mucus decreases.

You can collect a sample of mucus by using a piece of toilet paper to wipe the entrance to your vagina. However, you will get a more reliable result by collecting a sample internally. After washing your hands, carefully insert your finger into your vagina and collect a sample from around the cervix. Note the quantity and appearance of the sample. Stretch the sample between two fingers to check consistency. Check your cervical mucus daily, recording your findings on a chart. Although the first day of menstruation is day one of your menstrual cycle, start your chart on the day after the last day of your period, and continue until the first day of your next period.

OVULATION PREDICTOR KITS

If you find it difficult to monitor the natural fluctuations of your menstrual cycle, an ovulation kit may be worth trying. Although these kits come at a cost, they are one of the most reliable means of predicting fertility, as they measure levels of luteinizing hormone (LH) in your body. This is possibly the most important sign of ovulation; it is responsible for stimulating ovarian egg release itself. Fertility-indicating LH surges can be detected up to two days prior to ovulation, giving you plenty of warning as to when you are most likely to conceive. The kits work by measuring the amount of LH present in your urine. You can either collect your urine sample in a cup or hold a stick in your urine stream. Results appear as colored bands on a test card or on the stick, indicating the level of LH.

Infertility

If you've had regular unprotected sex for a year (or six months, if you're over 35) and are concerned that you have not yet conceived, seek advice from your doctor. It's possible that you or your partner, or both of you, have a fertility problem.

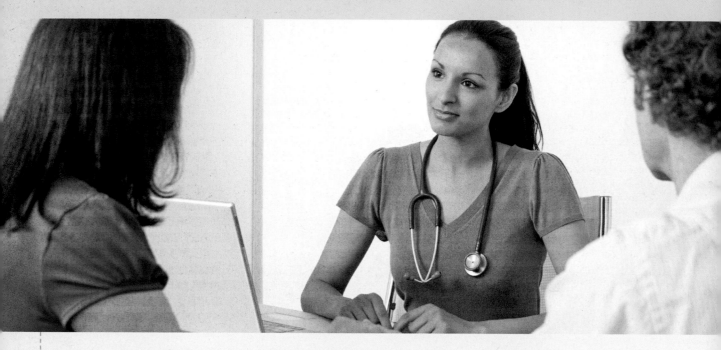

TALK TO YOUR DOCTOR
There are now many options for couples who have difficulty conceiving. Establishing the reasons that you haven't become pregnant is the first step to addressing problems and exploring the treatments available.

When you finally voice a concern that you, your partner, or both, have a fertility problem, you may already have been through difficult times. The future may also present challenges. You and your partner should be prepared to undergo tests and investigations that could be lengthy. Depending on the results, treatment may enable you to go on and conceive naturally. If not, techniques to help you conceive are available.

Seeing a doctor

When you seek help for a fertility problem, your doctor will ask you both lots of questions about your health—such as whether you've had any health problems in the past—and about your current state of health. You will also be asked about your lifestyles, and your sexual habits. It might feel as though the most private and intimate areas of your life are being invaded. However, it's important for your doctor to find out whether your problems could stem from a lifestyle issue, such as stress, or whether there might be an underlying problem preventing conception.

The doctor will probably carry out a physical examination and do some basic tests. If necessary, you will be referred to a fertility specialist for further investigations, which can be used to try to establish the cause of fertility problems. Both you and your partner will need to be tested.

Common causes of infertility

About a third of all fertility problems are due to problems with the woman and another third are due to problems with the man. The remainder are caused by a combination of problems in the man and woman, or else the cause cannot be identified. Some of the more common reasons for infertility in both men and women are detailed below.

FEMALE INFERTILITY
• Problems with ovulation.
The most common reason for female infertility is failure to release an egg during some or all cycles. This is often due to polycystic ovarian syndrome (PCOS), in which small cysts develop in the ovaries. It can also be due to thyroid or pituitary gland problems. Age is a major factor: After 35, the body becomes less effective at producing mature, healthy eggs. Lifestyle factors also affect ovulation, including smoking, alcohol, stress, obesity, being underweight, or using recreational drugs and some types of medications.

• Damaged or blocked fallopian tubes.
The fallopian tubes can be damaged or blocked as a result of sexually transmitted diseases, severe abdominal infections, such as appendicitis, or previous surgery. Damage can also be caused by severe endometriosis, in which tissue like the uterine lining (endometrium) grow elsewhere inside the abdomen, such as on the ovaries.
• Problems with implantation.
An egg may be unable to implant successfully if the lining of the uterus has been damaged, sometimes caused by operations such as surgical termination. Fibroids or polyps can distort the uterus, making it difficult for an egg to implant.
• Antibodies to sperm.
Some women have antibodies to sperm in their cervical mucus, which prevents sperm from being able to get through.

MALE INFERTILITY
• Sperm problems.
A low sperm count, abnormally shaped sperm, or sperm with poor movement can all lead to infertility. Varicose veins (varicocele) in the scrotum (the sac containing the testes) are a common cause of a low sperm count. Other causes of sperm problems include undescended testes, infections, a low testosterone level, and some long-term illnesses. Lifestyle factors such as alcohol, smoking, using certain medications and recreational drugs, or wearing tight clothing may also be responsible.
• Blocked sperm ducts.
Damage to the tubes that transport sperm can prevent sperm from reaching the female egg. Causes include an infection such as mumps, injury to the testes, birth defects, or a vasectomy. Sexually transmitted diseases, such as chlamydia, are also linked to such problems.
• Erection and ejaculation problems.
Sperm cannot enter the vagina if a man is unable to achieve or maintain an erection or if he has retrograde ejaculation, in which sperm are ejaculated into the bladder.

TESTS FOR YOU
You may be asked to have blood tests to check your hormone levels, and to see whether or not you are ovulating. In particular, levels of follicle stimulating hormone (FSH) and estrogen will be measured in a small blood sample. Blood tests can also assess the function of your ovaries, to help determine how many eggs you have in reserve.

One test, known as the "Day-3 FSH and estradiol test" measures the level of these hormones on the third day after your last menstrual period (LMP). High levels of FSH are a sign that the function of the follicles in your ovaries has deteriorated. An ultrasound through the vagina may be arranged to check the pelvic organs. You may also be offered specialized x-rays, which use contrast dyes to check the uterus, and rule out any blockages in the fallopian tubes. An operation called a hysteroscopy may be suggested. These procedures use cameras, inserted through tiny incisions in your abdomen, to diagnose and treat fertility problems. MRI (magnetic resonance imaging) and CT scans may also be recommended to check the health of your reproductive organs.

In many cases, no problems are noted or those that are can be quite easily addressed with minor interventions. You may be surprised to learn that male fertility problems are at the root of more than a third of all cases of infertility, so your partner will be investigated, too. Happily, scientific developments have ensured that there is a host of treatments available to address almost everything nature brings up.

TESTS FOR YOUR PARTNER
The first test for a man is often a semen analysis. Your partner will be asked to provide a semen sample by masturbation, after a few days' abstinence, usually on the morning of the test. This is then analyzed (normally within one to two hours of production) to count the number of sperm, and to see if they appear normal in shape and are able to swim normally.

If your partner's sperm count is low or his sperm are abnormal, other investigations may be done, such as blood tests to check hormone levels.

If a blockage in the reproductive tract is suspected, an ultrasound scan will be arranged. A more invasive test known as "vasography" is also used to detect obstructions, and involves injecting a radioactive dye into the vas deferens (the tube that transports semen). An x-ray is then used to examine this tube for blockages. A testicle biopsy, in which tissue is extracted under local anesthetic, may be recommended if there is a suggestion that the sperm-producing cells are not working properly.

Chromosomal abnormalities in the sperm are sometimes at the root of infertility, and genetic testing may be suggested to establish risk factors.

Treating fertility problems

Several different treatments are available to increase your chances of getting pregnant. The one that is best for you will depend on the reasons you can't get pregnant. It's important to understand that there are no guarantees that pregnancy will happen with any of the fertility treatments available. Your doctor can give you more information about the success rate of each treatment.

MEDICINES AND SURGERY

If you aren't ovulating, you may be offered medicines that can stimulate your ovaries to produce eggs. This is called ovulation stimulation or induction. In men, medication may help if sperm quality is affected by hormone problems or if there are problems with ejaculation. Surgical procedures can be used to repair damaged or blocked fallopian tubes, and to treat fibroids and endometriosis. In men, an operation may be able to remove blockages of the ducts that store or transport sperm.

ASSISTED CONCEPTION

Treatments that help you conceive by controlling the way that the sperm and the egg are brought together are known as assisted conception. The simplest type of assisted conception is intrauterine insemination (IUI). IUI involves taking fast-moving sperm and placing them inside the womb near the time of ovulation. This is usually the first method offered to couples who have unexplained infertility. It can be used for women who have mild endometriosis. IUI is also useful for men who have ejaculation problems or mild problems with the quality of their sperm. IUI can be combined with ovulation induction. The other main type of assisted conception is in vitro fertilization (see pp.40–41).

COMPLEMENTARY THERAPIES

If you are considering using a complementary therapy, it is important that you first get a diagnosis through conventional medical channels. A few complementary therapies may offer some help with fertility problems. Acupuncture seems to alter blood flow in the pelvis and may help healing of reproductive organs damaged by infection or endometriosis. Acupuncture may also have some effect on regulating

ACUPUNCTURE
Studies have found that acupuncture may improve the health of the endometrium and enhance sperm quality and quantity.

SUPPORTING EACH OTHER
Being unable to conceive can be very stressful, so offer support and take comfort in your partner at this time.

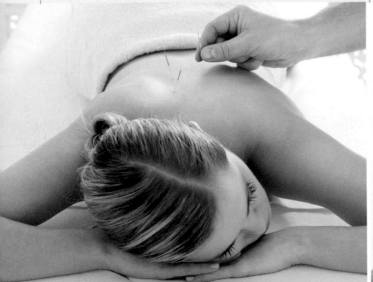

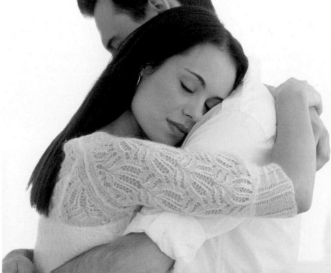

hormones and improve thyroid related infertility problems. Nutritional supplements can help women with eating problems or those who may have nutritional deficiencies for other reasons, for example, illnesses such as celiac disease. Some studies suggest that homeopathy may help improve fertility in both men and women.

Coping with emotions

During this time, you may feel you are on an emotional seesaw. Through all this remember that your first and best support is each other. It can also help to connect with others who have been through the situation themselves. Do seek support from online groups or ask your doctor for help such as counseling.

Stress comes with any medical procedure, and with assisted conception this is especially true because anxiety and hope can run high. You may feel low and despondent at some points while at others you may be optimistic that you are doing something constructive about having the baby you long for. The way your feelings alternate can be unsettling, as at times you allow yourself to imagine having a baby while at others you attempt to squash that idea to avoid future disappointment. All these emotions are a normal part of fertility treatment—but you don't need to manage them on your own. Use the support of those who love you, and ask for professional help along the way, too.

THE MIND-BODY LINK

Stress levels are known to have an effect on how quickly you become pregnant. Stress can also be a natural reaction to not conceiving as soon as you planned.

If possible, try to make changes in your life to reduce stress. Speak to your partner to find solutions together. If you feel that tension is being created by the frustration of not conceiving, talk about your feelings with your partner, but also set aside times when the subject is off-limits and you focus on other topics.

You can help counteract your stress by increasing feel-good activities, such as gentle exercise, meetings with friends, and finding time for hobbies and interests. If your stress is significant, you may find relief through talk therapies such as counseling. Practical assistance with debt is also available; credit counselors can offer advice and strategies on managing your money situation if this is causing anxiety.

> "Stress comes along with any medical procedure, and with assisted conception this is especially true because anxiety and hope can be running high"

How irregular menstrual cycles can affect fertility

The length and regularity of your menstrual cycles can affect the likelihood of getting pregnant. Your cycle is within the normal range if it's between 24 and 35 days. A short cycle—less than 24 days— does not usually pose problems in getting pregnant. In fact it can mean that you are ovulating more often than average and so have more chances to get pregnant. The only time a short cycle could be a problem is if you also have an unusually short luteal phase (see p.27). This is the phase of your cycle that occurs after ovulation, and if the luteal phase is too short, menstruation could wash away a fertilized egg before it has time to implant. If you have a short cycle, you may want to monitor how many days your ovulation and menstruation are apart.

A long cycle can make getting pregnant more difficult because you will be ovulating less often. Irregular periods can also make conceiving more difficult because it is harder to predict when ovulation will occur. One way to find out when you are ovulating is to use the cervical mucus test (see p.35). Recording your basal temperature can also be a helpful way to understand what is going on in your menstrual cycle. If you think that you are not ovulating, you need to see a specialist to find out why.

No matter what kind of cycle you have, if you are ovulating but still not pregnant after a year (or six months if you are over 35), consult your doctor.

IVF

If you have fertility problems, one option may be to have in vitro fertilization (IVF) treatment, where eggs are removed from an ovary and mixed with sperm in a laboratory. Once the eggs have been fertilized, they are placed in your womb.

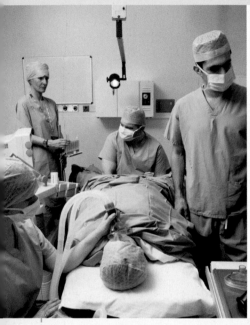

HARVESTING EGGS
Guided by an ultrasound, a long, thin needle is passed through the vagina to the ovaries, drawing in fluid and eggs.

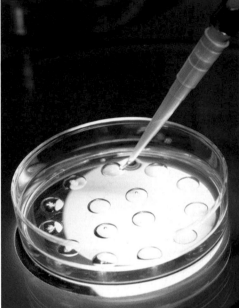

MIXING SPERM AND EGGS
Sperm is placed in a petri dish with the eggs, and incubated at the same temperature as a woman's body.

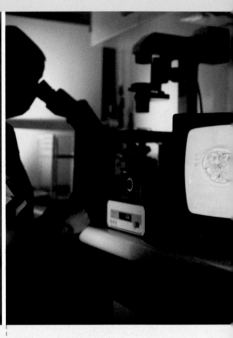

MONITORING EGG DEVELOPMENT
The sperm and eggs are left to mix for a period of 14 to 18 hours. They are observed closely to see if fertilization has occurred.

If your infertility is unexplained, your fallopian tubes are blocked, or other techniques such as fertility drugs or intrauterine insemination (see p.38) haven't worked, you may be advised to have IVF treatment.

IVF is now widely available, and your health insurance may cover some costs. IVF can be carried out with your own sperm and eggs or with donor sperm or donor eggs. The sperm and embryos can also be frozen for future use, although there can be ethical dilemmas about the fate of your unused frozen embryos, if you have more than you need. You should discuss this scenario with your doctor now.

How it works

You will need to take medication to control the timing of your monthly cycle accurately so that the eggs can be removed and fertilized on a specific day. A normal monthly cycle produces only one egg, but with this method you will produce several mature eggs at once. This is called supra-ovulation, and it increases your chances of a pregnancy. Initially you will be given injections for two weeks that encourage your ovaries to produce multiple eggs. This will be monitored with regular ultrasounds to ensure the ovaries are responding adequately to treatment. At midcycle, you will receive another drug, which helps ripen the eggs. A few days after this second treatment, the eggs will be collected while you have an ultrasound. A thin needle is passed through your vagina and into your ovary to withdraw the eggs. This is done as an outpatient procedure, usually under a local anesthetic and light sedation so you won't need to stay overnight in the hospital. On the morning of egg collection, your partner will be asked to produce a semen sample after a few days of abstinence. The sample is washed and spun at high speed so the healthiest sperm can be selected. If you're using donated sperm, it is taken from storage and prepared in the same way. Sperm and eggs are mixed in the laboratory and left for a few days. Successful fertilization can be seen with a microscope after about 16 to 20 hours. If you're under 40, one or two of the resulting embryos are transferred into your womb using a soft plastic tube passed through your vagina. Up to three embryos may be transferred if you're 40 or over. It is important to avoid twin pregnancies, as they are less likely to result in a live birth.

SUCCESS RATES

The success rate varies, with age being one of the main determinants of success. IVF really does depend on the quality of eggs, which is better in younger women. Generally each cycle carries a 30–50 percent success rate. IVF can be expensive, but some parts of the treatment may be funded by your provincial or territorial health insurance. You may need more than one cycle for success, but some of the initial embryos that have not been implanted may be frozen for the subsequent cycles.

Risks and side effects

No medical treatment is entirely free from risk, and infertility treatment is no exception. However, while it is important to have information about the risks of

The ICSI option

ICSI, or intracytoplasmic sperm injection, is similar to IVF. However, in ICSI a single sperm is selected and injected carefully into an egg in the laboratory. Once the egg is fertilized, the resulting embryo is transferred into the womb, and hormonal treatment is started in the woman to help maintain the pregnancy. This fertility treatment can be used when there is a shortage of healthy sperm or if problems between the egg and sperm prevent fertilization. It is often used when a man has had a vasectomy. The success rate is around 30–50 percent.

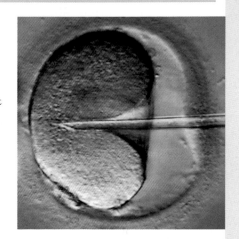

treatment, it is also important to appreciate that most women go through IVF and other assisted conception treatments without serious problems.

DRUG SIDE EFFECTS

A primary side effect of medicines given during IVF or ICSI treatment (see box) is called ovarian hyperstimulation. This is an overreaction to the medication used to stimulate the ovaries. Up to 1 in 20 women have mild nausea and abdominal discomfort that generally improves after a few days. A few women become very ill. If you have any of the following symptoms, contact your fertility clinic or doctor immediately: nausea and vomiting; severe pain and swelling in your abdomen; shortness of breath; feeling faint; and passing a small amount of urine compared to normal. You'll need to be treated in the hospital. Most women recover completely in one to two weeks.

COMPLICATIONS

Having fertility treatment increases the chances of having a multiple pregnancy (such as twins or triplets). This is why

your doctor may limit the number of embryos that are transferred into the womb. A multiple pregnancy increases the risk of health problems for both your baby and you. Miscarriage, early labor, and health problems in pregnancy, such as high blood pressure, are all more likely if you are having more than one baby.

The chances of having an ectopic pregnancy (see pp.44–45) may be higher in women who have IVF or other fertility treatments. An ectopic pregnancy occurs when the embryo starts to develop outside the womb, usually in a fallopian tube.

Removing the eggs for IVF or ICSI involves passing a tube through the vagina and into the ovary. This means that there is a risk of infection, which can usually be treated with antibiotics.

ALTERNATIVES TO IVF

Sometimes donor eggs or donor sperm might be suggested in cases where IVF or ICSI have failed. If you would like to consider this option, you will be given a thorough medical check to make sure your uterus is healthy enough to allow the eggs to implant.

Miscarriage

Miscarriage, which is loss of a pregnancy before 20 weeks, occurs in 2 out of 10 pregnancies. Having a miscarriage doesn't mean that you won't be able to get pregnant again; most women go on to have a successful pregnancy in the future.

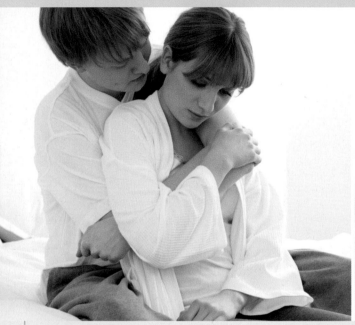

COMFORT EACH OTHER
Miscarriage can be a traumatic time for both men and women. Sharing your emotions and offering support to one another can help you to grieve and move on together.

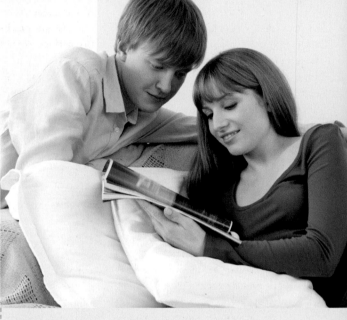

HAVING SOMETHING TO LOOK FORWARD TO
Try to remain optimistic, and plan some relaxing time together. In most cases women go on to have healthy pregnancies and babies. Reducing stress is one of the best ways to achieve this.

Most miscarriages—about 75 percent—happen in the first 12 weeks of pregnancy and are due to a "one-off" chromosome fault. Late miscarriages, occurring after 12 weeks, are usually caused by an underlying problem with the health of the mother, or are due to a serious health problem with the baby.

While a miscarriage does not usually seriously affect a woman's physical health, it can have a significant emotional impact. Knowing that it's a common occurrence doesn't make it any easier if it happens to you.

Why does it happen?

Early miscarriages are usually due to a problem in the way your genetic material (chromosomes) combined, when your egg and your partner's sperm joined during fertilization. This is more likely to be a chance event than caused by any underlying problem with either you or your partner.

However, some factors are known to increase the risk of miscarriage. Age has

the greatest effect, because egg quality decreases as you get older. At 30, your risk of miscarriage is one in five. At 42, your risk is one in two. Lifestyle factors associated with greater risk are drinking alcohol, smoking, or misusing drugs (particularly cocaine) during pregnancy. There is some evidence that consuming more than two cups of coffee or tea per day makes miscarriage more likely.

Women are more likely to miscarry if they are overweight or have a long-term health condition such as diabetes or high blood pressure. Some infections can cause miscarriage if you catch them while you're pregnant, including rubella (German measles) and toxoplasmosis (caught from pets). Other rarer risk factors are an imbalance in pregnancy hormones; structural abnormalities of the uterus; or a weak cervix. These can be causes of recurrent miscarriages.

There isn't enough evidence to show whether or not stress is a risk factor for miscarriage, but it's a good idea to take time during the day to relax. Doing moderate exercise or having sex while you are pregnant doesn't increase your risk of miscarriage. You're slightly less likely to have a miscarriage if you previously took the contraceptive pill.

SYMPTOMS OF MISCARRIAGE

A common symptom of miscarriage is vaginal bleeding. This can vary from light spotting to bleeding that is heavier than your period. You may also see blood clots, a brown discharge, or other tissue that isn't clearly identifiable. Other common symptoms are cramping and pain in the pelvis or back. You may find that the usual pregnancy symptoms, such as breast tenderness, nausea, and having to pass urine more frequently than usual, stop unexpectedly. Sometimes there are no symptoms, and miscarriage may only be discovered in a routine ultrasound.

If you have vaginal bleeding at any time during pregnancy, you should contact your doctor or midwife immediately for advice.

HOW IT'S DIAGNOSED

Your doctor will ask about your symptoms and any past or current illnesses, and whether you have had a miscarriage before. You may have an internal examination.

If further tests are needed, your doctor should be able to evaluate your situation in her office, using the equipment on hand. You may have blood tests to look for levels of hCG (the pregnancy hormone) and ultrasound scans of your uterus. These can show whether miscarriage has occurred and, if so, whether the fetus has been completely expelled (called a complete miscarriage) or whether there is still some remaining tissue in the uterus (an incomplete miscarriage). About two-thirds of miscarriages are incomplete.

Investigations into the cause of a miscarriage are not usually undertaken unless you have had three miscarriages in a row. This is because even two miscarriages are more likely to be due to chance than any underlying problem.

HOW IT'S TREATED

If the miscarriage is complete, then no further treatment is needed. However, if you had an incomplete miscarriage, you may need medication or surgery to remove the remaining pregnancy tissue.

Medicine is given orally or vaginally to help the uterus expel the tissue, which may take a few days. A quicker treatment option is a surgical procedure called D&C (dilation and curettage), which can be done in the doctor's office or a hospital, under general or local anesthesia. The cervix is dilated, and the doctor removes tissue from the uterus with a special tool or suction. Some women prefer to let nature take its course and choose expectant management. This involves waiting for the tissue remnants to be expelled while being regularly monitored by a healthcare professional.

After a miscarriage

The physical effects of a miscarriage tend to clear up quickly. Bleeding usually settles down within seven to ten days. It's best not to use tampons at this stage, to reduce the chance of infection. Your next period is likely to follow four to six weeks later.

Some couples decide that they want to begin trying for another baby right away, while others feel that this is too soon and need longer to recover emotionally. There's no right or wrong thing to do, and you need to do what you feel is best for you. You will usually be advised to wait until you have had at least one period before trying again, although it's safe to have sex when the bleeding has stopped and you both feel ready.

Coping with loss

You may have a range of strong feelings including sadness, grief, guilt, and self-blame, and you will be suffering the physical effects of your loss, too.

● Miscarriage is very common. Be reassured that you are likely to become and stay pregnant in the future.

● This is a time to look after yourself and rest, not to put pressure on yourself to get back to work, or to be cheerful for others' sake. Let your loss sink in, and find comfort with your partner until you are ready to take support from others.

● Every individual handles miscarriage differently. Sometimes, when an early miscarriage occurs, it may help to think of it as "meant to be." Some women are consoled by the thought that the miscarriage was due to a chromosomal abnormality that would have made having a healthy baby impossible. They feel more able to move on after making peace with a rational explanation.

Ectopic pregnancy

A fertilized egg that implants outside the uterus is known as an ectopic pregnancy. Early diagnosis and treatment—which means ending the pregnancy—is important, because the condition is potentially life-threatening.

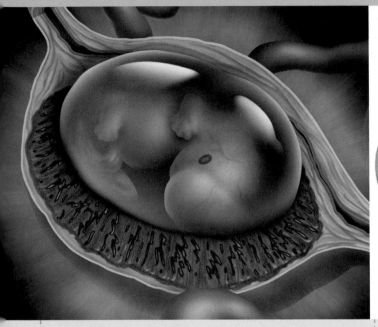

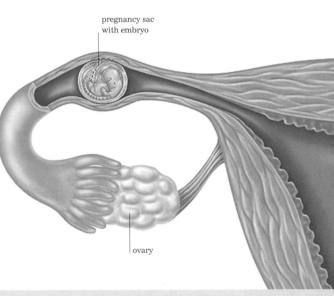

pregnancy sac
with embryo

ovary

ECTOPIC PREGNANCY
In an ectopic pregnancy, a fertilized egg implants and grows outside the womb. It is a life-threatening condition, despite medical advances. Once diagnosed, the egg must be removed.

EMBRYO IMPLANTING IN FALLOPIAN TUBE
An ectopic pregnancy usually occurs in the fallopian tube, which is stretched and sometimes ruptures as the fertilized egg grows and develops into an embryo.

Almost all ectopic pregnancies take place in a fallopian tube (called a tubal ectopic pregnancy). Only rarely do they occur in an ovary, in the abdominal cavity, or in the cervix.

An ectopic pregnancy cannot be transplanted into your uterus and, sadly, the only option is to end the pregnancy. If the embryo continues to grow inside a fallopian tube, the tube will eventually rupture, resulting in severe bleeding into the abdominal cavity. This can damage the fallopian tube and, if the bleeding is not treated promptly, can be fatal. Most ectopic pregnancies are found in time and safely treated with medication or surgery. Early diagnosis and treatment offer a woman the best chance of going on to have a normal pregnancy.

Risk factors

An ectopic pregnancy can happen to any sexually active woman, but the following factors make it more likely to occur.
• Previous ectopic pregnancy.
• Damage to a fallopian tube. This can prevent the fertilized egg from being able to pass along the tube. Instead, the egg implants in the wall. Damage to the tube may have been caused by a previous infection, often as a result of a sexually transmitted infection such as chlamydia.
• Becoming pregnant despite having had a tubal ligation (surgical sterilization).
• Having an intrauterine contraceptive device in place when you get pregnant.
• Taking medication to stimulate your ovaries, as part of fertility treatment.

Diagnosis and treatment

Most ectopic pregnancies are discovered when a woman has symptoms at about five to seven weeks. This is usually around two weeks after a missed period. You may not even be aware that you are pregnant. In some cases there are no symptoms, and the pregnancy is only discovered during a routine examination.

SYMPTOMS

A common symptom is pain low down on one side of the abdomen. You may also have vaginal bleeding, which you may think is a late period. However, the bleeding is usually different from that of a period. It may be intermittent and heavier or lighter than usual, and the blood may be dark red or brown.

Shoulder tip pain, which can be felt where the shoulder meets the top of the arm, may develop, especially when lying down. This is due to irritation of nerves by internal bleeding, causing pain that travels up the nerves to the shoulder.

Other symptoms include diarrhea, vomiting, and pain when passing urine or opening your bowels. If you have any of these symptoms, contact your medical practitioner. It's important to diagnose and treat ectopic pregnancy early to prevent rupture.

If the fallopian tube ruptures and causes severe internal bleeding, this is very serious. You'll develop signs of shock, which include pale, clammy skin, dizziness or fainting, and a racing heart. Call 911 immediately—you'll need emergency surgery.

HOW IT'S DIAGNOSED

If your symptoms suggest this type of pregnancy, you will undergo several tests.

If you are not sure whether you are pregnant, you'll be given a pregnancy test. If the test is positive, your doctor will feel your abdomen to check for a mass. You may then have an ultrasound scan using a small probe inserted through your vagina to look for the location of the pregnancy. You may also have blood tests to check levels of hCG (the pregnancy hormone), which are lower than normal in an ectopic pregnancy. If the diagnosis is still not confirmed, you may need a laparoscopy. This involves passing a viewing tube through a small opening in the wall of your abdomen so that the uterus and fallopian tubes can be directly examined. The operation is carried out under general anesthesia.

HOW IT'S TREATED

An ectopic pregnancy that is discovered before the tube has ruptured can be treated by surgery or medication. The choice you'll be offered depends on how clear the diagnosis is, and the size of the embryo. If a fallopian tube ruptures, you will need emergency surgery.

Surgery to remove the embryo is the most common treatment for an unruptured ectopic pregnancy. It is usually performed by keyhole surgery, in which a tiny camera and instruments are passed through incisions in your abdomen. Part or all of the fallopian tube may need to be surgically removed. If an ectopic pregnancy is diagnosed very early, it can be treated with methotrexate, a medication that stops the growth of embryo cells. The drug is given by injection. You will need to be closely monitored for several weeks and have repeated ultrasounds and blood tests to make sure the drug has worked.

If you do not have symptoms or they are mild, the doctor may recommend a "wait and see" approach. Many ectopic embryos die naturally without the need for surgery or drugs and cause no further problems. You will be closely monitored in case treatment becomes necessary.

If a fallopian tube ruptures, you will need emergency surgery to stop the bleeding and repair or remove the fallopian tube. The operation is carried out under general anesthesia and involves making an incision in your abdomen to open it up.

AFTER AN ECTOPIC PREGNANCY

It is common to feel anxious or depressed for a while after treatment. Worries about a possible future ectopic pregnancy, the effect on fertility, and sadness over the loss of the pregnancy are normal. Talk with a doctor and your partner about these and any other concerns following treatment. If you find it hard to get over these feelings, you may want to consider seeking further help from a qualified counselor.

Ectopic pregnancy and fertility

Your risk of having another ectopic pregnancy increases if you have previously had one. So it is important to see your doctor early in future pregnancies so that ultrasounds can be arranged and you can be closely monitored. Even if one fallopian tube is removed, you have about a 7 in 10 chance of a future normal pregnancy. That's because the other fallopian tube will still usually work. However, if one of the tubes was ruptured or badly damaged, your chances of conceiving again may be reduced.

If you have not conceived after a year of trying, then treatment is needed. The good news is that you are an excellent candidate for assisted conception techniques, such as IVF (see p.40).

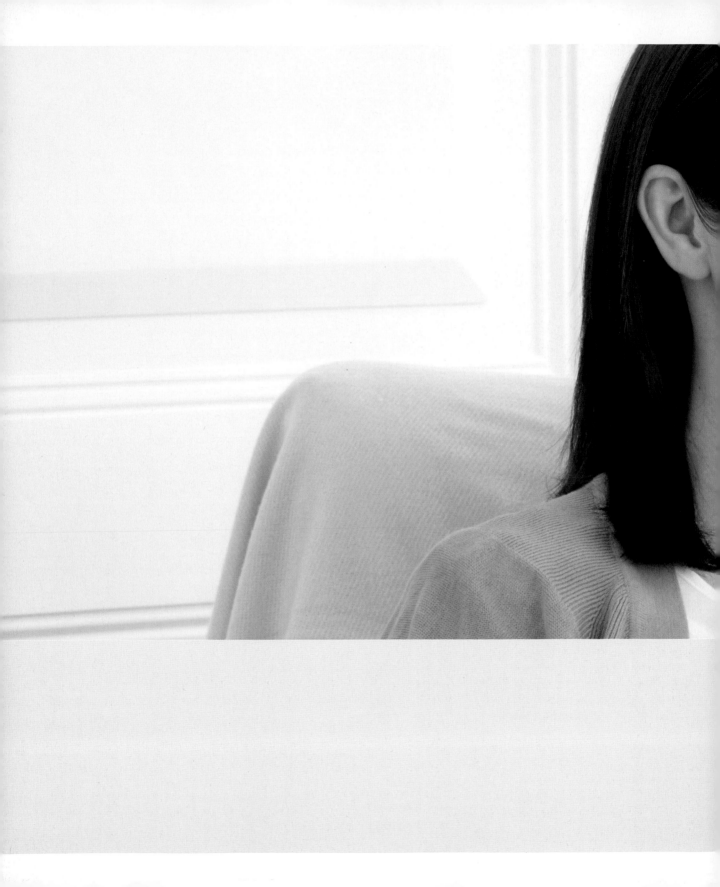

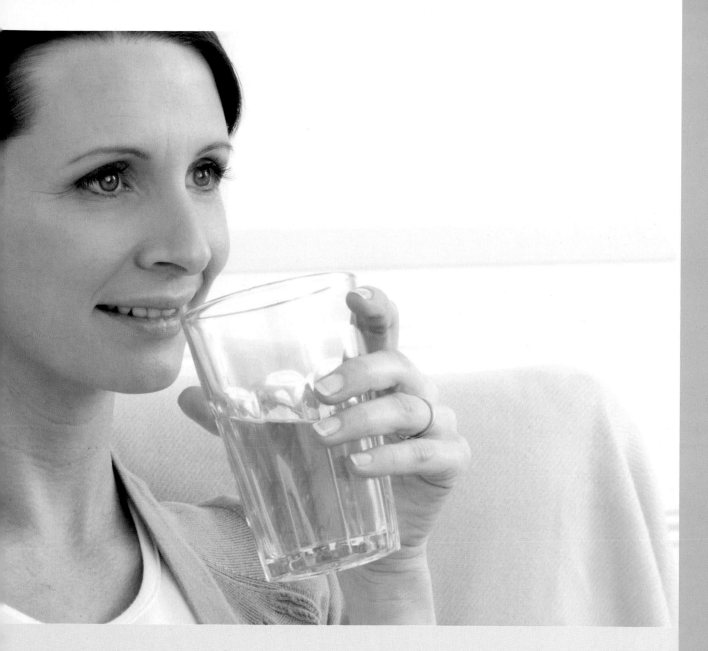

My health and lifestyle

By making positive changes to your lifestyle, you can protect yourself and give your baby the best possible start.

My pregnancy diet

The food choices you make during pregnancy have a direct impact upon your baby's health and development, as well as the way you feel. A good diet can help you stay fit, prepare your body for the birth, and maintain your energy.

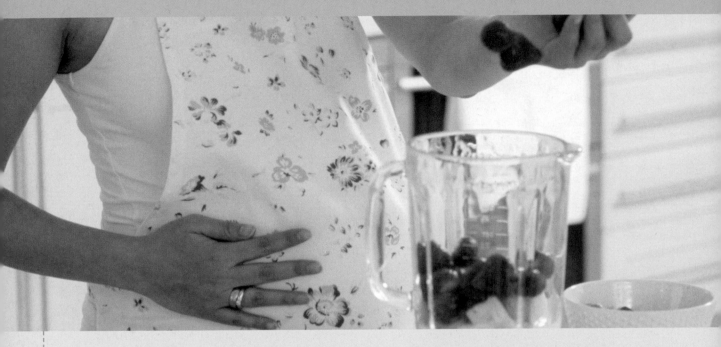

DELICIOUS SMOOTHIE
A breakfast smoothie is the perfect way to start the day. Fresh fruit is an excellent source of vitamin C, and adding a dollop of plain yogurt will provide you with protein and calcium.

You don't need to change your diet radically during pregnancy, but now it's even more important than ever to eat a wide range of healthy, nutritious foods so you and your baby have all the nutrients you need.

Natural goodness

The best way to improve your diet is to cut back on the amount of refined and processed food you eat and opt for a greater variety of whole, fresh foods. These are foods that are closest to their natural state; in other words, fresh or frozen fruits and vegetables, fresh meat, fish, and poultry, high-quality cheeses, yogurt and milk, whole-grain bread and pasta, brown rice, nuts, seeds, and legumes, such as chickpeas and lentils. These foods are particularly nutritious because their vitamin and mineral content is not reduced by processing. Eating more natural whole foods helps encourage healthy weight gain, and also minimizes the consumption of additives and chemicals that are often present in processed foods, which could harm your baby's development.

DON'T EAT FOR TWO
Gone are the days when moms were encouraged to eat twice as much as they did before pregnancy. In fact, your body becomes more efficient when you're pregnant and makes even better use of the energy you get from your food.

Your needs will depend on your pre-pregnancy weight and level of physical activity, but you may need to increase your calorie intake by about 350 calories in the second trimester and 450 calories in the third. This amounts to a sandwich or a few pieces of fruit, so it certainly isn't a great deal more food. Try to take care that the calories you do eat throughout pregnancy are nutrient-dense; in other words, the food you eat should contribute to the health and well-being of you and your baby. Your appetite is probably the best guide to how much food you need: Eat when you are hungry and choose the right foods, and you shouldn't have to worry about counting calories.

LITTLE AND OFTEN

Eating little and often helps keep blood-sugar levels steady and sustains your energy through the day, while helping to ease nausea and dizziness. A good breakfast is the ideal start to the day, while a small snack before bed can encourage restful sleep and help prevent nausea when you get up in the morning.

Key vitamins and minerals

The best way to get the vitamins and minerals you need is by eating a healthy diet. However supplements can sometimes be beneficial, for example if you suffer from severe pregnancy sickness or are unable to eat balanced meals for any other reason. Check with your doctor, midwife, or pharmacist before taking supplements other than folic acid, because an excess of some nutrients can be harmful.

VITAMIN B12

Vitamin B12, found in meat, fish, eggs, milk, soy, and fortified breakfast cereals, plays an important role in making new cells (especially blood cells) and building the nervous system. Meat-eaters should get adequate levels in their diet, but if you are vegetarian or vegan, you may need a supplement.

FOLIC ACID

Folic acid (a B vitamin) has been shown to prevent neural tube defects such as spina bifida. You need 0.4 to 1mg per day, in tablet form, from the time you are trying to conceive and throughout your whole pregnancy (see p.19). It's also important to eat foods containing folic acid, including fortified breakfast cereals, legumes, brown rice, leafy green vegetables, peas, beans, citrus fruit, and potatoes.

VITAMIN C

Vitamin C helps your body absorb iron from the food you eat, promotes healthy skin, bones, and joints, and fights infection. It is needed for the development of your baby's bones, skin, cartilage and tendons, and her immune system. During pregnancy, you will need at least 85mg per day, and the best food sources are citrus fruits, tomatoes, broccoli, peppers, currants and other berries, potatoes, mangos, and kiwi fruit.

VITAMIN D

Vitamin D helps to keep your bones and teeth healthy and promotes the healthy development of your baby's bones. Our bodies make vitamin D when exposed to sunlight, so it's important to spend at least 15 to 20 minutes outside each day. Your doctor may also recommend a supplement (usually around 5 to 10mcg per day), because there is increasing evidence that many women do not get enough vitamin D in their diets. A little vitamin D is found in fortified foods, such as margarine and some breakfast cereals, and in eggs, fish, and red meat.

CALCIUM

Calcium is essential for your baby's bones and teeth, and for healthy development of her heart, nerves, and muscles. It is required for her to develop a normal heart rhythm, and for her blood to clot. If you don't get enough calcium in your diet, your baby will use stores from your own bones, which can put you at risk of osteoporosis (thinning of the bones) later. You need 1g (1,000mg) per day while pregnant. The best sources are dairy products, soy, leafy green vegetables, dried fruits, almonds, and fortified products such as orange juice and bread.

IRON

Iron is essential in pregnancy to help your red blood cells transport oxygen around your body and through your placenta to your baby. It is also required to produce bones, cartilage, and other connective tissue. Many women don't get enough iron in their diets to sustain them during pregnancy (pregnant women need 27mg per day; non-pregnant women need only 18mg). There are two main types of iron: Heme iron, found in "animal" foods such as eggs, lean meats, poultry, and fish, is the most easily absorbed. Non-heme iron, found in "plant" foods such as leafy green vegetables, dried fruit, nuts, oats, legumes, and fortified breakfast cereals, is harder for the body to absorb.

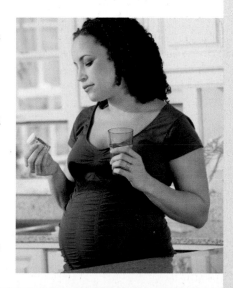

Fresh fruit, vegetables, nuts and seeds, yogurt, cheese, plain popcorn, and even half a sandwich or a bowl of vegetable soup are ideal snacks.

In the early stages, you may find that you develop an aversion to certain foods, which may be your body's way of helping you to avoid foods that may not be ideal for a healthy pregnancy. For example, some women find that they lose interest in coffee, fatty foods, and alcohol.

Getting the balance right

The key food groups that you'll need for a healthy pregnancy diet include:

UNREFINED CARBOHYDRATES

In general, these are carbohydrates that are not "white," since they have not been through the refining process. Not only are these foods richer in nutrients, but they also provide a sustained source of energy that can keep your blood-sugar levels stable. Whole-grain bread and pasta, potatoes (in their skins), spelt, quinoa, brown, red, and wild rice, sweet potatoes, oatmeal, corn, and legumes are ideal choices, and they will provide you with fiber and a little protein, too. Carbohydrates are your main source of easily accessible energy, and also play a role in body functions such as blood-clotting, cell communication and development, and your immunity. You'll need at least one or two servings at every meal.

FRESH FRUIT AND VEGETABLES

These should form the mainstay of your diet, not only because they are rich in important vitamins and minerals for a healthy pregnancy—and baby—but because they provide fiber, a sustained source of energy, and folic acid (see p.19). What's more, they'll fill you up without overloading your digestive system or encouraging unhealthy weight gain. Go for a wide variety in an array of different colors to get the greatest number of nutrients, and aim for seven or eight servings a day. Fresh is best, after which frozen, canned, dried, and juiced are good options.

PROTEIN

Protein provides the building blocks for your baby's growth, is a good source of iron, and is involved in a host of different body processes. This is one food group you simply can't do without, and you can get it from animal or plant sources. Fish, eggs, dairy, and lean meat are all animal proteins (containing essential amino acids). Legumes, quinoa, beans, whole grains, and seeds are plant sources.

Mixing and matching different forms of protein within meals, and across the day, will ensure that you get what you need. In particular, fish, seeds, and nuts offer omega oils (essential fatty acids; see right). Aim for at least two or three servings a day.

HEALTHY FATS

Fat is required for the development of your baby's brain, nervous system, and eyes—both before and after birth. It

---

PROTEIN
Lean meat is a good source of protein, which plays a key role in your own health and your baby's development.

CARBOHYDRATES
Important sources of vitamins and fiber, carbohydrates such as bread will probably form the basis of your diet.

VEGETABLES
A vegetable stir-fry is a healthy choice, because the quick method of cooking preserves the nutrients in the ingredients.

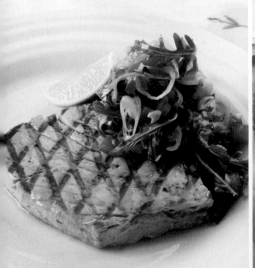

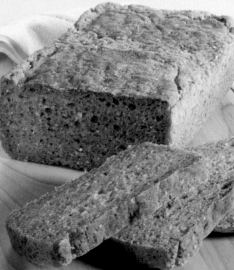

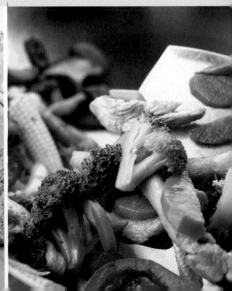

encourages the health of your placenta and the growth of many tissues in the body. There are three main types of fats: monounsaturated fats (found in olives and olive oil, nuts and nut butters, and avocados), polyunsaturated fats (in soy beans, nuts and seeds, flax and cold-water fish, such as salmon and mackerel), and saturated fats, which are best eaten in moderation (found in meat, dairy produce, and tropical oils, such as palm or coconut). The most important oils are the "omega" oils (also called essential fatty acids, or EFAs), which are crucial for the development of your baby's brain. Good levels of polyunsaturated fats and, in particular, nuts, seeds, and oily fish, will give you all you need.

There is another type of fat to avoid if you can: These are "trans fats," which are created when fats are "hydrogenized," or made stable and spreadable at room temperature. Trans fats are found in many different products, from margarines to baked goods like cakes and cookies, and can damage health and lead to obesity. Try to avoid any product that contains the word "hydrogenized" in the ingredients list.

MILK AND DAIRY PRODUCTS
Cheese, milk, yogurt, and butter provide calcium, protein, and vitamin D, which are needed for strong bones and healthy teeth. Calcium is essential in pregnancy for building your baby's bones, teeth, muscles, heart, and nerves, and for blood clotting. However, dairy products are high in fat, so you may wish to opt for low-fat or skim milk and reduced-fat butter, spreads, and cheeses—all of which contain the same nutrients as higher-fat versions. Aim for three portions a day.

FIBER
Fiber, or "roughage," as it used to be known, helps to keep your bowel movements regular and aids the efficient absorption of nutrients, as well as keeping blood-sugar levels steady. It is found in whole foods, including grains, fruit, vegetables, and legumes. Aim for about 1oz (25–30g) of fiber per day.

"Eating a balanced diet containing all the food groups will ensure that you get plenty of nutrients"

FRUIT
Red berries, such as raspberries, make a delicious snack, and are also high in antioxidants and useful vitamins.

DAIRY
To get all the calcium you and your baby need, try to have a couple of servings of a dairy product, such as cheese, every day.

IRON
Eggs are rich in iron, so omelets and frittatas are a good choice for a quick meal. Make sure the eggs are well cooked.

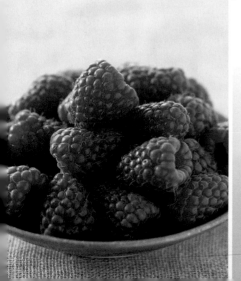

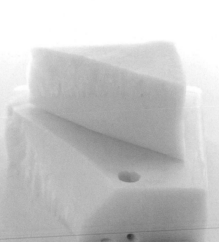

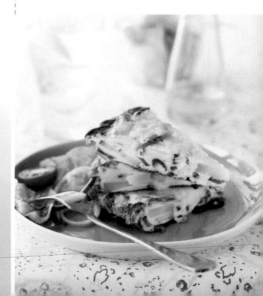

Special diets

Whether your diet is limited for religious or ethical reasons, or you suffer from a health condition or allergy that makes it impossible for you to eat certain foods, it is important that you find ways to get all of the nutrients you need.

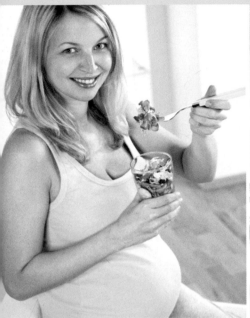

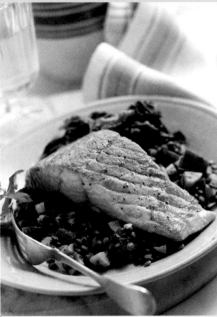

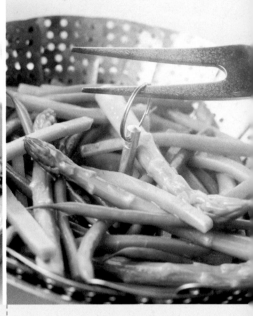

HEALTHY SALADS
Leafy greens, including salad leaves, are a source of iron. Spinach, arugula, and watercress are particularly nutritious.

KEEPING UP THE PROTEIN
Vegetarians who eat fish are likely to get all the protein they need. Non-fish eaters need to consume plenty of legumes, grains, and nuts.

STEAMING VEGETABLES
Boiling vegetables reduces their vitamin content, so try to steam them whenever possible to preserve iron and other nutrients.

If you have a restricted diet, you are probably more aware than most people of what you eat. However, you may need to take steps during pregnancy to ensure you're getting sufficient nutrients to meet your own and your baby's needs.

Vegetarian/vegan

Some vegetarians are happy to eat fish, eggs, and/or dairy, which means that their diets are likely to be fairly well balanced. One area that may need to be

addressed is iron intake. Although there are many good sources of "non-heme iron" (see p.49), this form is not as easily absorbed by the body, and you may require iron supplements in pregnancy to make up for the shortfall. Look for iron in whole-grain cereals and flours, leafy green vegetables, molasses, legumes such as lentils and kidney beans, and some dried fruits, such as raisins and apricots.

Furthermore, it is important to ensure that you are getting enough protein. Vegetarian sources of protein (such as seeds, nuts, whole grains, and some

vegetables) are known as "incomplete," which means that they do not contain all the amino acids (building blocks) required for optimal health and development. One solution is to add quinoa to your diet; quinoa is one of the few plant sources of protein that contains all the essential amino acids, and it is also high in omega oils, which are good for your baby's nervous system and brain. Alternatively, eating a wide range of different legumes, grains, and vegetables can help to ensure that you get a good balance.

If you don't drink milk or eat dairy products, you may need to work a little harder to get adequate levels of calcium. Look for fortified products such as orange juice and soy milk, and eat plenty of leafy green vegetables, almonds, dried fruit, and tofu or other soy products.

You might also need to increase your intake of vitamin B12 during pregnancy; it is essential for making tissue and cells. The recommended daily target is 2.6mcg. Vegetarians who eat eggs will have no trouble meeting this (one egg provides about 50 percent of your daily needs); however, there are few reliable plant-based sources. If you are vegan, include vitamin B12-fortified foods (such as enriched soy milks and breakfast cereals) in your diet; Talk to your doctor about your B12 levels if you're vegan. If all else fails, you may need a supplement.

Dairy-free

If you are intolerant to the sugar in milk (lactose) or have an allergy to the proteins in milk, dairy products are very likely to be off the menu. The main benefits of dairy products are their high calcium levels and the fact that they are a good source of healthy fats and protein. Adopting some of the tips for vegetarian diets (see box, below) should ensure that you get enough of these. Your doctor may recommend a calcium supplement for the duration of pregnancy and while breastfeeding, to protect your bones and teeth, and those of your baby.

If you are intolerant rather than allergic to lactose, you can purchase lactose-free dairy products, such as butters, cheese, and milk. If you can tolerate a little dairy, mix it with other foods, such as whole grains or cereals, which make it easier to digest. Yogurt, aged cheeses, such as cheddar, Parmesan, and Swiss, and buttermilk, are more easily tolerated.

Gluten-free

Wheat contains the protein gluten, which cannot be tolerated by anyone suffering from celiac disease—an auto-immune condition in which gluten causes the immune system to produce antibodies that attack the delicate lining of the bowel, which is responsible for absorbing nutrients from food. If you have celiac disease, you need to continue eating a strict gluten-free diet in pregnancy, choosing gluten-free alternatives to your favorite foods and eating a range of other grains, fruit, and vegetables, dairy products, and plenty of iron. However, well-controlled celiacs encounter few problems in pregnancy.

The bowels of celiacs cannot absorb enough iron for the demands of pregnancy, and you will probably need a supplement. In addition to this, high doses of folic acid, which needs to be prescribed by a doctor, should be taken until at least 12 weeks of pregnancy, ideally from three months before conception. This reduces the risk of spina bifida, miscarriage, and cleft lip/palate.

Wheat intolerance

Wheat is a good source of B vitamins (including folic acid), some protein, and, in its unrefined state, fiber. If you are sensitive or intolerant to wheat, you may find that you are absolutely fine eating a wide variety of different grains, such as rice, corn, quinoa, millet, and buckwheat. These will provide you with the nutrients you need.

Eating well on a restricted diet

Eating a wide variety of food will help you get a good balance of nutrients; every food contains different combinations of vitamins and minerals—as well as other essential nutrients, such as EFAs (see p.51)—which are required for optimal health and development. The greater the variety in your diet, the more likely it is that you will get what you need.

• A vegan (and sometimes vegetarian) diet can be low in calories, which can leave you feeling tired, hungry, and even nauseated. Getting plenty of high-protein foods, such as grains, nuts, seeds, and legumes, can help rectify this. Choose soy creams and margarines to add flavor and calories and, most importantly, eat whenever you are hungry.

• Untreated celiac disease can lead to difficulty becoming pregnant and also miscarriage, so don't take any chances. Talk to your doctor about nutritional supplements, and be scrupulous about avoiding foods that contain gluten.

• The calcium in fruit and vegetables is not as easily absorbed as it is from milk products. You'll need 1,000mg per day while pregnant, so it may be necessary for milk-allergic and lactose-intolerant moms to take a calcium supplement.

• Eat a piece of fruit or drink some orange (or other fruit) juice with meals, so that iron in your food is better absorbed. Avoid drinking tea with iron-rich foods because it contains tannin, which reduces iron absorption.

Off the menu

While most foods are safe to eat during pregnancy, there are some that should be avoided because they contain bacteria that can cause food poisoning or are otherwise potentially harmful to your health and that of your baby.

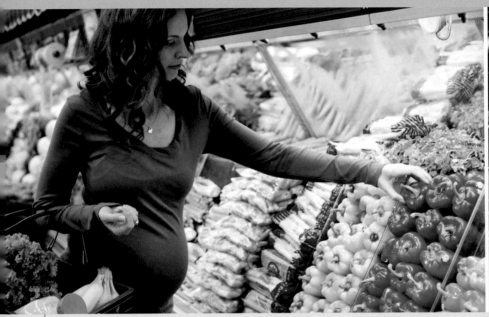

FRESH IS BEST
Fresh fruit and vegetables are bursting with nutrients that will keep you and your baby healthy. Wash them carefully, to remove traces of chemicals and bacteria.

CHECK THE TEMPERATURE
Use a thermometer to ensure that poultry and meat is fully cooked, and any bacteria or other food-borne illnesses are destroyed.

Eating certain foods puts you at greater risk of coming into contact with listeria, salmonella, parasites, pollutants, and other threats that are particularly important to avoid during pregnancy. Keeping these off the menu can help keep you and your baby safe and healthy.

What to avoid

In general, you should steer clear of unpasteurized foods, raw eggs, unwashed fruit and vegetables, some prepared foods, liver, and some fish and seafood.

SOFT CHEESES

Avoid soft, unpasteurized cheese, such as brie, goat cheese, camembert, feta, and blue cheeses, *unless* the label states that they are made with pasteurized milk. Unpasteurized dairy products can contain listeria, a harmful bacteria that causes listeriosis, which can cause miscarriage, premature delivery, and even the death of your baby.

Other potential sources of listeria include packaged meals (unless they are cooked to piping hot all the way through), prepared salads, such as potato salad and coleslaw, and pâté. Pasteurized

cream cheeses are fine, and homemade salads using fresh ingredients are perfectly acceptable, as long as they are kept chilled before serving.

UNCOOKED EGGS

Foods containing raw or partially cooked eggs (such as homemade mayonnaise, or soft-boiled or lightly scrambled eggs), can carry salmonella, another bacteria that can cause food poisoning. Although it is unlikely to harm your baby, it can make you very ill, so it is best to err on the side of safety. You can also get salmonella from unpasteurized dairy products, undercooked meat and poultry (particularly those made of ground meats, such as sausages and burgers), and buffet foods that have been left uncovered in a warm environment.

UNWASHED FRUIT AND VEGETABLES

The soil on fruit and vegetables can contain a parasite known as *toxoplasma gondii*, which causes a serious condition known as toxoplasmosis. This can lead to miscarriage and serious health problems in your baby. The parasite can also be found in undercooked or raw meat, raw cured meats such as salami or prosciutto, unpasteurized goat milk and cheese, and cat feces (see p.59).

LIVER

Although liver is a rich source of vitamin A, an important nutrient in pregnancy, high levels can cause a buildup that can harm your baby, leading to birth defects and developmental problems. Liver is now believed to contain too much vitamin A to be healthy in pregnancy, and should be avoided. For the same reason, you should avoid taking vitamin A supplements during pregnancy.

SHARK, SWORDFISH, AND MARLIN

Oily fish is rich in essential fatty acids that are now known to encourage the health of your baby, and the development of her brain and nervous system. However, these fish can also play host to certain pollutants, such as dioxins and PCBs, which can damage your baby's health. Shark, swordfish, and marlin are most likely to contain high levels of mercury, and should be avoided completely during pregnancy. Other fish, such as fresh tuna, mackerel, sardines, salmon, and trout, can be eaten once or twice a week, which will give you plenty of the omega oils your baby needs.

RAW SEAFOOD

Oysters should be avoided, since they can contain a bacteria that can make you ill (known as *vibrio vulnificus*). Cooking kills this bacteria, so cooked oysters are fine. Raw seafood and fish can contain hepatitis A or parasites that may also cause ill health; however, freezing destroys these, and makes the seafood safe to eat. Store-bought sushi should be fine, since it will have been frozen at –4°F (–20°C) for at least 24 hours. If you make your own sushi at home, freeze the fish for at least 24 hours before using it.

Some raw fish used to make sushi, such as smoked salmon, doesn't need to be frozen before it's used; smoking kills any parasites in the fish. Other methods such as salting and pickling can also make raw foods safe to eat.

ALCOHOL

In the first few weeks of pregnancy, your baby is extremely vulnerable to the effects of alcohol, tobacco, drugs and other toxins. Alcohol *does* cross the placenta and enter your baby's own bloodstream, where it can affect brain development and the health of her liver, among other things. For this reason, it is recommended that pregnant women avoid alcohol completely during this period. After 12 weeks, the risk of damage to your baby is slightly reduced. After this point, a small quantity (one small glass on very special occasions) may be acceptable, but the truth is that we do not know for sure what constitutes a safe level, and this level seems to differ between women. We do know that binge and heavy drinking can cause something known as "fetal alcohol spectrum disorder," in which your baby can suffer serious mental and physical defects.

Research has found that one in ten pregnant women drinks more than the recommended limit, so it is important that you are clear about what constitutes a unit. About 8oz (.5 pint) of beer, or a small glass of wine (4oz/125ml) is considered the maximum for a single sitting. You may find that you naturally lose interest in alcohol during pregnancy, but if you don't, try to cut down—or exclude it completely. After all, it's only nine months. . .

Cutting back on caffeine

While coffee boasts some powerful antioxidants that are beneficial to health, it also contains caffeine, which, in excess, can cause problems during pregnancy. Coffee isn't the only culprit; cola drinks, energy drinks, dark chocolate, and brown and green tea also contain caffeine.

Current guidance is to have no more than 300mg of caffeine per day during pregnancy (about two 8-oz/237-ml cups of coffee), because higher levels are linked to miscarriage and low birthweight. What's more, caffeine promotes the release of adrenaline, a hormone involved in the stress response. We know that babies who experience maternal stress in the womb can become anxious and receive a reduced blood supply for a short period, which could harm growth. Furthermore, caffeine affects your heart rate and metabolism, which can not only make you feel jittery and perhaps "out of sorts," but may also have the same impact on your baby.

The good news is that new research has found that having less than 300mg of caffeine per day poses no threat to babies, nor does it increase the risk of miscarriage or early labor. Drinking your coffee or tea with milk can help reduce the short-term impact of caffeine, so this might be worth considering. Avoid drinking caffeinated beverages with meals, since doing so can prevent the absorption of nutrients.

Food hygiene

Taking care to prepare, cook, and store your food properly can significantly reduce the risk of food poisoning, which could put your baby at risk. A few small changes to the way you do things may be all it takes!

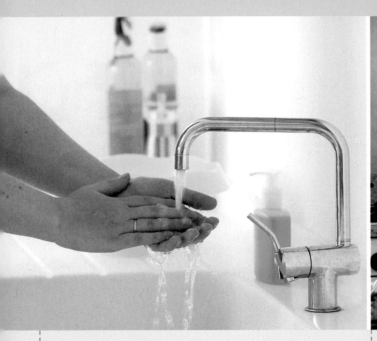

FREQUENT HANDWASHING
Wash your hands religiously with soap and water, particularly before, during, and after you prepare food, to prevent the spread of bacteria, viruses, and other germs.

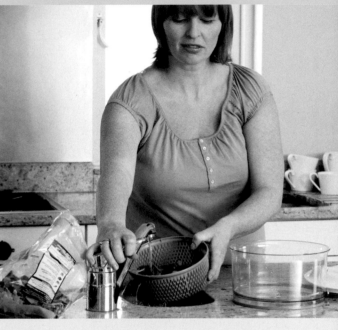

RINSING PRE-PACKED SALAD
Although pre-washed salads are safe to eat—if you keep them in the fridge in a sealed bag and eat before the use-by date—it is a good idea to wash them again, to remove any traces of listeria bacteria.

Sensible food hygiene is important in pregnancy for many reasons. First of all, your immune system is under extra pressure during pregnancy, and you will be more susceptible to food poisoning, such as salmonella and E. coli, to name just two. Secondly, there is a risk that food-borne illnesses can affect the health of your baby, so it pays to be cautious.

WASH YOUR HANDS

Wash your hands carefully and regularly, with hot water and soap. Make sure they are completely dry before preparing food, since bacteria spreads more easily on damp skin. It's particularly important that you wash your hands after any contact with raw meat, fish, or eggs.

REFRIGERATE FOOD

Keep food in the fridge until you plan to prepare it, and refrigerate or freeze leftovers as soon as possible (ideally within one to two hours) after preparing. The longer they are left at room temperature, the more chance there is that bacteria will breed. Eat any leftovers within two days, except for cooked rice, which you should eat within one day to avoid food poisoning. If you're having a party or making a buffet, leave the food in the fridge until people are ready to eat. Generally, don't leave food out of the fridge for more than four hours. Finally, make sure your fridge and freezer are at the right temperature (below 41°F/5°C and below 0°F/ 18°C, respectively), and keep raw and cooked foods well away from each other. They should ideally be on different shelves, with raw food on the lowest shelf, and carefully sealed to prevent leaking.

"Eating out is perfectly safe as long as you take steps to avoid any foods that are not considered appropriate during pregnancy"

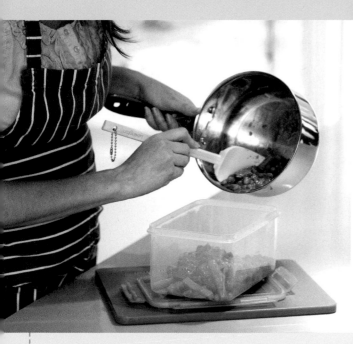

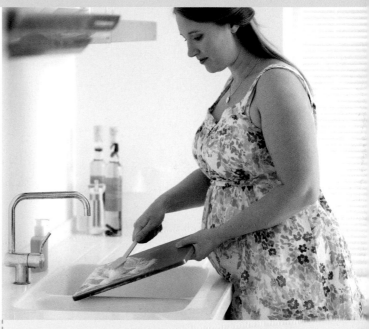

STORE LEFTOVERS IMMEDIATELY
Freeze or refrigerate leftovers as soon as possible to prevent the buildup of harmful bacteria. Use sealed containers to prevent cross-contamination with other foods in the fridge.

CUTTING BOARD HYGIENE
Get into the habit of using different boards for meat, bread, and vegetables. Washing them carefully after use in hot, soapy water will ensure that bacteria do not multiply on the surface.

KEEP IMPLEMENTS CLEAN
Wash cutting boards, knives, spoons—and anything else that comes into contact with raw food—immediately after use, so that they don't have time to cross-contaminate other items in your kitchen. Better still, put them in the dishwasher, where the high heat kills bacteria and parasites.

Use different knives and cutting boards for preparing raw foods, and clean your work surfaces carefully before beginning to prepare food and then immediately afterward.

SERVE FOOD PIPING HOT
Everything you eat should be cooked thoroughly before serving. Always serve food piping hot, because germs can start to multiply rapidly when it is lukewarm. This is particularly important if you eat packaged or frozen meals. Foods are properly cooked only when they are heated long enough and at a high enough temperature to kill the harmful bacteria that cause illnesses. Food should have reached a temperature of: 145°F/63°C for roasts, steaks, and chops of beef, veal, and lamb; 160°F/71°C for pork and ground beef; 165°F/74°C for ground poultry; 180°F/82°C for whole poultry. Use a meat thermometer to check.

EATING OUT
It's obviously impossible to control the preparation, cooking, and storage techniques used in a restaurant, but you can play it safe by asking for food to be cooked until well done, avoiding buffets or any salads with mayonnaise (such as potato salad and coleslaw), and avoiding salads and raw vegetables that may not have been properly washed.

Environmental hazards

What's best for you and your baby is also best for the environment, so now's the time to get rid of any potentially harmful chemicals that might lurk in or around the home, and to avoid exposure to toxins or harmful pests.

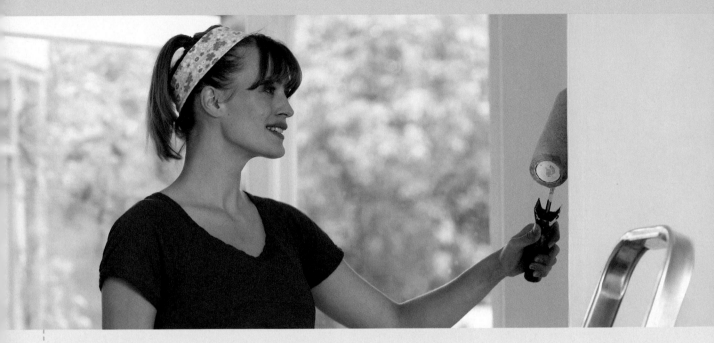

WHILE YOU ARE NESTING
Protect yourself from airborne pollutants by selecting low-VOC paint and varnishes and by keeping the room well ventilated.

Most of us use chemicals in and around the home, in the form of personal products such as deodorants and hairspray, and in cleaning agents, such as detergents, bleach, and air fresheners. We may also come into contact with parasites in the garden or when caring for pets that could be dangerous for a developing baby. While the risks are minimal, many women choose to minimize exposure to harmful chemicals while pregnant and opt for natural products instead.

Chemical hazards

Some chemicals, including lead and pesticides, should be avoided completely during pregnancy because they are

known to increase the risk of premature birth, developmental problems, birth defects, and miscarriage. Lead, for example, can be found in old pipes and paints, so if you plan to decorate or live in an old house, you may want to hire an expert to check whether lead is present.

HOUSEHOLD CLEANERS
Most household cleaners contain chemicals. Although these are considered safe during pregnancy, it is unclear whether high levels of exposure can affect the health of your baby. As a precaution, it is recommended that you avoid products with ammonia (found in some glass and window cleaners) and chlorine (found in some bleaches). It's also a good idea to give aerosols and air

"Protect yourself and your baby from potential household toxins, and you'll also protect local water sources and the marine environment"

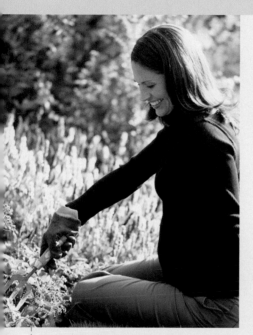

IN THE GARDEN
Gardening gloves are a must during pregnancy because of parasites in the soil. Try to limit exposure to pesticides, as well.

fresheners a pass (other than those using natural products, such as essential oils), as these products tend to release more chemicals into the air.

Limit your exposure by making sure that the space you are cleaning is well ventilated, avoid using toxic oven cleaners (or putting your head in the oven when cleaning it), wear rubber gloves to avoid absorbing chemicals through your skin, read the labels on all products and pay attention to toxicity warnings, and avoid combining products, which can create toxic fumes. The good news is that there are many eco-friendly cleaning products now available, which are also kinder to the environment.

DRY CLEANING
Although dry-cleaning relies on chemicals to clean clothing without water, there is no known risk to either you or your baby—in moderation. However, it may be sensible to remove the plastic from your clothing when it is returned, to allow chemicals to escape.

PAINTING AND DECORATING
Many moms enjoy decorating, especially when preparing the home for a new baby, but it's important to avoid contact with some paint-strippers and brush-cleaning fluids, which can contain the volatile organic compounds (VOCs) that have been linked with birth defects. Stripping paint is best left to someone else, since some paints contain lead. Choose low- or zero-VOC paints; better still, go for natural paints, made from ingredients such as water, clay, chalk, and plant dyes.

Home and garden

During pregnancy it's important to have fuel-burning appliances serviced. That includes gas stoves, all forms of fire and heating boilers, plus their flues, vents, and chimneys. This is very important in winter, when windows and doors are shut, as it reduces your risk of exposure to the toxic gas carbon monoxide, which is absorbed more easily by pregnant women and their unborn babies and harms the developing brain. Secondhand smoke also increases carbon-monoxide levels. If people smoke at your home, they should do so well away from the house.

Always wear sturdy rubber gloves when digging and planting. Soil can harbor the same harmful toxoplasmosis parasite as the one found in cat feces (see below). Avoid using lawn treatments and moss or weed killers (which often contain pesticides). For the same reason, avoid artificial fertilizers and preserved wood for fences and decking; instead opt for untreated hardwoods and linseed oil or water-based wood treatments.

PETS AND PESTS
Wash your hands with soap and hot water after handling your cat, and give litter-box duties to someone else, especially in the first trimester. Toxoplasmosis is a parasite transmitted to humans through contact with infected cat feces, and is harmful to an unborn baby.

It's also a good idea to stay away from pets after they have been treated for pests: flea collars and other treatments can contain harmful pesticides. So, too, can routine sprays used to kill pests in buildings and weeds outdoors.

Mosquito and tick bites can sometimes lead to infection, so it's a good idea to use a good insect repellent. Avoid those that contain the insecticide DEET, which has been linked with birth defects, and go for natural repellents.

Safety at work

Apart from tiredness, most women don't find it tricky to keep working through pregnancy. But in specialist professions, such as hairdressing and dentistry, it pays to make yourself aware of the risks—and how you can overcome them.

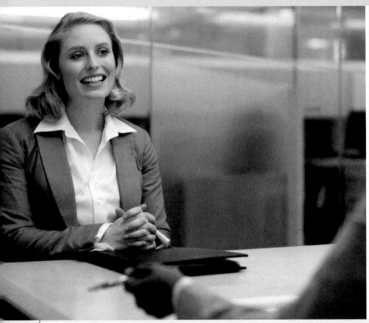

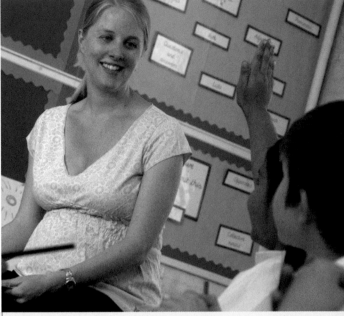

TALKING TO YOUR BOSS
It's a good idea to let your employer know that you are pregnant as soon as you can, so that you can talk about and plan any changes that may be needed to keep you safe at work.

STANDING FOR HOURS
If your work involves standing for long periods, try to take regular breaks or find ways to rest while you are working. It's also important to wear comfortable, flat shoes.

It's up to you to decide when you want to tell your employer about your pregnancy. Most women wait until after the first trimester, when the risk of miscarriage is greatly reduced, but some women who are experiencing severe symptoms of morning sickness feel that they must divulge the information sooner, to explain their behavior. If you're concerned about safety issues at work, you may want to tell your supervisor about your pregnancy sooner rather than later, and find out whether accommodations can be made for you.

It is completely safe to continue working in most jobs and companies; however, it is important to be aware of the potential risks to you and/or your baby, and make the appropriate adjustments.

The purpose of a workplace risk assessment is to identify any areas or work practices that could pose a threat to you and/or your baby. You can undertake this on your own, or ask someone from your human resources department to evaluate your work space with you. Most employers are eager to ensure that you are well protected.

Assessing risks

Make sure that you are not exposed to fumes, chemicals, or radioactive rays, required to lift or carry heavy loads, or spending lots of time on your feet. Make sure your work station is comfortable. If you work with the public, your employer can help you assess the risk of having to deal with unruly customers, or the threat of violence. Other potential risks include:
• Working with animals, which may put you at risk of E. coli, tularemia, and other infections and diseases.

"If you need help in changing your working conditions, talk to someone—your personnel department, union rep, or an advice helpline"

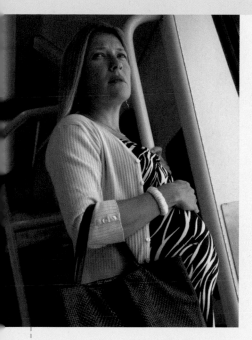

CHANGING YOUR COMMUTE
If you can't get a seat on buses or trains, can you shift your working day slightly to avoid the rush hour?

viruses including childhood illnesses (see p.21), which may harm your baby.
• Inadequate facilities, such as lavatories and a place to rest during breaks.
• Excessive working hours.
• A tightly fitting uniform; this may seem silly, but it can make you uncomfortable and make pregnancy symptoms worse. Reevaluate your workstation several times during pregnancy, as your needs and abilities change.

COMPUTER SCREENS
There is no research to suggest that using computers, even for long periods, is risky during pregnancy. But do make sure your keyboard and monitor are at the proper height, and take hourly breaks to rest your eyes and stretch your legs.

TRAVELING
If your job involves long hours in a car, train, or plane, you may need to make some changes. Flying after about 28 weeks is discouraged; after 36 weeks, it's best not to travel at all. It's wise to keep car trips to no longer than five or six hours and take regular breaks (particularly if you are driving; see p.85), and to walk around planes or trains in transit. Always wear seatbelts, with the lap belt fitting snugly over your hips, not your bump, and shoulder belts across your chest and over your shoulder. Avoid traveling to high altitudes, where oxygen levels are lower.

To ease the discomfort of commuting to work, especially later in pregnancy, try to get a seat when you can, or rest against a partition so you're reasonably secure when the train or bus stops and starts. Hold on tight. It's easy to lose your footing with your altered center of gravity. Keep a bottle of water in your bag to stay hydrated, and a healthy snack to keep blood-sugar levels stable.

• Chemicals, such as those used in medical, dental, or pharmaceutical occupations, and in painting, cleaning, farming, dry-cleaning, gardening, beauty salons, pest control, and carpet-cleaning. Check the safety data of chemicals on the packaging, or online.
• Food hazards, such as listeria, E. coli, and salmonella, which can be acquired by handling raw food.
• Slippery floors.
• Viral hazards, particularly in medical settings, or even childcare facilities, where you may be in contact with

Changing how we worked

During the first three months of my pregnancy I was so tired that occasionally I would grab a mat from the children's play area at work. I would sneak into a spare room and have a nap instead of a lunch break. CH

I was already into health and fitness, having run a marathon not long before my first pregnancy, but my job was getting in the way of a healthy lifestyle. I was in my final year of my pediatric residency and not getting enough sleep or finding enough time to eat—I would just grab whatever I could find when on overnight call. Once I became pregnant, I worked harder to make sure (if only somewhat successfully) that I had time to rest, sleep, shop for groceries, and prepare healthy meals. LJ

Keeping fit

Exercise has a host of benefits during pregnancy, for both you and your baby. Choose activities carefully, exercise gently and regularly, and you'll feel better for doing it. Being fit also gives you more energy for labor and life with a baby.

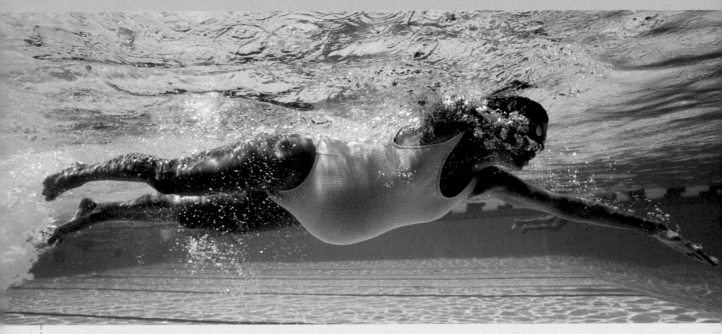

SWIMMING
It's safe to continue swimming from the first trimester. Vary your strokes and build some relaxation into every session.

Exercise has immediate health benefits for you, your baby, and the placenta, and women who exercise tend to have fewer pregnancy-related discomforts. It also releases endorphins—feel-good chemicals—that improve your mood. Exercising regularly has longer-term benefits, too—it helps prevent too much weight gain during pregnancy, boosts energy levels, and prepares you physically for labor and delivery. Exercising in pregnancy is associated with a faster labor and swifter recovery.

Experts recommend that healthy pregnant women should aim for about 2.5 hours of low-impact aerobic exercise every week. If you aren't a natural athlete, it's never too late to begin a gentle fitness program.

Enjoying exercise

Anything that keeps you active will encourage a healthy pregnancy. Gardening, housework, and even chasing a toddler fall into this category. The secret to sustaining an exercise routine is to choose activities you enjoy and that fit easily into your day. You don't even have to leave home to keep fit; regular home stretching sessions or routines from a pregnancy workout DVD can help to keep you in good shape for the months to come.

The best form of exercise for you depends not only on what you enjoy, but on how fit you were before you became pregnant. If you run marathons, you may feel like running through most of your

"To build motivation, think about the example you'd like to set for your child—there's none better than regular exercise and great nutrition"

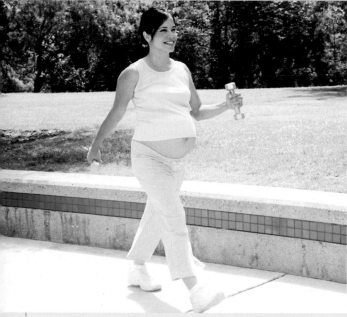

STRIDING OUT
From strolling with the dog to power-walking with weights, this is the perfect form of exercise throughout your pregnancy, and you can tailor what you do to your level of fitness.

PRENATAL EXERCISE CLASS
Prenatal fitness classes can help you improve muscle strength, posture, and cardiovascular fitness as well as make friends—all of which put you in good stead for labor, birth, and beyond.

pregnancy. But if you haven't trained before, build up slowly. A gentle daily walk is perhaps the best place to start.

JOGGING AND RUNNING
Easy, inexpensive, and available wherever you live, this form of exercise works the cardiovascular system (heart and lungs) while strengthening the lower body. If you ran or jogged regularly before getting pregnant, it's safe to keep running or jogging through most of your pregnancy. Just make sure you wear a good pair of supportive shoes and don't

push yourself too hard. Run on level ground now, and take along a bottle of water. You may need to modify your routine as the weeks pass; listen to your body and when you feel uncomfortable or very tired, slow down and stretch. If you haven't run before, don't start now. Try gentle walking, then slowly increase your pace and build up to power-walking.

CYCLING
This provides a good cardiovascular and lower body workout, and it's a great way of spending more time in the fresh air,

but using an ordinary bicycle increases your risk of falling, since your center of gravity shifts during pregnancy. It's much safer to use a stationary bike at the gym. The bicycle supports your weight while you exercise—the benefits of this become clear as the weeks go on!

SWIMMING
An ideal way to keep fit and flexible during pregnancy, swimming shares the cardiovascular benefits of running or cycling, but the water aids buoyancy, supporting your growing weight and

vulnerable joints. Exercising in water helps many people feel more relaxed and breathe more deeply, and it suits those who tend to overheat in the gym or while jogging. It also increases endurance, preparing you for labor. If you have groin pain or symphysis pubis dysfunction (see p.387) breast stroke can worsen it, so alternate strokes or use a kickboard and just kick your legs.

YOGA AND PILATES

When taught by a teacher trained to work with pregnant women, yoga and Pilates can strengthen your abdominal and pelvic floor muscles, and build stamina without placing undue strain on your joints or spine. The poses and exercises improve flexibility, too, which can enhance your balance and posture. You will also find out how to relax fully and control your breathing. For more details, see pp.72–75.

STRENGTH WORK

Although training with heavy weights is not recommended during pregnancy, you can continue to work out with weights throughout pregnancy. Just switch to lighter weights, reduce the number of repetitions, and increase rest periods between sets. If you use weight machines, be careful: They can be safer than free weights because they help you maintain good posture and stability—but don't train too hard. If you attend a gym or exercise class, talk to a trainer or the teacher about modifying your workout.

Exercising safely

The key to exercising safely while pregnant is to think "mild and moderate." Don't attempt to get super-fit, train for a big event, or think about losing weight; just aim to keep everything moving.

Start slowly and build up incrementally—15–20 minutes five days a week is a good starting point for beginners. You should always be able to carry on a conversation while exercising; if you can't talk, slow down. Stop if you experience any discomfort and pay attention to achy joints—in pregnancy, increased levels of the hormone relaxin loosen ligaments and joints, making them less stable (see p.172).

You may be aware of pressure on your bladder, which can make rigorous exercise somewhat challenging, but make sure you are well hydrated before you start and take water breaks. If you feel you're overheating, slow down and sip some water.

To minimize injuries, don't start any new activity or rigorous regime until you have talked to your doctor or midwife. If you enjoy a regular activity, talk to your teacher, coach, or trainer. He or she will help you adapt your routine to account for your changing center of gravity and looser ligaments and joints.

TRIMESTER BY TRIMESTER

In the first trimester, it is not advisable to exercise strenuously or to start a new activity. Instead, focus on resting and conserving energy until the fetus is well implanted. If you want to stay active, stick to a little walking, gentle stretching,

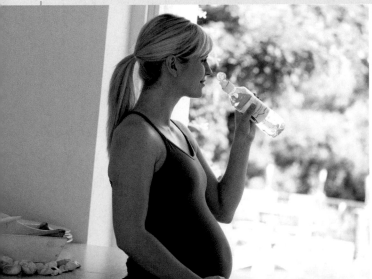

KEEP HYDRATED
Drink water before, during, and after an exercise session—it's important to keep your body well hydrated.

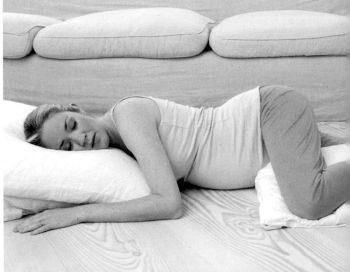

AND RELAX
After a period of exercise, rest for a while to allow your body and mind to adjust and absorb the benefits.

and slow swimming. Keep well hydrated and watch that you don't overheat.

In the second trimester, you may feel your energy and enthusiasm for exercising returning. After 12–14 weeks, it's safe to go back to any form of exercise you enjoyed before your pregnancy (just avoid dangerous sports), but start gently and keep the level moderate. Alternatively, look for an exercise class specially devised for pregnant women. Your center of gravity will be shifting now, so be aware of changes in your balance. Avoid lying on your front from now on, and do not twist deeply or try any form of movement that compresses or strains the abdomen. Stop exercising on your back after 12 weeks, or earlier if you feel nauseated or dizzy.

In the second and third trimester (earlier in some women) avoid exercising on your back. If you take yoga or Pilates, tell your teacher that you're pregnant so she can show you how to adapt your position using blocks, bolsters, and folded blankets. When walking, be mindful of the changes in your center of gravity, and expect your balance to change as your pregnancy progresses. If you haven't tried a prenatal yoga class yet, now is a good time to sample the breathing and relaxation techniques.

WARM UP, COOL DOWN

Warming up and cooling down are especially important when exercising during every stage of pregnancy, to help prevent injury. When starting an exercise session, spend five to ten minutes warming up by walking around, moving your arms and legs to warm your muscles, and gradually increasing the intensity until you feel slightly out of breath. Then stretch out for 10 minutes— focus on the front and back of your arms, your calves, and the front and back of your thighs. Now you're ready for aerobic activities.

After finishing a session, cool down by walking around again for five minutes, taking the pace down until you are no longer out of breath. Then stretch out the muscles you have worked for another 10 minutes, paying attention to your calves and thighs, chest, shoulders, and arms.

WHAT TO AVOID

Some high-risk activities are no-nos during pregnancy: extreme, strenuous, or high-impact sports, such as waterskiing, horseback riding, downhill skiing, scuba diving, snowboarding, and rock climbing. Weight-lifting and other exercises that involve standing in one place for long periods may decrease the flow of blood to your baby and make you feel dizzy.

If you feel very hot, nauseated, short of breath, or tired, stop the session and cool down. Stop immediately and contact your doctor if you notice any of the following symptoms:
- chest pain
- rapid heartbeat or palpitations, even while resting
- dizziness or faintness
- headache
- muscle pain or weakness
- pain or swelling in the calf (could indicate a blood clot)
- pain in the back or pelvis
- contractions
- fluid leaking from your vagina
- vaginal bleeding.

BEING CAUTIOUS

Aerobic exercise (which works the heart and lungs, raising your heart rate and encouraging blood to circulate more quickly around the body) is generally safe in pregnancy. However, it is not recommended if you have any of the following conditions:
- heart or lung disease
- high blood pressure
- severe anemia
- diagnosis of incompetent cervix (IC)
- persistent bleeding in the second or third trimester
- placenta previa
- pre-term labor
- your water has broken
- preeclampsia.

Discuss which activities may be suitable for you with your doctor or midwife.

Keeping active during pregnancy

I did very little in the way of physical activity in the first trimester, because I felt too tired—and also pretty nauseated at times. After my first ultrasound (around 12 weeks), when I felt better and had more energy, I started yoga again and swam twice a week. Even then, I was careful to alternate my strokes to avoid straining muscles and prevent pelvic pain. I also went for walks outdoors when the weather was good. TL

My pediatric residency schedule kept me working long, sleep-deprived hours, and I had little spare time for formal exercise. I continued using my home stair-climbing machine in a low-impact way, but wasn't using it as often as I wanted to. So I made a point of taking the stairs at the hospital whenever I could. Of course, it could make colleagues and visitors nervous to come across a very pregnant woman short of breath while determinedly climbing several flights of stairs! LJ

I enjoyed water aerobics before I became pregnant, and I kept it as part of my weekly routine throughout my pregnancy. I liked that it was a low-impact form of exercise, and that I could work out each time at a level that suited how I felt. CH

Exercises for a fit pregnancy

There are some key exercises that are particularly helpful when you are pregnant because they strengthen muscles in the legs and pelvis, build core strength to support your posture, and enhance flexibility and coordination.

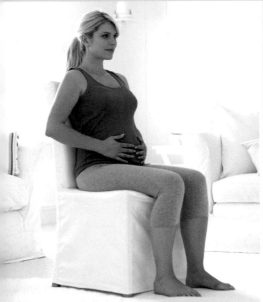 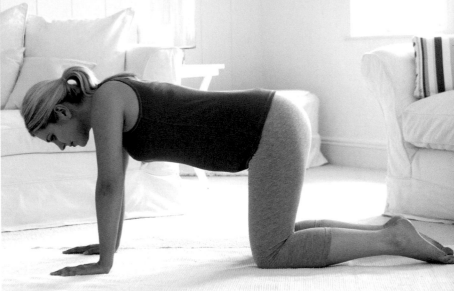

ABDOMINAL PULL
Sit, back supported, feet hip-width apart, palms on your bump. Breathe in. Exhale, and feel the abdominal muscles pull your bump toward your back. Relax and inhale, repeat.

ALL FOURS
Kneel with knees hip-width apart, palms beneath your shoulders. Exhaling, draw your bump toward your back and tilt your pelvis forward slightly. Inhaling, relax the space between your shoulder blades but maintain the table-top position. Release and repeat.

Done regularly, these exercises not only give you more stamina, but also stretch, strengthen, and relieve tension in the major muscles that alter in pregnancy.

Target areas

The exercises on these pages use gravity and your body weight to provide resistance—the safest option as pregnancy progresses. They target key areas during pregnancy—the lower back, arms, and thighs—and safeguard a good range of movement in the hips, neck, and upper back.

SEATED EXERCISES
These support your growing weight and allow you to focus your attention on important areas of the body: the upper back, neck, and shoulders. As your weight moves forward, the muscles around the spine have to work harder to keep your shoulders and head back, leading to aches and pains—especially in the lower back and base of the neck, which could lead to headaches. Seated exercises counter this by safely lengthening the muscles around the lower back and building strength in the core muscles of the abdomen that keep the body upright.

ALL-FOURS POSITION
As your belly swells and drops lower, the backs of your legs and gluteal muscles in your buttocks have to work hard to keep you upright. Exercising in the all-fours position can relieve the strain. It also focuses attention on the back of your body, which is often neglected during pregnancy. From this position you can

"As you practice these exercises, visualize your breath filling the back of your body, from the kidneys to the back of the ribs"

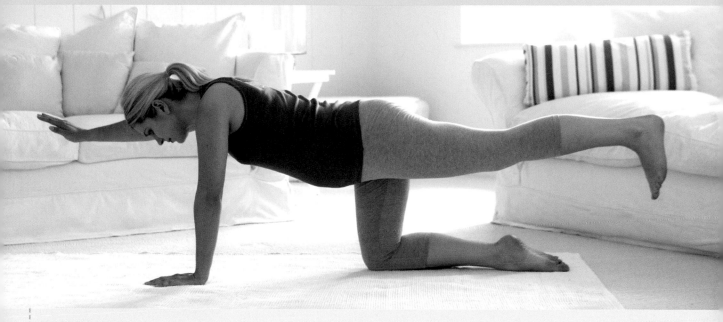

SUPERMAN POSE
From all fours, stabilize your weight over your left palm and right knee. Holding the table-top position, stretch your right arm forward. If you feel stable, stretch your left leg backward. Hold briefly, and lower. Repeat on the other sides.

safely strengthen the muscles on either side of your spine and keep your hips mobile. It's a good position in which to practice push-ups to strengthen your arms, and helps the baby settle into a good position for birth.

STANDING EXERCISES
Combine seated and floor exercises with standing exercises to improve balance and strength in your legs. Try standing in front of a chair to practice squatting—work with your feet facing forward, then with feet turned out at 45 degrees. Avoid

squats later in pregnancy if your baby isn't in the right position (if, for example, he is breech or transverse, see p.272).

PELVIC FLOOR EXERCISES
Also known as "Kegels" after the doctor who designed them in the 1940s, these exercises can be practiced anywhere, as often as you can remember to do them. To find your pelvic floor muscles, try to stop your urine flow mid-stream, using the muscles in the vaginal area. (Don't do this too often, though: It can push urine back up into the bladder and lead

to infections and bladder weakness.) Slowly contract the muscles to draw up your pelvic floor. Hold for a count of five, then gently let it down again. Repeat several times a day, until you can hold the count for 15. If you lose control partway through, start again, ensuring you can feel the muscles being released as you "let down" your pelvic floor. Do two sets, then rest for a minute. Now tighten and release the pelvic floor muscles as quickly as you can. Do this 30 times, then rest. Do two sets of these fast exercises. This completes the session.

My pregnancy workout

So what are the components of a safe but effective workout during pregnancy? Exactly those of a regular workout: aerobic activity to exercise the heart and lungs, strength work to target key muscles, and stretching for flexibility.

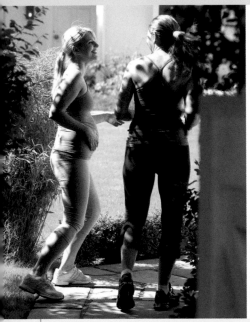

JOGGING
If you like jogging, there's no reason not to continue in pregnancy. Take a friend and keep the pace gentle.

GYM WORKOUTS
During aerobic workouts in the gym, it's easy to monitor your heart rate to maintain a safe level of exertion.

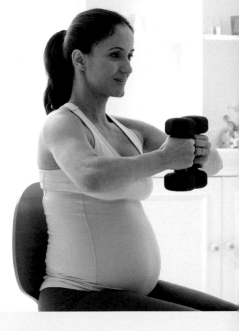

USING FREE WEIGHTS
It's a good idea to use slightly smaller weights during pregnancy, and to keep the movements slow and controlled.

What changes in pregnancy is the level of intensity you work at. Listen to your body: If a workout feels too strenuous, slow down or stop. Watch your technique, too—quality matters more than quantity. Aim for slow, well-executed movements, with good posture, balance, and control.

Types of exercise

There are three main elements of a good pregnancy workout: aerobic activity, strength training, and flexibility work.

AEROBIC FITNESS
Also known as cardiovascular training, aerobic activity is anything that raises the heart rate to 65–85 percent of its maximum and forces the lungs to work harder to deliver oxygen to the body. You should be able to sustain the activity for 20 minutes or longer. This builds stamina and endurance. These activities usually work the large muscles of the arms, legs, and chest as well as the heart and lungs. Swimming, jogging, and cycling are good examples. Aim to include at least 15–20 minutes of aerobic activity in every

exercise session, after your warm-up. Just bear in mind that your heart is already working harder than normal in pregnancy. The average woman's heart rate is 70 beats per minute, but during pregnancy it increases to 85–90 beats, or higher if you're expecting more than one baby. In the last trimester, your heart rate can increase by 10–20 beats. If any exercise makes you feel breathless or lightheaded, take it down a notch. As a general rule, don't allow your heart rate to exceed 140 beats a minute (use a heart-rate monitor).

"Listen to your body while you are exercising, and if any activity feels too intense, simply slow down or stop"

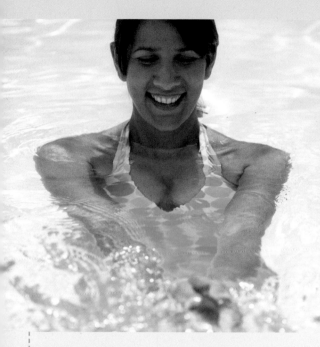

WATER RESISTANCE
Water workouts are fantastic because your weight and joints are supported while you build strength.

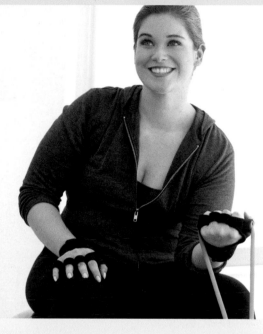

USING RESISTANCE BANDS
Resistance bands are a safe, effective way to strengthen your leg and arm muscles. Ask an instructor to demonstrate the best exercises for pregnancy and to suggest how many repetitions you should aim for.

The safest form of aerobic activity in pregnancy is low impact, meaning that at least one foot is on the floor at all times, so there's less jarring on your joints. If you enjoy classes, reduce the intensity or the height of the step; when swimming, cut the number of laps and focus on quality strokes.

STRENGTH AND FLEXIBILITY
Strength training can use any form of resistance—free weights or weight machines, water, rubber bands, your body weight, gravity—to make your muscles work harder than they usually would. This strengthens the muscles, ligaments, and tendons, builds bone mass, and can improve the way in which joints work. Work on muscle strength after the aerobic part of your workout, and always stretch afterward. Strength training targets specific groups of muscles. In pregnancy, focus on building your arm muscles (you'll need strong arms to carry your baby!) and your legs (to help support your growing belly, and to help you to push more effectively during labor). Don't do too many repetitions, and keep movements well controlled. Resistance bands are also useful to isolate movement in the correct muscle group. Exercising in water is ideal for strengthening your arms and legs while your weight and joints are fully supported.

The more flexibility you have, the greater your range of movement. Add a stretching routine to every session—a quick one after warming up and a longer one after cooling down (see pp.70–71). Stretching lessens the risk of injury, encourages circulation, and relaxes you.

Stretching out

Stretching reduces muscle tension, boosts coordination, and increases your range of movement, relieving pregnancy aches, pain, and discomfort. It also encourages circulation and enhances relaxation—good for you and your baby.

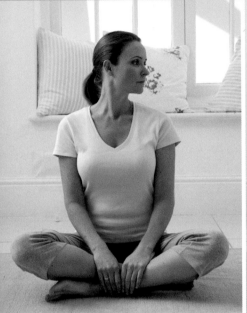

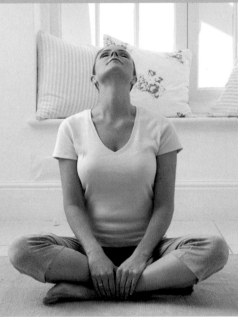

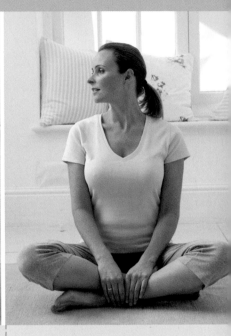

NECK RELEASE, LOOK LEFT
To relax tense neck and shoulders, sit with legs crossed. Relax arms and hands. Sit tall and look forward. Exhaling, turn to look over your left shoulder. Relax your right shoulder away from your ear. Inhaling, turn to center.

NECK RELEASE, LOOK UP
Very carefully lift your chin and look up. Keep the back of your neck long and shoulders down; make sure you do not crunch or jam your neck backward. Then lower your chin and lengthen the back of your neck.

NECK RELEASE, LOOK RIGHT
Exhaling, turn smoothly to look over your right shoulder. Relax your left shoulder away from your ear and feel the stretch. Inhale, then slowly turn your head back to center.

Stretching exercises feel so good in pregnancy because they help increase space for your baby, which makes you feel more comfortable—especially as you move toward the final stages of pregnancy or if you are carrying more than one baby. Stretching also makes you much more aware of your posture. This awareness encourages you to stand and sit well, allowing more room for your baby in every activity you undertake. Sitting and standing correctly can also influence your baby's position in the uterus, helping to prepare you both for a good labor. Various stretches can help shift the weight of your baby away from your back as pregnancy progresses, which brings great relief.

Stretching encourages you to focus your awareness inside, which helps you feel more connected to your body and how it's changing as you move through pregnancy. This also makes you more aware of your shifting center of gravity, and helps you adjust accordingly to keep yourself active and prevent injury.

Focusing inside also gives you welcome time to "connect" with your baby.

When and how

There are no rules about when and how to stretch—just listen to your body and have a stretch whenever you can. Don't confine your stretching to a 10-minute warm-up or cool-down in an exercise session (although it's always a good idea to incorporate stretching as part of a

"You don't have to be flexible or able to touch your toes to benefit from stretching; it boosts health and well-being on all levels"

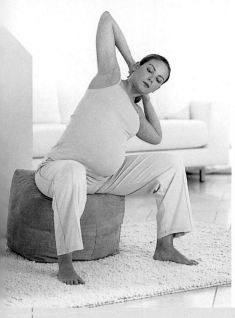

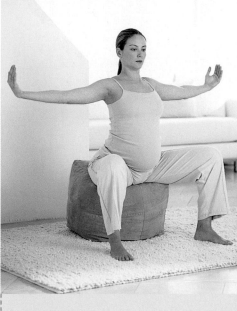

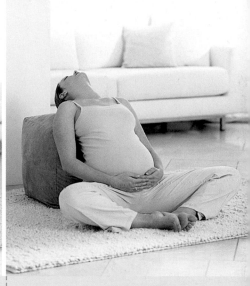

SIDEWAYS STRETCH
Place feet flat on the floor, cradling the back of your head in your palms, elbows wide. Exhaling, lengthen your right side, from hip to elbow; lower your left elbow. Inhale, lift back to center. Repeat on other side.

CHEST OPENER
From the same sitting position, stretch your arms wide. Relax your shoulders. Inhaling, take your arms back slightly, without compressing your lower back. Lift and open your chest. Hold for a few breaths, then relax.

GROIN STRETCH
Sit on the floor with a support behind you. Bring the soles of your feet together. Lower your back to the support. If you feel strain, sit upright. Rest your palms on your bump. Relax for a few breaths, then sit up.

workout). During pregnancy, the more often you can stretch, the better; it brings benefits on so many levels.

Try to do a little every day—find a general class (be sure to tell the teacher you're pregnant) or one especially for pregnant women, or follow a prenatal DVD or book at home. If you can't find time every day, try to practice once or twice a week. You may find you are stiffer first thing in the morning, but stretching will make you feel better and is a great way to start the day. At the end of the

day you may feel tired, achy, or sore, but a good stretch helps to ease all these problems. Your body will respond especially well if you have spent long hours at a desk or in a sedentary job. You may also want to incorporate meditation or visualization techniques into your stretching, to really help yourself wind down after a long day.

STRETCHING SAFELY
Don't stretch to your maximum potential while you are pregnant; hold back a

little. Work to the point at which you feel a comfortable stretch, but don't push yourself to the limit, and if your muscles start to shake, ease off! The hormone relaxin makes your ligaments more flexible, and reduces stability in the joints. So although you can stretch more easily during pregnancy, your joints may not thank you for doing so.

Avoid groin stretches (above) if you have symphysis pubis dysfunction (SPD) or any pain in the groin area (see p.387), since they may exacerbate the condition.

Prenatal yoga

The benefits of yoga during pregnancy are the same as stretching, but magnified: Yoga teaches breathing techniques that calm and focus the mind and provide tools for coping during labor, or indeed, any of life's stressful situations.

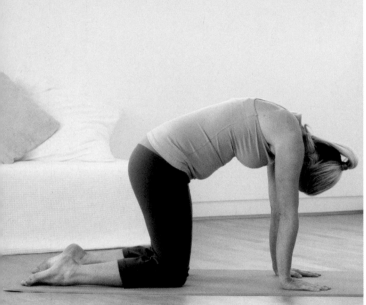

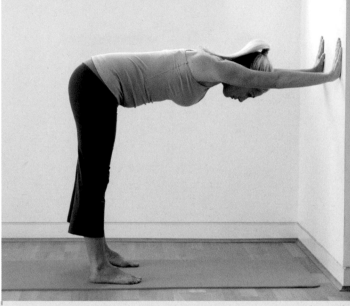

CAT STRETCH
Press your hands on the floor, fingers spread out and tops of feet pressing into the floor. Exhaling, tuck your chin into your chest and round your back; as you inhale, flatten your back to a neutral spine. Imagine you are hugging your baby in toward you with each exhalation, and try to round a little more each time. Repeat 10 times.

SPINE STRETCH
Stand with your feet hip-width apart, hands pressing against the wall, and make a right-angle shape with your legs and body. Press back through your heels and forward through your hands and press your hips back. This helps lengthen your spine and take the weight of your baby off your back. Hold for 5–10 slow, deep breaths.

Like all exercise, yoga promotes health and well-being, reduces tension and painful muscles, boosts circulation, and releases endorphins, the feel-good hormones that lift mood and relieve pain.

Benefits of yoga

Even better, during pregnancy, yoga strengthens the muscles that help you to support the weight of your growing baby.

The standing *asanas*, or yoga postures, help to build core stability by strengthening the back and abdominal muscles. Other techniques help you strengthen the pelvic floor muscles (see p.67). Many asanas create more space in your pelvis for your baby, which makes you feel more comfortable and can ease a bad back. Others encourage the pelvis to widen in preparation for labor, and guide the baby into the optimal position for delivery. A recent study found that

pregnant women who practice yoga have less risk of developing high blood pressure during pregnancy, and of going into premature labor. Yoga may even help to speed up labor. After the birth, it can help speed recovery.

What differentiates yoga is the focus on *pranayama*, or breath-control techniques, which can be an invaluable aid during labor. It's helpful to take your birth partner along to some classes so that he or she can remind you of the

"Yoga is one of the most nurturing activities during pregnancy, since it calms the mind while preparing the body for labor"

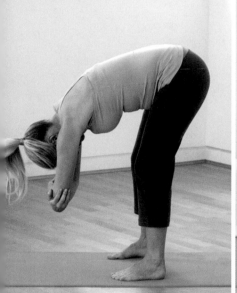

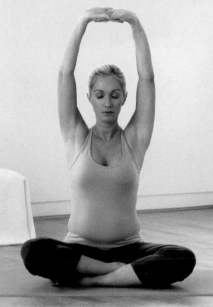

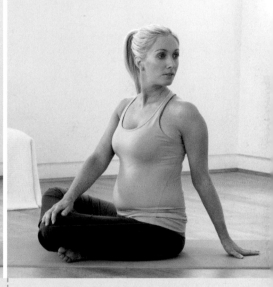

FORWARD FOLD
Feet hip-width apart (or so), bend your knees, hold elbows with hands, and hang forward. Feel your neck and upper back release and the stretch through the backs of your legs, straightening them if you want to stretch the hamstrings.

ENERGIZING ARM STRETCH
Sit cross-legged (or straight-legged) on the floor or a cushion, interlace your fingers, and stretch your arms up, palms up. Feel the stretch all the way up the body, creating space for your baby. Take 5 breaths. Slowly release your arms as you exhale.

SEATED SPINAL TWIST
Place your right hand on your left knee and your left fingers on the floor behind you. Look over your left shoulder, easing the shoulder back and down. Lengthen through the spine as you inhale and twist a little more as you exhale. Hold for 3–5 breaths, release, then change sides.

breathing techniques during labor. Above all, many women value the time a yoga session devotes to relaxation and meditation, especially if they have busy lives or older children. In this quiet time, yoga allows you to connect to your body and baby, allowing you to prepare psychologically for the birth.

CLASSES OR HOME PRACTICE?
Both ways of practicing yoga have their benefits. Classes for pregnant women are especially valuable because they provide you with a ready-made network of other new and more experienced pregnant women, who can offer advice, practical tips, friendship, and even a support network now and after the birth. Often, yoga for pregnancy is taught alongside birth-preparation in classes endorsed by midwives, which cover subjects such as natural pain relief, labor breathing techniques, and positions for an active labor. This is the best way to learn yoga if you are new to the form. But if you can't get to class, doing yoga at home with a DVD or book specially created for pregnancy is often the easiest way to fit yoga into a busy schedule or home life.

If you are new to yoga, it's best to start with a special prenatal yoga class, or an instructor who has trained in pregnancy yoga and who can give you the one-on-one attention you need. She will know how to adapt the standard poses to suit the different trimesters.

Pilates for pregnancy

The Pilates system of low-impact exercises was devised to develop a balance of strength and flexibility in the body's muscles and heighten poise and body-awareness. It shares many of the benefits of stretching and yoga in pregnancy.

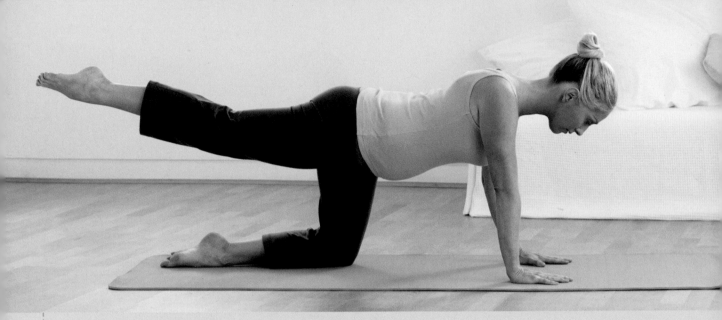

STRENGTHENING THE LOWER BACK
On all fours (wrists below shoulders and knees below hips), extend your right leg behind, keeping the leg straight at about hip height. Hold for one breath, then release back down to all fours and change sides. Look down so that your neck is in line with your spine. You can continue to straighten alternate legs or try extending the opposite arm in front at the same time as you extend the leg back.

Pilates is a physical fitness system invented during the 20th century by Joseph Pilates in order to restore balance to the body. You can practice Pilates on mats using a series of floor-based exercises, or you can use Pilates machines known as "reformers," which use spring tension to work different muscle groups. The technique is favored by dancers for promoting posture, strength, flexibility, and control, and also by athletes seeking to recover after injury.

The benefits

The controlled movements taught by Pilates teachers develop strength in the central, or core, muscles of the abdomen and pelvis that stabilize the body while increasing flexibility throughout. The method focuses awareness on the way in which your body moves and it also introduces breathing techniques and emphasizes the importance of relaxation. The precise exercises—which increase in difficulty—isolate different parts of the body without putting strain on the joints or spine.

In pregnancy, any form of exercise that strengthens the core muscles is useful—for increased stability, to improve posture and circulation, and to help prevent backache. Pilates also incorporates pelvic floor exercises (see p.67), which are essential during pregnancy to support the weight of your growing baby. When these muscles are

"Pilates builds core strength to support you through pregnancy and birth, and is a great way to get your figure back afterward"

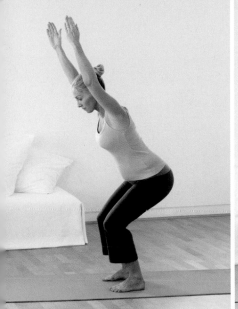

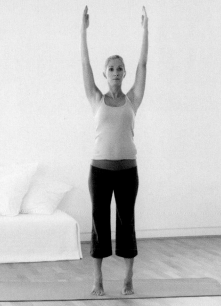

STRENGTHENING THE LEGS
Stand, feet hip-width apart and parallel. Raise your arms up, keep your shoulders down, and sink down through the hips to sit into an imaginary chair. Hold for 3-5 breaths, stand up straight again and lower your arms. Repeat a few times.

GIVING FEET AND BODY A LIFT
Stand, feet hip-width apart, arms by your sides. Lift up on the balls of the feet, raising the heels high, and raise your arms up (keep your shoulders down). This strengthens the inner arches of the feet, and is energizing. Hold for about 5 breaths; repeat a few times.

the method, and the mat exercises taught in these classes are very effective in tackling backache and postural problems. However, general classes won't be able to deliver the specialist program you need during pregnancy. It's best to search out a dedicated prenatal Pilates class (there are also postpartum classes) or a teacher who has trained in prenatal Pilates. She or he will know which exercises you should avoid, and be able to give you the one-on-one attention you need.

This is even more important if you are new to the method. Once you have a good knowledge of the mat exercises and which movements to adapt and avoid, it's easy to continue practicing Pilates at home or with a DVD or book specially created for use in pregnancy.

toned, you are likely to experience a more comfortable pregnancy and may have an easier delivery and speedier recovery, too. Because Pilates targets the stomach, back, and pelvic floor muscles without straining other joints, these exercises can work particularly well for you during pregnancy.

Many Pilates exercises are performed on your hands and knees, which is an ideal position for pregnancy. Adopting this position can take some of the strain off your back and pelvis, and, toward the end of your pregnancy, may help to get your baby into the right position. Some Pilates exercises can also be useful in labor, to help keep you focused and mobile.

Where to practice

General Pilates classes are the first port of call for most people who are new to

Staying safe

During pregnancy, you should avoid the reformer or use it with caution under expert instruction. The springs and cords might exert too much pull on the hip flexor and groin muscles, leading to groin strain or pelvic pain (SPD, see p.387). As with all forms of exercise, after the first trimesters, avoid exercising on your back. You won't be able to work lying on your abdomen after the first trimester; a teacher can demonstrate modified moves. Use a Pilates exercise ball only under the supervision of an accredited instructor.

Taking care of my appearance

Looking after yourself can lift your spirits, making it easier to cope with aches, pain, and other symptoms of pregnancy. And what's not to like about the glowing skin, thick hair, and glossy nails that pregnancy can promote?

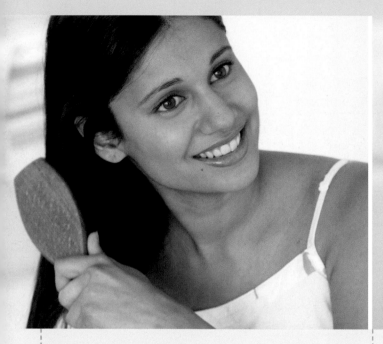

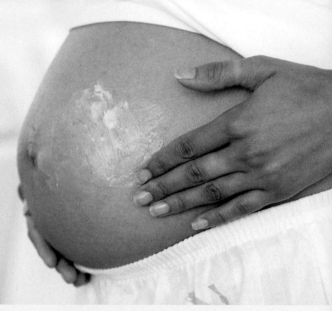

CARING FOR YOUR HAIR
Hair remains in a growth phase during pregnancy, which means it will likely be thicker and glossier than usual. If your tresses become unmanageable, you may need to try different products to tame them.

MOISTURIZING ESSENTIALS
Using a stretch-mark cream or belly oil specially formulated for pregnancy morning and night makes your skin feel smoother and more hydrated—even if there's no guarantee that you'll avoid marks.

Whether you're concerned about looking good or simply want to avoid appearing tired, it makes sense to devote a little extra time to self-care essentials during these important months. Your skin, nails, hair, and teeth will thank you!

Skincare basics

Most women find that their skin changes during pregnancy. Many report that their skin is better than ever, with fewer breakouts and greasy patches, plus that fabled glow. Others find that pregnancy hormones result in more pimples, especially in the first trimester, or that their skin feels extra-sensitive and tight or itchy as pregnancy progresses.

If your skin becomes more sensitive during pregnancy, you might want to consider switching to products formulated for sensitive skin, which are free from parabens, chemicals, and preservatives, such as formaldehyde and phthalates. Chemicals and formaldehyde can irritate sensitive skin, while parabens concern some experts because they mimic estrogen. Phthalates can be toxic to the reproductive system and fetal development. Visit the Environmental Working Group's Skin Deep cosmetics safety database (cosmeticsdatabase.com) to check the products you use. If you're looking for something new, try shopping in a health-food store for products that are based on organic ingredients.

Some pregnant women insist on not applying to their skin anything they wouldn't eat, given that some 60 percent of what we rub into the face or body is absorbed transdermally (through the

"When your bump grows and you can no longer see your feet, a pedicure really is the perfect treat"

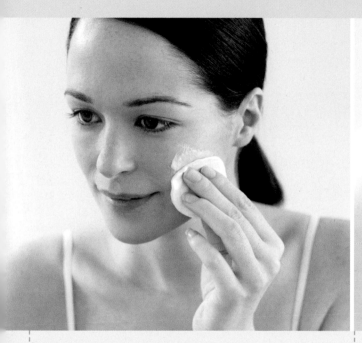

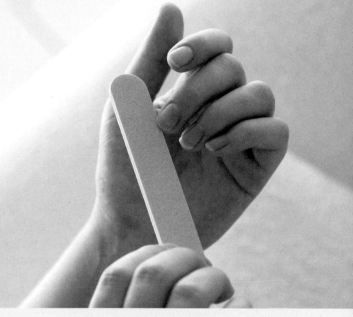

CHANGING YOUR SKINCARE PRODUCTS
Consider swapping your regular skincare essentials, such as cleansers and toners, for organic products to cut down on the number of chemicals you are exposed to during pregnancy.

NATURAL NAILS
Your nails grow faster during pregnancy, so you may need to file them more regularly. You can use natural products, including buffers and oils, to bring out their natural beauty.

skin into the bloodstream). Anti-aging and acne creams containing retinoids (a form of vitamin A) are not recommended in pregnancy for this reason, since high doses of vitamin A can be harmful to an unborn child, as can salicylic acid, found in some facial and body peels.

It might be best to do a patch test when trying a new beauty or hair-care product—dab a little on an area of delicate skin (behind your knee or ear) and wait 24 hours to see if your skin reacts. If it does, avoid that product. You can also look in your fridge and pantry for safer skincare treatments: an oatmeal paste to treat oily skin, yogurt or milk instead of your normal facial cleanser, cooled green tea or rosewater as a toner, and mashed banana and avocado as a face mask.

STRETCHING SKIN
As your belly and breasts balloon, you may find that your skin feels tighter, thinner, and more itchy than usual. Moisturizing morning and night can help. It's also worth switching from a standard to an organic laundry detergent for your clothes. If itching is still intense after 28 weeks, consult your doctor.

Stretch marks can occur when the skin expands rapidly and most often appear on the belly, breasts, thighs, and buttocks. They are said to affect 90 percent of pregnant women, hence the huge number of stretch-mark products on the shelves. While creams may make you feel better, whether or not you get stretch marks, and their color and extent, depends largely on genetic inheritance—some people just have stretchier skin.

Try moisturizing those areas that are prone to stretching morning and night. A number of everyday oils make great natural moisturizers: olive oil suits very dry or inflamed skin, while sunflower oil is light and easily absorbed, and grapeseed oil is considered a powerful skin healer. Rosehip oil is valued for repairing scarred and sun-damaged skin. Rub the oil in while your skin is moist, after a bath or shower. But whatever you rub onto your skin, be aware that stretch marks never fade entirely, so try to think of them as a badge of honor!

SUN PROTECTION

Pregnant women have higher levels of the hormone that produces the pigment melanin, which is responsible for darkened nipples and the dark line (linea nigra) that may appear down the center of your abdomen. Because of this extra pigment, you may develop facial discoloration known as chloasma or melasma (the so-called "mask" of pregnancy), when you expose your face to the sun. This is characterized by blotchy pigmentation around your cheeks, forehead, and neck, which becomes darker in light-skinned women and lighter on darker skin.

Don't, however, be tempted to avoid sunlight completely. The rays of the sun are important for your body to produce vitamin D, which encourages the healthy development of your baby's bones and teeth, and also prevents weakening of your own bones. Just try to avoid strong direct sunlight (usually between 10am and 2pm), and wear a broad-brimmed hat and sunglasses.

Wear sunscreen, but go for one with an SPF of 20 to 25, which allows some beneficial rays to penetrate your skin. Natural sunscreens are best, since they contain fewer chemicals. Many use sun reflectors, such as zinc oxide, to deflect the sun rather than act as a barrier. Avoid using anything that contains "nano" particles, which are associated with a host of health problems. Tanning beds are not recommended in pregnancy. Some types may cause overheating, which can harm your baby, and there is evidence that their UV rays may lower levels of folic acid in your body, increasing the risk of birth defects.

NAIL BASICS

During pregnancy, your nails remain in a growth phase, often looking and feeling very healthy and strong. Equally, however, you may find that they split or become dryer than usual. A little olive oil, rubbed into the nails and the nailbed daily, will help to rehydrate them and encourage healthier growth. Keep them well trimmed to avoid tearing.

Many women are concerned about chemicals found in nail polish and nail-polish removers, but there is no evidence that these pose any significant risk. Some experts recommend avoiding them in the first trimester, when your baby is most vulnerable to toxins. It also makes sense that any pedicures or manicures should take place in a well-ventilated room. Choose water-based polish, or check the label to make sure that your polish doesn't contain dibutyl phthalate, also referred to as

CARING FOR YOUR TEETH
Pregnancy hormones soften your gums, so it's important to brush and floss at least twice a day to keep gum disease at bay.

APPLYING MAKEUP
You may find that you need to apply makeup differently, to accommodate skin changes and coloring. You may also need no makeup at all!

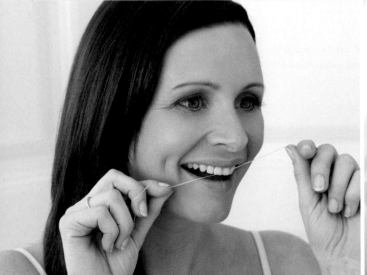

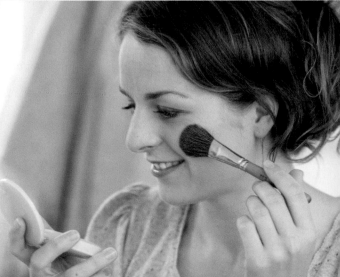

DBP, and other potentially harmful ingredients, such as toluene or formaldehyde.

If you wish to play it safe, simply shine your nails with a nail buffer, and massage with a little olive or jojoba oil to keep them looking healthy.

As your bump grows, you'll find that your toenails are increasingly neglected. Why not ask a friend to come over for a pampering session. A foot bath can feel deliciously decadent when you can no longer see your feet—cool water soothes hot, swollen feet at the end of the day, while warm water eases soreness. If you can persuade your partner to give you a foot massage, all the better!

HEALTHY HAIR
Hair usually looks fantastic during pregnancy; increased estrogen

encourages a consistent cycle of hair growth, meaning that fewer strands fall out. As a result, your locks may look remarkably thick and glossy, so it's worth taking advantage of this to experiment with a new, hassle-free haircut.

If your scalp becomes dry or sensitive during pregnancy, try switching to an organic shampoo made without harsh detergents, and avoid anything containing sodium laureth sulphate (SLS), which can irritate the skin and eyes. Organic shampoos won't lather as much, but they're just as effective.

If you color or perm your hair regularly, you might be concerned about the safety of the products applied to your scalp, but studies suggest that occasional treatments (every six weeks or so) won't have an adverse effect on your health or that of your baby. Even so, many women wait until after the first trimester to get a treatment, and do so at a reputable salon, often choosing high- or lowlights, instead of an all-over color. There are many organic hair salons, too, which use natural, chemical-free dyes and colors. If you use colorants at home, follow the safety instructions on the box. Semi-permanent, vegetable, and wash-out colors pose less risk, and henna is safe during pregnancy.

If you have older children, you may be familiar with head lice or "nits." It's best not to use any insecticide treatments during pregnancy, either on you or any other family member. Instead, slather hair in conditioner and use a fine-toothed comb to trap the insects. Employ this method every three days or so until you are all clear.

DENTAL CARE
Everyday care of your teeth is even more important than usual during pregnancy, since hormones can soften your gums and lead to gum disease (gingivitis). Gum disease is a known risk factor for

premature birth, so scrupulous attention to oral hygiene is essential. Book an appointment with your dentist or hygienist when you become pregnant, and get a good overall cleaning to remove any existing plaque. Brush regularly with a soft toothbrush, which won't irritate your gums, and pay attention to the area where your teeth meet your gums. Rinse regularly with a teaspoon of salt in water to prevent plaque build-up, reduce bacteria, and soothe sore gums, and floss daily, even if this is a little uncomfortable at first. Bleeding gums are not uncommon, but if you are uncomfortable or there are signs of inflammation or infection, such as swelling and pain, see your dentist.

Making time for yourself

Looking after yourself is not only relaxing and rejuvenating, but it can also elevate your mood and make you more confident about and comfortable with your changing appearance. A little self-nurturing goes a long way toward promoting a positive self-image, which is one step toward becoming the confident mom you will soon be. What's more, there is an undeniable link between mood and overall health. If you feel great, you are less likely to experience the annoying symptoms of pregnancy, and more empowered to deal with them.

Treat yourself to a little pampering from time to time—sink into a scented bubble bath, invest in a conditioning treatment for your hair or a great new cut, book a relaxing massage, experiment with natural goodies to make your skin glow, and, above all, enjoy time for you. It won't be long before the demands of motherhood take priority and time for yourself is a distant memory.

Looking good

Sometimes it was the basics that made me feel better, such as soaking in a bath then setting aside enough time to get dressed. I found that those little indulgences really boosted my mood. CH

I got my hair cut and colored as near to my due date as I dared. It made me feel great and I hoped would distract from the bags under my eyes. VB

No matter what stage of pregnancy I was in, in the end I found that looking good—to myself and others—came from within. It's that personal confidence, the glow of knowing that you are carrying your baby, and appearing comfortable in yourself that shines through. LJ

My pregnancy wardrobe

Your growing bump gives you the perfect excuse to experiment with what you wear—and have fun doing it. You won't need new clothes at first, but a few key items later on will help see you through pregnancy in comfort and style.

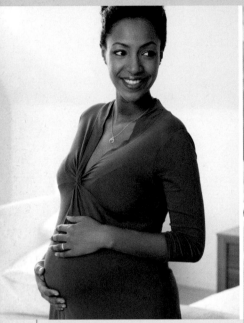

GLOWING AND GLAMOROUS
When you feel and look good, you perform better. This makes a pregnancy work wardrobe particularly important.

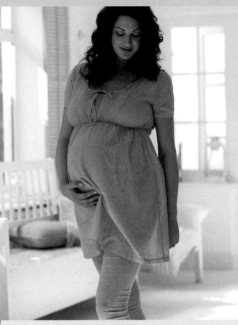

DRESSING FOR COMFORT
In the summer months choose natural fabrics, such as linen and cotton. Loose-cut dresses and pants will help you stay cool.

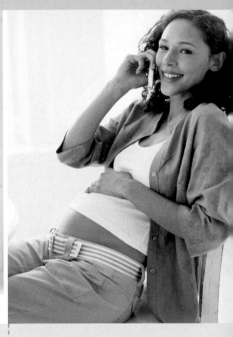

LOW-RISE EASE
Low-slung pants sit neatly under your growing bump and allow you to get by in regular clothes during the early months.

There's no doubt that being pregnant requires an adjustment to the way you view your body. At a time of such huge change, especially in the first trimester, it's easy to slip into feeling fat and frumpy—but there's no need to think this way. These days, there's such a vast choice of maternity wear available that it's much easier to look great, and to be as fashion-conscious and comfortable as you were pre-pregnancy.

Indeed, many women welcome this rare opportunity to step away from the tyranny of the sizing system. There's no point in coveting those size-zero outfits now, so why not embrace the new curvy you and dress to flaunt your assets?

A liberating new look

It's important to separate pregnancy weight gain from the attitudes we have about regular weight gain. All too often, doctors and midwives have to listen to newly pregnant women worrying about putting on weight. But the weight you gain now is not about getting fat. Although you don't have license to live on pies and cakes, as long as you have a healthy lifestyle (eating well and exercising regularly), you don't need to worry about how many pounds you are putting on, nor compare yourself with others. Weight gain in pregnancy differs from woman to woman, governed partly by whether you were a healthy weight, overweight, or underweight when you got pregnant. So enjoy being liberated from the tape measure and scales.

"What's in your wardrobe right now says a lot about how attractive and self-confident you feel"

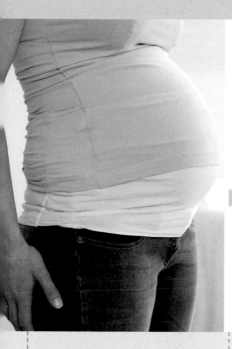 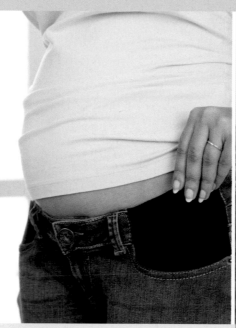 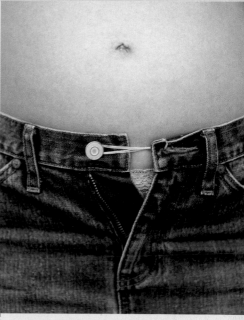

BELLY BAND
This is a tube of stretchy fabric that can fill the gap between jeans or skirts and tops that ride up as you get bigger.

PREGNANCY JEANS
Specially designed pregnancy garments are made to fit your new shape and will make you feel stylish and confident.

MAKE DO AND MEND
Don't want to ditch your favorite jeans? In the first trimester, use every means necessary to keep them comfortable.

THE EARLY DAYS
One of the best pieces of practical advice for newly pregnant women is not to rush out and buy a whole new maternity wardrobe. You can probably adapt what you have in those first three months, making the most of clothes made from stretchy fabrics or those with elastic waists, or improvising by not doing up every button or zipper.

As you progress through the second trimester, you'll need to rethink your wardrobe a bit and invest in a few key pieces that can accommodate your bump.

It's well worth investing in a pair of maternity jeans, for example, because they're comfortable and look great. Most have expandable waistbands, so you can adjust them as your belly grows. Flowing tops and dresses, and those that nip in under the bust and then flare out, are also very flattering.

Buy the basics as you go along, rather than in one shopping spree, so you can adapt to the seasons, as well as your shape. The clothes you wore earlier in pregnancy will also come in handy after you have your baby. Your skinny jeans

won't fit immediately after delivery—in fact your pre-pregnancy clothes may not fit for a few months afterward, so keep anything you bought early in the second trimester; you will probably be able to recycle it once your baby is born.

VERSATILE BASICS
You may decide to pay a bit more for good quality maternity wear if you want it to last—especially if you fully intend to use your maternity clothes at least once more in the foreseeable future! It's true that you are going to be wearing

these items for some time—at least four or five months in this pregnancy anyway—and quality fabrics and finishes will wear and wash well. On the other hand, you may prefer to save money by buying cheaper or second-hand clothes, since fashions change quickly and you'll only be wearing them for less than a year. Whichever route you take, start by investing in a few staple items as soon as you need them and then add one or two items each month to revive these everyday staples.

As well as comfort, keep your personal style in mind. If you weren't happy in dresses or tailored jackets pre-pregnancy, you are unlikely to be so now. That said, do try an empire-cut dress (the waistband sits below the bust). It will see you through most of your pregnancy, and can be dressed up or worn over jeans.

For work, purchase a few neutral pieces in simple shapes, then accessorize with scarves, jewelry, and pretty sweaters. For everyday wear, it's worth investing in a good pair of maternity pants—something stretchy, like you might wear to a yoga class—with an adjustable waist. Or choose low-slung hipster pants, teaming them with an oversized shirt to cover the gap. You can purchase a "belly band," which is designed to fill the gap between skirts or pants and your usual-length tops as your waistline expands.

BUMP ON A BUDGET

You need plenty of clothes that make you feel great during pregnancy—trying to get by on a few favorites can leave you feeling unattractive. But that doesn't have to mean a huge expense; it's worth cutting corners wherever you can. For one thing, you'll be so sick of maternity clothes by the end of your pregnancy, you may never want to wear them again!

BEGGING AND BORROWING

Not everything has to be new when you are pregnant. Like baby clothes, most maternity wear is in great condition because—thanks to changing seasons and body shapes—they are worn only for a limited time. Make the most of this by looking for second-hand garments. Don't hesitate to accept offers of maternity clothes from friends and relatives—it's worth organizing a clothes swap for pregnancy and postpartum clothes. Try vintage shops and garage sales. Also look online at auction sites. You might hit the jackpot and find a whole maternity wardrobe for a fraction of the cost of an entirely new one.

Even if your second-hand garments are not right for the office, wearing them at home will allow you to spend a little more on work clothing. Try raiding your partner's closet, too—large T-shirts or dress shirts and comfortable cardigans can be ruched in with a low-slung belt. Men's clothes tend to be cut more loosely and therefore may be more comfortable.

ADAPT AND SURVIVE

Look at your regular wardrobe with a creative eye to see whether you can adapt old favorites. If you've got an old pair of jeans that are ready for recycling, cut out the front and sew in an elasticized panel—look online for free

---

VERSATILE WARDROBE
Try neutral pieces in basic shapes. This look can take you from the office to social situations.

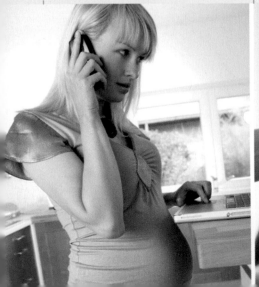

THE RIGHT FIT
It's important to be measured by a professional every six weeks or so, as your breast size can change dramatically.

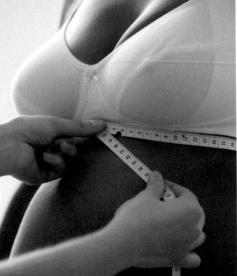

CHOOSING SWIMWEAR
One-piece swimsuits are always flattering, or you can show off your bump in a tankini, with a long-length top.

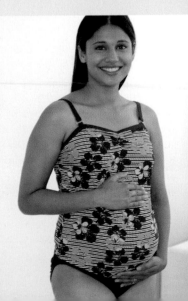

patterns and tips. If you're handy with a needle and thread, try making stretchy cotton Lycra tube skirts that will grow with you or a wrap skirt with a waist tie that expands and also sits neatly under your belly. There are plenty of tutorials online on craft websites and blogs.

SEASON-SAVVY SHOPPING

Figure out the seasons in which you'll be pregnant to avoid stocking up on long-sleeved tops when you'll be heavily pregnant in summer. It's worth investing in maternity swimwear after the first trimester if you have a vacation planned or you've made swimming part of your regular exercise regime. There's nothing more demoralizing than having to squeeze into a pre-pregnancy bathing suit in public. And having a great suit that fits beautifully can help you maintain the motivation for swimming after the initial enthusiasm wanes.

Think twice before investing in a winter coat for pregnancy. You are likely to feel very warm in your third trimester, and may find it more comfortable to wear plenty of layered knits rather than one warm coat or jacket. Consider wearing your usual coat with a long scarf hanging down to fill the gap, or purchase a large shawl or wrap, which will see you through the winter months and keep you and your baby warm when she arrives.

Choosing shoes

Since your center of gravity changes when you are pregnant, as your weight shifts forward, very high heels can be dangerous—not to mention uncomfortable. Look for elegant flats or shoes with a low or kitten heel instead. Supportive shoes, such as cross-trainers or those with a contoured footbed, will feel good; flimsy pumps that don't

provide too much support can lead to tired, achy feet. If your regular size feels tight, get the length and width of your feet measured professionally. During pregnancy your ligaments loosen, thanks to the effects of the hormone relaxin, and the bones in your feet can spread so much that your pre-pregnancy footwear may feel tight or no longer fit.

Although your feet haven't actually grown, the effects last after the birth, meaning that you'll need to invest in shoes a half or whole size larger. It's worth the expense to spare the discomfort of ingrown toenails, bunions, and calluses. Fit can also be affected temporarily by swelling feet.

Buying bras

You may think of maternity underwear as an unnecessary expense—after all, who sees it? But your breast size as well as your belly and chest can increase hugely during pregnancy, which makes

buying new underwear a legitimate expense. The item that you will need more than any other maternity garment—and early on—is a maternity bra. It might look like a piece of scaffolding, if you are used to light wisps of lace, but it will transform the way you stand, make your clothes fit and hang better, and give your shape more definition. You will also feel much more comfortable. You may also find it comfortable to wear a light bra at night later on or if you have a large bust. Invest in two good-quality maternity bras at first, to accommodate your changing size, and don't be surprised if they need to be replaced in a few months time. Always get measured by a professional.

When your milk comes in a few days after the birth, your breasts will grow again. You will need a nursing bra. Professional bra fitters will be able to predict which size you'll need from 36 weeks of pregnancy, so get re-measured then rather than trying to get out to the store after your baby is born.

Making the most of our pregnancy shape

I found clothes that flowed and felt light on my skin made me feel most comfortable, and that in turn gave me confidence in my shape. Empire-waist dresses gave me room to move without looking like I was wearing a tent. CH

My best maternity buy was two pairs of nice black maternity pants with waistbands that I could expand as my bump expanded. I also bought a long, loose dress for when I did not want restrictions on my tummy. It was not even a maternity dress, but I was able to wear it right up to delivery—and I got good use out of it after the birth, too. Since my bump was so small, I managed in non-maternity clothes for longer than some other moms. NK

Yoga pants are the best for feeling comfortable and unrestricted. My sister-in-law wore hers nearly every day of her pregnancy. TL

I hit the jackpot during my pregnancy when I came across a garage sale. Some new mom had recently had her last child and put her entire maternity wardrobe on sale. LJ

In my first pregnancy, I found that, suddenly, none of my usual clothes fit. I bought a box of maternity clothes with a dress, tunic, shirt, and leggings all in one color that seemed a big investment at the time, but I wore them all the time with different accessories. They saw me through the next pregnancy, too, and a few of my friends'! VB

Travel and vacations

If you're experiencing a problem-free pregnancy, it's perfectly possible to travel up to about 36 weeks. Just take a few sensible precautions, try to be prepared for the unexpected, and enjoy a well-deserved stress-free break.

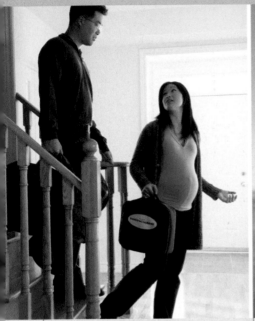

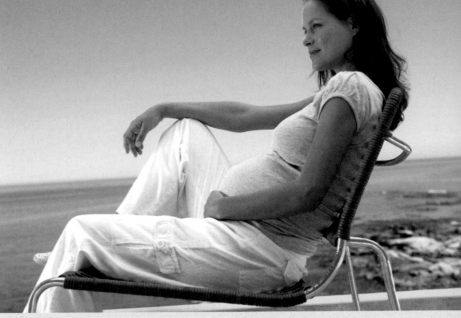

CARRY-ON ESSENTIALS
Make sure you keep everything you need for the trip, such as travel-sickness aids or any medication, in your carry-on bags.

RELAXATION TIME
Don't plan too many activities while on vacation when pregnant; give yourself time to sit and relax, read, or just watch the world go by. When you're a new mom, you'll realize what a luxury this really is!

Most women have the greatest energy for traveling in the second trimester, after nausea has settled down and while they still feel mobile and energetic. Take the opportunity to get away on a vacation if you can, especially if this is your first baby: It might be your last opportunity for a while to completely relax, take in some sights, and spend quality time alone with your partner.

If you want to travel by plane, bear in mind that you may not be able to fly late in pregnancy without your doctor's permission (see opposite). After 36 weeks, it's best to stay within an easy drive of the place where you intend to give birth.

Where to go

Very hot, long-haul destinations and active holidays probably won't feel as relaxing as they once did. Closer destinations, comfortable surroundings, good food, and plenty of opportunities for relaxation will be much less stressful.

It's advisable to avoid traveling to parts of the world where there is a high risk of disease, or where the emergency services are not reliable. Although shots for tetanus, hepatitis, and the flu are considered safe in pregnancy, live vaccines, such as chicken pox, measles, mumps, and rubella, are not usually recommended at this time, and oral vaccines to protect against yellow fever, typhoid, polio, and anthrax are contraindicated. However, if you do need to travel, your doctor may decide that the risk of the vaccine is lower than the risks associated with contracting the disease itself. In countries where the water is not safe to drink, rely on bottled water, even to brush your teeth. Only eat fruit you peel yourself and avoid ice in drinks, and leafy greens and salads, which may have been washed in contaminated water.

Planning your trip

Before you book anything, consult your doctor to discuss any potential risks particular to your pregnancy, and any medical reasons why it might not be safe to go away. If you have a history of miscarriage, ectopic pregnancy, premature labor, or placental abnormalities, you will be at increased risk of complications, which you would probably prefer to be managed at home, should they occur. Some women with high blood pressure, heart disease, a history of thrombosis, or severe asthma may be advised not to travel at all. Your doctor will make an assessment according to your individual needs. Check that your insurance policy covers travel to international destinations, if

you're planning to venture abroad. You may want to invest in travel insurance, although some companies consider pregnancy to be a pre-existing condition, making coverage tricky to obtain. To be safe, you may want to bring along a printed list of medical facilities at your destination, in case you have an emergency or problem. Don't forget to get a photocopy of your pregnancy file to bring along in your carry-on bag, and bring your health-insurance information.

TRAVELING BY PLANE
Check with your airline before booking a ticket, and tell the ticketing staff or travel agency about your pregnancy. Some airlines are wary of flying with women in their last month of pregnancy; in fact, some will not allow you to fly after 36 weeks without a letter from your doctor, written within a 72-hour period, that confirms your due date and your fitness to fly.

When booking your flight, reserve an aisle or bulkhead seat—both give extra leg room. Pack in your carry-on bags everything you might need for the trip, from snacks and drinks that stave off nausea to travel-sickness aids suitable

for pregnancy. Don't forget any regular medication; you may not find what you need at your destination. Then you can relax in the knowledge that you have enough to get you through both traveling and your time away.

Pregnant women are more prone to blood clots (thrombosis) and varicose veins, so it's particularly important to keep your blood flowing on long trips—whichever form of transportation you take—by moving your feet and legs.

Remain as mobile as you can (without risking losing your balance), and get out of your seat every hour or so to stretch and walk around. Wearing support stockings or socks will help, as will drinking plenty of fluids.

CAR TRIPS
Car trips are notorious for inducing travel sickness and fatigue, so drink regularly, eat energy-giving foods (such as fruit and nuts), and stop often for breaks. Wear your seat belt with the shoulder strap between your breasts and the lap belt under your bump, rather than across your belly. Keep a window open and share the load with someone if you are driving, to help you stay alert.

Enjoying a hassle-free trip

Being well prepared can make any trip more relaxed. Consider the following tips when planning your trip:

• Take a pillow and blankets so you can prop yourself in different positions. An eye mask and relaxing music on your MP3 player can make sleep more likely, and a pair of cozy socks is comforting if your feet tend to swell when you remove your shoes.

• If you are traveling by car, ensure that someone else lifts your luggage into and out of the trunk.

• Your luggage should be light enough to be carried easily or pulled. A few smaller bags may be better than one large one, which will require help to transport.

• Take several pairs of comfortable shoes. The best shoes or sandals have a contoured footbed to help prevent aches and a thick, skid-resistant sole.

• Choose hotels or other accommodation with good access to transportation; you may feel full of energy now, but travel can be exhausting, and you may need to return to your room frequently to relax.

• Although you may be a seasoned traveler and used to organizing accommodation and an itinerary at the last moment, it is a good idea to plan ahead during pregnancy. You may need to investigate activities to ensure that they are suitable for pregnant women.

• Pack plenty of loose clothing that can be layered or easily removed according to the temperature. Stick with separates, which will help accommodate frequent trips to the bathroom. Breathable, wrinkle-resistant fabrics will be more comfortable and convenient.

Getting enough sleep

Restful sleep can seem an elusive commodity, particularly as pregnancy progresses; however, it's important to get as much as you can. Being well rested improves your mood and energy levels, and helps you cope much better with labor.

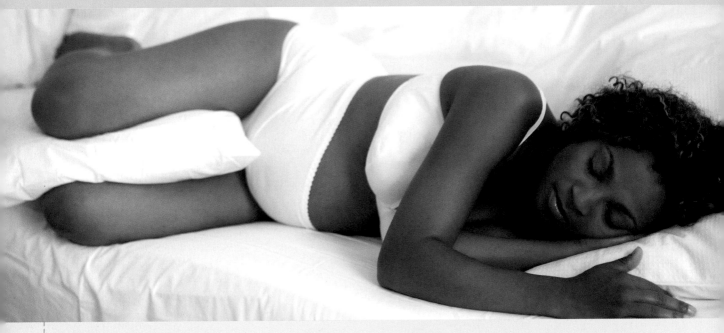

GETTING COMFORTABLE
Using pillows to support your back and knees can help to ease minor aches and pains, and encourage more restful sleep. Sleeping on your back is not recommended during late pregnancy.

There are several reasons why sleep may be more disturbed than usual during pregnancy. Most obviously, you may need to get up to go to the bethroom in the middle of the night. The significant increase in blood circulating through your system forces the kidneys to work harder to filter the volume, creating more urine. Then there's the pressure on your bladder from your expanding uterus.

Aches and pains can also disturb restful sleep, the result of hormonal and physical changes as your body adjusts to your expanding uterus. Emotional issues—stress, nervousness, anticipation—all affect sleep, and don't be surprised if you experience very vivid dreams. They can be triggered by disrupted sleep patterns, physical and emotional changes, and hormones. If you are worried by your dreams, talk to your partner or doctor.

Many pregnant women experience restless legs syndrome (RLS), when their legs feel "twitchy" and have to be moved constantly. No one is sure what causes it, but it may be linked to hormones, circulation, and possibly a deficiency of folic acid or iron. Eating healthily can help, as can plunging your feet into a cold bath to ease symptoms. When you return to bed, raise your feet on a pillow.

Feeling tired?

Fatigue is extremely common in the first few months of pregnancy, as you begin to adjust to the physical and emotional demands. You are effectively "growing" an entire human being in just nine months, so your body is hard at work nurturing this process. It's also possible that you haven't yet adjusted your lifestyle to suit your condition.

Being tired is your body's way of telling you that it's time to slow down and get more rest. Ideally, you need at least eight hours sleep a night, so if you're getting less than this, you may feel lethargic during the day. Or you may simply feel tired because you cut down on caffeine when you discovered you were pregnant. Fatigue can be a symptom of a lack of the coffee/cola buzz, but will soon pass. Not drinking enough water can also leave you feeling drained. Fluid demands increase tremendously during pregnancy, so make sure you drink enough from early on.

The good news is that fatigue generally lessens after the first trimester and your energy levels should improve.

Improving sleep

Your bedroom needs to be conducive to sleep, so try to make sure that it's quiet, technology-free, and a comfortable temperature. Take time to unwind before you attempt to go to sleep. Regular daytime exercise will ensure you are physically tired enough to nod off and reduces the impact of stress. Aim for at least 30 minutes a day. If you are fit, you are also less likely to experience backache and other nighttime pains.

Avoid caffeine and other stimulants in the afternoon and evening, since they can discourage sleep and make you feel restless and anxious. Then just relax. If you begin to panic that you'll never get to sleep, you probably won't! Even if you can't sleep, rest is important. Get to bed early and relax until you drift off.

Relaxation exercises can ease you into sleep. Starting with your toes, flex (tighten) and then relax the muscles in your body, all the way up your legs, through your abdomen, chest and arms, and to your face. Ask your partner to give you a massage before bed to ease away any tension that could be preventing restful sleep.

SLEEP SOLUTIONS
These simple tried-and-true strategies can help you to relax before bed, encouraging restful sleep:
• eat foods containing the amino acid tryptophan, which encourages the body to produce serotonin, since this aids restful sleep. Have a glass of milk, a bowl of yogurt, or an egg or tuna sandwich.
• take a warm (not hot) bath before bed.
• dim the lights in your home during the hour before bedtime to help your body get the message that it's time to sleep. If you're taking a bath, consider doing it by candlelight.
• turn off your television and computer an hour before bedtime; the bright light can affect your ability to nod off.
• sip a cup of chamomile tea before bed.
• avoid getting too hot; have your own set of sheets and blankets so you can peel off layers without waking your partner.
• if you suffer from heartburn, eat a slice of fresh pineapple after your evening meal, which helps to neutralize the acid—but try not to eat or drink for a couple of hours before bed.

GETTING COMFORTABLE
Invest in some firm pillows to support your bump. As pregnancy progresses, try placing one pillow between your legs to support your hips and another under your lower back to relieve pressure. Experiment to find a position that works for you. If heartburn keeps you awake, sleep propped up on a nest of pillows or, better still, get your partner or a friend to raise the head of your bed by about 4–8in (10–20cm) by placing large books or blocks of wood under the legs.

Sleep strategies that worked for us

Difficulty sleeping is sometimes more about what's in the mind. I got worrying thoughts or lists of things "to do" out of my head by jotting them down before turning off the light. CH

The baby would wake up and give me a good kick just as I lay down to sleep. In the end I came to see it as comforting, because it told me that all was well. FF

Listening to a self-hypnosis CD in bed certainly sent me to sleep—and had the added benefit of preparing my body and mind for birth. The messages go into your subconscious while you sleep. TL

I was up every hour or two to empty my bladder. It was exhausting, but perhaps I coped with the first few months of a baby better because of it?! VB

Taking naps

If you aren't sleeping well at night, try napping during the day. Naps are amazingly reviving, but some women find it difficult to doze in the daytime. Practice during pregnancy to help prepare you and boost your energy levels for life with a new baby, when there's no guarantee of an undisturbed night. And remember that a poor night's sleep can be disruptive and exhausting, but it's not the end of the world.

Time to relax

Reducing stress is one of the best ways to maintain health and happiness at any stage of life. But it's even more important during pregnancy, when the effects of stress on your body systems may also affect your baby.

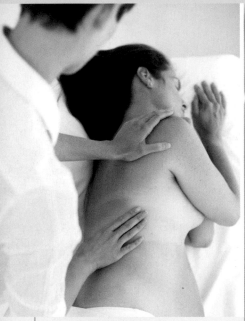

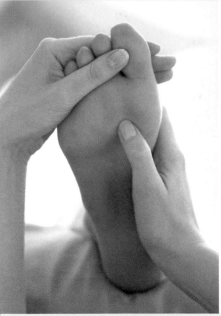

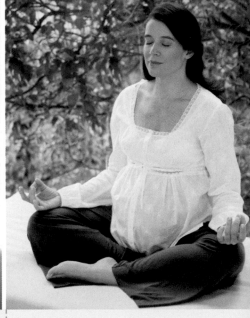

MASSAGING AWAY TENSION
A masseur can target body areas where you hold tension. Look for a professional who specializes in prenatal massage.

REFLEXOLOGY TREATMENT
Therapies such as reflexology can encourage relaxation and overall health, and also be used to control symptoms of pregnancy.

MORNING MEDITATION
Finding a few minutes in the morning to sit still and calm your mind can improve your mood for the entire day.

Being stressed out occasionally is an accepted part of everyday life and may increase quite naturally during pregnancy, since all change, however positive, brings with it some extra challenges. And don't forget that we all need some level of stress in our lives for its valuable activating effect—for example, feeling stressed can motivate you to address issues at work, or in a relationship. However, being exposed to the effects of stress for a prolonged period is known to increase health risks—it is associated with high blood pressure, digestive problems, and emotional difficulties—and is among the top three reasons for taking sick days.

How stress affects your body

A stressful situation has a physical impact because it triggers the release of the hormones cortisol, adrenalin, and noradrenalin. These prepare your body to take action to defeat or get away from the "stressor." For example, by diverting blood flow to the muscles and giving you a surge of energy, your body equips itself to successfully fight or run away. However, most stressful everyday situations—from being stuck in traffic to work deadlines—cannot be remedied by the quick physical action these hormones prime us for. So the hormones continue to circulate and our body systems cannot return to their pre-stressed state. Over time, this can make us more susceptible to health risks including increased blood pressure.

"Spend more time doing anything that makes you feel calm, and also try methods such as yoga that train your body and mind to relax"

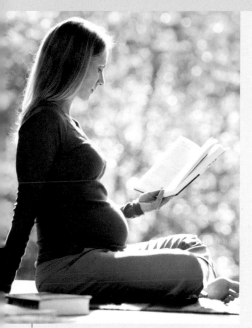

TIME OUT TO READ
Taking some time to read a good book, perhaps sitting outside in the sun if it's a nice day, can help relax you.

STRESS IN PREGNANCY
Studies are still underway into the effects of stress on unborn babies during pregnancy, and much is unknown in the early stages of investigation.

However, the most reliable studies suggest that high stress levels during pregnancy may increase the risk of babies not sleeping well in the first two years of life and suffering from behavioral and mental health difficulties when they are older. Reassuringly, experts report that there is no evidence to link stress and miscarriage.

Stress doesn't only affect your baby; it can increase your risk of suffering from anxiety and depression. While this does not mean that you need to lead a completely stress-free life during pregnancy, it does mean that it's worth taking action when your stress levels rise.

Ways to relax

What can you do to counter stress? A little gentle exercise and some regular relaxation are the best everyday strategies to reduce its effects, boost your mood, maintain a positive state of mind, and safeguard your physical health. Exercise allows the stress hormones to activate your body systems as intended. It also increases endorphins—or feel-good hormones—in your body. Relaxation methods help you react to difficult situations with less tension, thereby reducing the levels of stress hormones released in the first place.

Swimming, walking, or other forms of exercise almost always help to reduce stress (to find the type of exercise most appropriate to your lifestyle and stage of pregnancy, see pp.62–65). Exercise can also relieve some of the uncomfortable symptoms of pregnancy that exacerbate stressful situations, from backache to constipation and insomnia.

The easiest way to relax is to find something you enjoy doing, and then simply spend more time each day doing it—whether that be reading, walking the dog, or knitting. However, it's also worth trying a pastime that actively trains you in ways to relax—yoga, tai chi, and meditation all offer useful approaches. Yoga classes, for example (see pp.72–73), teach a series of exercises and mental techniques that help to bring about a state of deep calmness. The teacher will show you how to relax into that state on your own, so that you can apply the technique whenever and wherever you meet potential stressors. This can make you less susceptible to a stress response. Relaxation or meditation CDs or DVDs can also be helpful for home practice. You might like to explore HypnoBirthing CDs, which, as well as being incredibly relaxing, prepare you psychologically for the birth.

HOME STRATEGIES
Assess how well you balance your work life with your home life. Start with your working day—you'll know if the number of hours you work or the timing of shifts makes you feel stressed. Think about talking to your employer and colleagues about ways to make your working day less frantic. When at home, try to make yourself unavailable after hours by turning off your phone and keeping away from emails.

Spending time with people who care for you is another good antidote to stress. Share your free time with people who have an optimistic attitude and tend to see the upside of situations; they can help you to stay positive, too.

How I'm feeling

Emotional ups and downs are normal during pregnancy. Although these months lead to a wonderful outcome, many women find them tough going, making it important to monitor your mood and take prompt action to beat the blues.

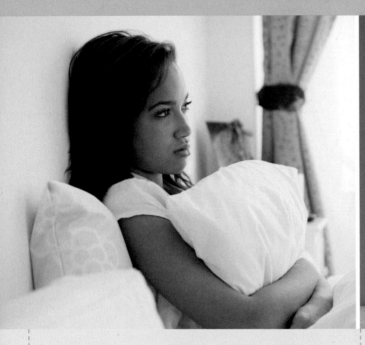

FEELING DOWN
Everyone feels low at points during pregnancy, whether it's due to hormones or worries about everyday life, but talk to your doctor if the blues last more than a couple of weeks.

SHARE THE EXPERIENCE
You are going through this life-changing experience together, so confide in your partner if you have concerns—supporting each other can help you both feel more positive.

Changes in your hormone levels during pregnancy can trigger a roller coaster of emotions and mood swings. It is important that you anticipate and expect some low times, but also that you don't brush off persistent emotional upsets or feelings of sadness.

Your hormones

During the first trimester, your body is adapting to being pregnant, and this means changes in two specific hormones: progesterone and estrogen. Before pregnancy, these hormones tend to counterbalance each other, keeping emotions largely on an even keel. However, changes in their levels in the first weeks of pregnancy can make you feel unusually positive and calm, or irritable, low, and anxious. This can be particularly noticeable during weeks six to ten of pregnancy.

Mood swings tend to even out in the second trimester, but even so, being quick to shed tears is a common characteristic of pregnancy. A sad movie or story on the news can have you in floods of tears in a moment. You may also crave more physical affection and reassurance; don't be scared to talk to your partner about this. By the final weeks of pregnancy, hormonal changes may lead to fairly intense mood swings again, as your body prepares for labor and delivery.

EMOTIONAL UPS AND DOWNS
Mood swings in pregnancy are not all about hormones. Realizing just how life-changing it will be to become

a parent can play havoc with your emotions, too. It is entirely normal to swing from elation that a new life is developing inside you, to feeling stressed and anxious about how you will manage the responsibilities that a new life brings. One moment you may be on a high about becoming a mom, and the next crave the return of your pre-pregnancy life and familiar body, and be wondering why on earth you thought having a baby was a good idea.

Even if being pregnant is the thing you want most in the world, there can be times when the blues take over. You might be concerned about work and your financial situation after the birth, worried about how your relationship, friendships, and family life will adapt to fit your new role, or wonder how you'll ever manage to learn all the new skills required to care for a tiny baby. All mothers-to-be share these worries.

There are useful practical things you can do to lift your mood, if you feel down or overwhelmed. A little gentle exercise is very effective, as is spending time outdoors in the natural world. Try to stick to a regular daily routine of working, resting, exercising, eating, and sleeping, and ask friends and family for their support. This could be something practical—such as cooking for you or cleaning the house once a week—or more emotional support, such as reassuring texts, phone calls, and hugs.

PRACTICAL SOLUTIONS
These simple tried-and-true strategies can help smooth out some of the common causes of mood swings and restore your peace of mind:
• Get some rest—worries seem less burdensome if you are well rested. Try to work shorter hours, take an afternoon nap, or make an appointment at a spa.
• Pamper yourself every day by building treats into your routine: spend 20 minutes with your favorite magazine, pick a bunch of flowers for your desk, or browse online for a flattering new dress or lipstick.
• Talk to your partner, who is probably feeling just as spooked as you are about this impending new life. Can you go out to dinner once a week? If you have older children, book a regular babysitter.
• Meet up with other moms-to-be for lunch and a laugh about your mood swings; knowing that everyone shares similar concerns is so reassuring.

Prenatal depression

Most women find that their mood lifts with a little practical help and one-on-one support. But for a small but significant number of moms-to-be, changes in mood can become more serious, leading to bouts of prenatal depression. You may find that a low mood will just not lift, be unable to motivate yourself to do things you usually enjoy, often oversleep or suffer from insomnia, or have frequent negative thoughts about your pregnancy and yourself, or even think of harming yourself.

If any of these symptoms describe your mood, visit your doctor. About one in ten moms-to-be require professional support to deal with depression. Talk therapies such as counseling and cognitive behavior therapy can work well, and in some cases medication might be needed. Your doctor will be able to advise you.

How we stayed positive

Doing some form of exercise daily—walking, swimming, yoga—kept me incredibly positive and helped even out my mood. Generally, I didn't suffer from mood swings. Instead, I found that the pregnancy hormones made me much more relaxed than usual, and I was in a better mood a lot of the time. Certain breathing techniques that we practice in yoga (like alternate nostril breathing) also helped to balance my emotions. TL

Buying beautiful baby clothes kept me feeling upbeat, as did losing myself in all the practical things, like choosing the color scheme and making curtains for the baby's room. NK

Because of my medical background I was fortunate enough to see pregnancy discomforts as a necessary means to a happy end—a beautiful baby—and so I just made an effort not to dwell on the bad points. LJ

I went to Feldenkrais (a movement therapy) prenatal classes and met a group of women who became my confidantes during pregnancy—and friends for life. CH

I wasted a lot of time in my first pregnancy preparing myself for a poor outcome because of what I'd seen as an obstetrician. It meant that I distanced myself from my baby. I was much more positive the second time around, which helped me to bond more quickly with my baby. When women have negative thoughts about pregnancy, I try to help them focus on the positives. The majority of pregnancies have a good outcome. VB

My relationship

Having a new baby is a huge adjustment for any couple, and your relationship is bound to change. Nothing is better than parenting with someone you feel is wholeheartedly in it with you, and now's the time to start reinforcing that bond.

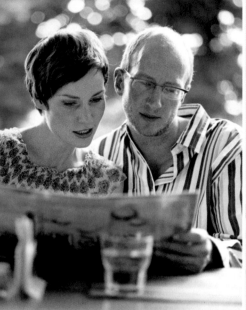

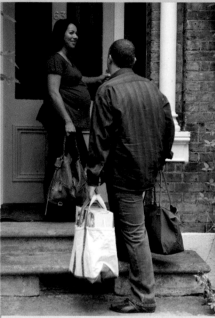

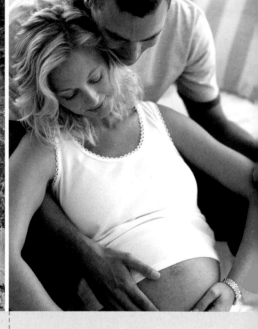

TIME TOGETHER
Give your relationship as much time as you can to reduce feelings of anxiety and build a strong and continuing bond.

SHARING THE WORKLOAD
The way you divide up household tasks has probably already changed. Think now about how you'll make things work after the birth.

LEARNING THE BASICS
Your partner may feel left out—attending prenatal classes together will make him feel more involved.

From the moment you know you are pregnant, alongside your joy will be some fears, and many of these fears may center around the ways in which your relationship will change. What if your partner feels left out of the mother-and-baby love-fest? What if neither of you adapts well to the interrupted nights? What if you feel trapped by the unending commitment of the new relationship? It's impossible to control the changes the future will bring. What you can do is talk about your concerns.

Time together

You know you are supposed to look after your health during pregnancy, but are you as tuned in to taking care of your relationship? Simply spending regular time together is the best way to nurture the bond you have as a couple, countering fears about change and further strengthening your relationship before the baby is born. If you are both working long hours and don't spend much quality time together, schedule at least one evening a week and some

time on the weekend to enjoy each other's company. Even stolen moments can keep you feeling close.

Try to maintain a softness of attitude toward each other and try to be honest about your feelings, especially when you feel tired or irritated. Share your plans, thoughts, and emotions for the future, and listen to your partner's ideas and concerns. Remind your partner that it's completely normal to have worries about what's to come. And remember each other's need for physical affection; a hug or gentle touch can be all that's needed to re-establish a loving connection at times of tension.

TALKING HONESTLY

We all tend to have strong opinions about how to parent, based on our own experiences and childhoods. So what if your ideas are at odds with those of your partner? To prevent future clashes, start talking about how you'll parent your baby well before she is born. Find out from each other your expectations of parenting. Perhaps you have very different thoughts on where the baby should sleep, on disciplining toddlers, on education, and even on names. What kind of mom do you plan to be? How does your partner envision fatherhood? Talk it over. Open up about your early experiences, whether your parents were affectionate, authoritarian, or easygoing, and how they handled discipline and shared the childcare load.

Your own upbringing is a significant influence on your parenting values, but you now have the chance to agree to a new way and formulate ideas about a joint parenting philosophy. This is a good time to read parenting books and discuss the options they suggest. Don't feel that you need to arrive at tidy conclusions; simply admitting that your opinions clash is a good way to start reaching a compromise.

SHARING THE WORKLOAD

How you'll divide up the day-to-day tasks of parenting and running a home is another area of contention to discuss before the baby arrives. Think about the demands of your jobs, where your skills and experiences lie, what you enjoy doing, and what you hate. From this, try to draw up lists of jobs, especially for the early weeks, when you are likely to spend much time in bed and in feeding. Talk about practical ways in which your partner can cut you some slack. Can you alternate diaper changes at night in exchange for daytime naps, for example? Shopping, cooking, and cleaning duties are sure to change; how can you plan for this now?

FEELING LEFT OUT

It is all too easy for partners to feel left out of pregnancy. Checkups, ultrasounds, and other people's interest can focus on you as the mom-to-be, and dads may be treated as a support rather than a full partner. Remedy this by discussing issues and making mutual decisions; schedule appointments that you can attend together, and be assertive if you feel the professionals are not including both of you in the decision-making process.

Birth-preparation classes are good for ensuring men feel included. Sessions will give your partner a clear notion of what happens at a birth, and how he can help practically—with massage and breathing techniques, for example. He may also increase his confidence to act as your advocate when talking to medical staff—perhaps about your birth plan and pain-relief options.

> "When you enter parenthood, your bond and lifestyle as a couple will alter; recognizing these changes and adapting together is a necessity"

How we involved our partners

I was fortunate that my husband and I were best friends for several years before we dated. So by the time we got married, we were already accustomed to working as a team and accommodating each other's schedules and needs. Having our first baby certainly posed a challenge to the way we did things, but we just had to figure out new ways to divide and conquer the chores, especially since we were both working long hours and spending every third or fourth night on call or at the hospital. LJ

Going to the ultrasound appointment together helped make my pregnancy a shared experience, as did choosing names together. We also took a HypnoBirthing course, where my husband had to visualize the birth and learn a few helpful techniques to use during labor! TL

My husband came with me to prenatal appointments whenever he could, and we also tried to cram in extra time for each other while I was pregnant. Those dinner dates and quiet nights together were worth the effort—we knew that we'd be focused on our baby after the birth. CH

My support network

While some women remain hugely independent during pregnancy, others take the opportunity to build a network of people to call on for practical and emotional support during these life-changing months and into the baby-rearing years.

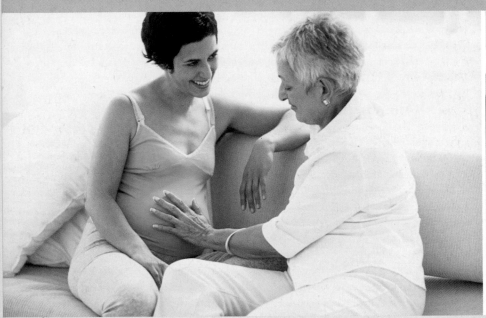

GRANDMOTHER-TO-BE
Your mother may become one of the most important people in your life once your baby arrives; it's worth getting closer through pregnancy.

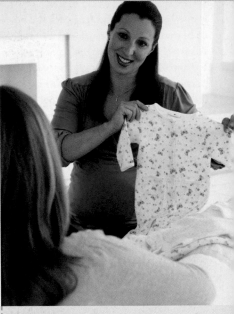

WHAT FRIENDS ARE FOR
Take a friend along to a checkup or to shop for newborn clothes. It can make you closer and help her understand your new world.

The physical and emotional changes of pregnancy make accepting a little help a necessity rather than a luxury for most new moms. Having support can keep your emotions on an even keel, which makes you feel more in control.

Help is important

Getting some help can allow you to keep doing the things that you know you should do every day to feel well, but that are so easy to ignore—eat well, exercise, relax, and rest. In particular, it's useful to have people on call—your baby's grandparents are a good place to start– to cover childcare for older children and to help you with lifting children and heavy work when your walking turns into an ungainly waddling toward the end of your pregnancy. In terms of emotional support, a friend who offers comfort when you feel tearful is invaluable, as is someone with a cheerful, dispassionate viewpoint when future prospects seem overwhelming. Receive offers of help gracefully, remembering that you can say "no" if assistance starts to turn into interference.

NEAREST AND DEAREST

Your family and friends will probably be eager to get involved with your pregnancy and your baby's life, so let them have the privilege of helping. Guide them by being clear about the most useful things they could do and delegate tasks so each person feels that he or she has a part to play. Don't be afraid to explain how you are feeling if you become overwhelmed by offers of help.

OTHER MOMS-TO-BE

Often, other pregnant women on the same journey as you provide the most

"Friends and family can be an invaluable resource during pregnancy, and even more so after your baby is born"

useful and reassuring support. After all, they are encountering similar obstacles, and negotiating the same twists and turns. Mothers with older children may be too busy in their own stage of parenting to remember the details of the experiences you are going through, or may even be dismissive of your concerns, while many non-pregnant friends just won't get it.

Where can you find these useful moms-to-be? At parenting and prenatal groups or pregnancy exercise classes. Many of the moms at these classes get together again for mother-and-baby classes after the birth, so the babies make friends, too. Look for cafés or parks where new moms congregate. You can also talk to your ob/gyn or future pediatrician—many doctor's offices and hospitals host breastfeeding or general postpartum support groups; get the details now so you know just where to go when you and your baby are ready for that first outing.

Internet sites and chatrooms on parenting are another great place to meet people and share queries and concerns, especially seemingly minor troubles that you might not want to own up to face-to-face. Regardless of where you live and the time of day or night, you'll be able to hook up with other women to brainstorm particular issues, and that forges strong bonds. It can feel like having your own exclusive community of moms-to-be.

PROFESSIONAL SUPPORT

The professionals in your life—your doctor or midwife and their nurses—offer a reassuring safety net throughout your pregnancy. They are with you for many moving moments, such as hearing your baby's heartbeat for the first time or seeing her tiny arms and legs waving around. They are on hand to answer your questions about physical or emotional health. Turn to them for expert opinions if you have concerns or questions.

GOING SOLO

If you are embarking on this journey without a partner, it's extra important to establish a special group of people whom you trust—parents, friends, and neighbors—to support you each step of the way, sharing the milestones of your pregnancy as well as sustaining you on days when it doesn't feel so good. You will be especially grateful for their support in the early days after birth, when parenthood can feel overwhelming.

Start planning practical assistance now. Is there someone who can help you figure out the financial logistics? Who could give you a lift to hospital appointments and bring you home afterward? When you need a hand with the grocery shopping or someone to look after older children while you take a rest, who could you call on? Once the baby has arrived, who do you trust to tend to the baby while you take a nap? Who could be relied on to help with the laundry, drop off a home-cooked meal, or do some dishes? Try to put some plans in place as soon as you can.

Respect from others means a lot, especially at times of emotional uncertainty such as pregnancy. Unfortunately, in many cultures single parents can be treated with disrespect, so ensuring that you have a close network of supporters who stand by you and challenge negative views is invaluable. You could also look online for single-parent support groups.

Who we relied on

In both my pregnancies I moved to a new area around two weeks before I delivered—really bad planning! It took a lot of effort on my part to find a network of new moms to socialize with, but it makes a huge difference in how you cope with the everyday stresses and strains of life with a new baby. I strongly encourage my patients to join prenatal and postpartum groups for this very reason. VB

I grew closer to my mom. I wanted to know how she managed when she was having me. Mom found a letter she had written describing my birth. My own daughter's birth was virtually the same. That felt reassuring. FF

Coping with symptoms

Many women sail through pregnancy, but early on, as your body adjusts to hormonal changes, you may experience some discomfort, including nausea. Physical symptoms from swelling to heartburn can also strike in the final weeks.

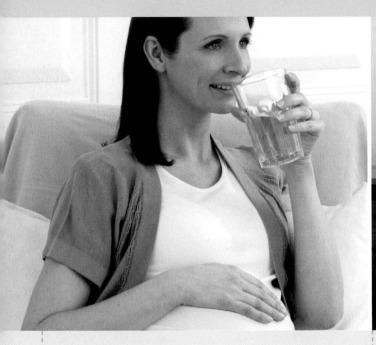

STAY HYDRATED
Drinking plenty of water throughout the day is one of the best ways to prevent constipation and feelings of nausea.

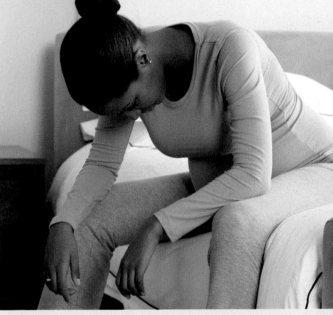

WHEN YOU FEEL FAINT
Lowering your head can help to prevent lightheadedness. From a sitting position, lean forward, resting your forearms on your knees.

It's unusual to go through pregnancy without experiencing at least one unpleasant symptom. Don't despair—there are lots of ways to cope.

Common problems

The good news is that most pregnancy symptoms usually pass after a few weeks. If you do succumb to some of the more common discomforts, try some of the tried-and-tested tips on these pages.

NAUSEA AND VOMITING

Pregnancy sickness (sometimes referred to as morning sickness, a bit of a misnomer since it can last all day) can be one of the most debilitating symptoms of pregnancy. In most women, symptoms are worse in the first trimester, settling down once hormone levels become more stable in the second trimester. For a few women, nausea and vomiting become more than just a nuisance. If sickness stops you from keeping meals down or does not subside after the first trimester, visit your doctor. For most women, a few strategies can ease the symptoms:

• Eat little and often—symptoms are often worse when you are hungry; eating frequent meals stabilizes blood sugar.
• Drink plenty of water—dehydration makes nausea worse.
• Eat a little *before* getting out of bed in the morning; plain dry crackers are good.
• Keep away from trigger foods—certain smells can bring on nausea.
• Avoid fatty and junk foods, which make symptoms worse.
• Invest in a motion-sickness wrist band—wear as directed, so the plastic button presses an acupressure point on your inside wrist.

"If you are well rested and able to relax, you are much less likely to suffer from the physical symptoms of pregnancy"

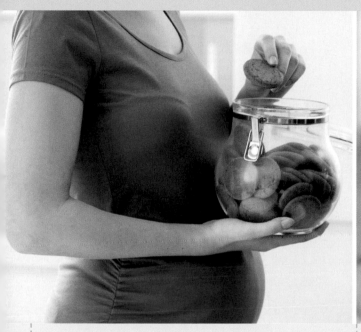

EATING GINGER COOKIES
Ginger is known to help relieve nausea by working directly on the digestive system.

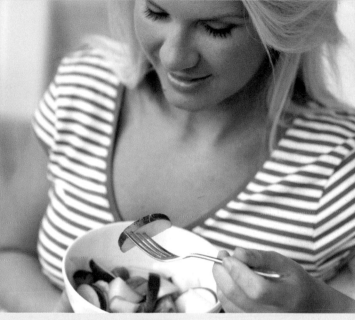

HEALTHY SNACKING
Eat small healthy snacks at frequent intervals to keep your blood-sugar levels stable; this will stave off nausea and even out your moods.

• Try a regular supplement of vitamin B6. Its deficiency appears to be linked with pregnancy sickness.

• Eat ginger—fresh, candied, in cookie form—to settle your stomach.

• Cooking may be a powerful trigger for nausea. If someone else prepares your food, there's a better chance you'll be able to eat it.

FAINTNESS
Feeling faint can be a result of an increase in blood volume and decrease in blood pressure. If you feel lightheaded when standing up or getting out of bed, stand up more slowly, giving your blood pressure time to adjust to the movement.

• Lie on your back with a cushion under your right hip and your feet raised and resting against the wall or on the seat of a chair until you feel better.

HEARTBURN AND INDIGESTION
The sphincter at the bottom of your esophagus relaxes during pregnancy, making digestive symptoms more common. Certain foods—tomatoes, citrus fruit, caffeine, spices, even chocolate—can aggravate symptoms. If all else fails, take a calcium carbonate antacid after meals, or as needed. This is safe in pregnancy. But first, try these remedies:

• Eat little and often, to avoid overfilling your stomach, and avoid fatty and fried foods, which take longer to digest.

• Eat a slice of fresh pineapple after every meal; its digestive enzymes prevent acid build up.

• Don't lie down after meals; it can cause acid to enter the upper digestive tract.

• Give up coffee, tea, and carbonated drinks, which make symptoms worse.

• Try not to drink during mealtimes—it increases volume in your stomach and pushes acid up into your esophagus.

HEADACHES

Many pregnant women report more headaches than usual, especially through the first and second trimesters. If you experience blurred vision or vomiting, see bright lights, or have a persistent headache, especially in the last trimester, see your doctor immediately. For less severe headaches, try the following:

• Drink some water—many headaches are caused by dehydration.
• Get gentle exercise—this encourages the release of pain-killing endorphins.
• Eat plenty of fresh, whole foods to prevent headaches caused by swings in blood-sugar levels.
• Apply a cold compress to the base of your neck.
• Acetaminophen, at the recommended doses, is safe in pregnancy.

EYE PROBLEMS

A drop in male hormones (androgens) during pregnancy can make your eyes dryer than usual, or you may experience sensitivity to light, itching, or excessive tearing. If you wear contact lenses, try switching to glasses for a while. These remedies can be helpful:
• Visit your doctor for eye drops and ointments suitable for pregnancy.
• Try a yoga "palming" exercise—rub your palms together until they feel warm, then rest the heels of your hands on the eye sockets and the palms gently over your closed lids; imagine the warmth bathing the "roots" of your eyes.

SWELLING AND EDEMA

During pregnancy, more water collects in the body, causing swelling, particularly in the legs and feet. If you experience discomfort, invest in a comfortable pair of shoes and put your feet up as often as possible. Try these remedies, too:
• Keep a bottle of water—the best natural diuretic—in your bag, and drink it.
• Exercise regularly, to encourage circulation and disperse built-up fluid.
• Put your feet up regularly to take the pressure off your circulatory system, and direct blood and fluid to your baby.
• Build natural diuretics into your diet—asparagus, pumpkin, onions, grapes, beets, parsley, green beans, pineapple, and garlic.
• Reduce your salt intake—it encourages fluid retention.
• Increase your intake of vitamin B, another mild diuretic, found in good levels in whole grains.
• Have a regular massage with a therapist specializing in pregnancy, to encourage circulation.

VARICOSE VEINS

The veins in your legs can bulge or darken during pregnancy when more blood flows through your veins and hormones cause the walls to lose elasticity. The condition generally improves after childbirth, but use these ideas as a preventative measure:
• Don't sit or stand for long periods.
• Try not to cross your legs and avoid sitting cross-legged or kneeling.
• Exercise most days—try yoga or a brisk walk.
• Lie with your legs up a wall if less than 28 weeks pregnant.
• After 28 weeks, if you feel faint or uncomfortable on your back, sit with your legs elevated on a chair, or partially recline in bed with your legs on pillows.

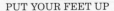

ASK FOR A MASSAGE
Regular massage loosens tension and eases discomfort in stiff or painful areas of the back.

PUT YOUR FEET UP
Take periods of complete relaxation. If you suffer from varicose veins or swelling, relax with your feet higher than your heart.

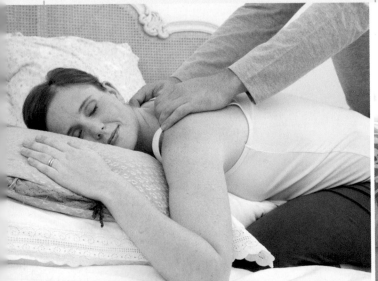

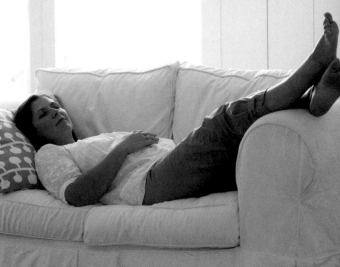

• Spend time lying on your left side (and sleep on this side)—to rest your inferior vena cava, the large vein running down your right side.

• Wear maternity support stockings to ease discomfort. Your doctor can write you a prescription for these special stockings, which may be covered by your health insurance.

LEG CRAMPS

Cramps in the legs and feet—especially at night—are caused by the effects of pregnancy hormones on your muscles and pressure on your veins, but can also be a sign of insufficient calcium, magnesium, or potassium. If the pain does not reduce or you develop a tender spot, contact your doctor, but for most women the following techniques help:

• Drink more water to boost hydration.

• Stretch your calves before bed—place your palms on a wall and step one foot back, pressing the heel to the floor until you feel a stretch in your calf.

• Point and flex the foot when you feel a cramp coming. If this doesn't ease the pain, go for a walk.

• Apply a hot water bottle to the muscle.

• Boost your intake of calcium and potassium by having a banana and some milk or coconut water (or a banana

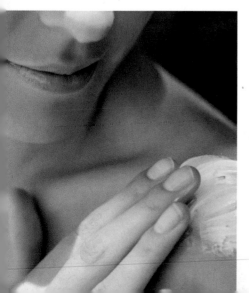

Dealing with pregnancy symptoms

I suffered leg cramps in the middle of the night that would make me sit up wide awake in pain. To stop my calf muscles from spasming, I'd have to stand up to stretch the muscle, then I'd have my husband massage my calf until it was less sore. I was also sensitive to smells, had a limited appetite, and threw up throughout my entire first trimester and up to 19 weeks. Simply avoiding trigger smells—coffee, tuna fish, the refrigerator—helped my nausea. Getting enough sleep made a difference, too. The sleep-deprivation associated with being up all night on call took a toll. I'd often throw up after being up all night. It would take me 24–48 hours to recover—just in time to be on call again! LJ

My prenatal yoga students swear by bananas and milk or coconut water for night cramps. They also recommend sparkling water for nausea and lassi (a yogurt drink) for heartburn. I found that reflexology eased my sore feet and helped me sleep better at night. TL

I found backache and swollen ankles very annoying toward the end of pregnancy. Putting up my feet as often as I could solved the first problem; using a maternity support belt helped with the other. CH

---

milkshake) before you go to bed.

• Add sources of magnesium to your diet—dates, green vegetables, apples—or ask your doctor about a supplement.

BACK PAIN

The extra weight and softened ligaments of pregnancy can mean back pain, particularly around the lower back. During the day, stay active to alleviate the pain, and try a maternity support belt. In bed, make yourself comfortable with pillows beneath your knees. Here are more suggestions:

• Shift position often, to avoid straining one part of your body.

• Place a footstool (or pile of books) under your feet to reduce pressure on your back while sitting.

• Raise your feet on pillows or cushions when lying down.

HEMORRHOIDS

These swollen veins around the anus are more common in pregnancy because of the pressure of the enlarged uterus on the vena cava. They may ache or itch and perhaps bleed a little after a bowel movement. Usually they clear up on their own after delivery. To ease discomfort, try the following:

• Avoid constipation by drinking plenty of water and including plenty of fiber in your diet (fruits, vegetables, and whole-grain bread, for example).

• Soak a cotton ball in witch hazel solution that you have kept in a fridge. Place this over the hemorrhoids to relieve pain and itching. You can buy witch hazel from your local pharmacy.

• Anesthetic creams and suppositories can be helpful. Speak to your pharmacist or doctor.

SKIN CHANGES

Skin changes can occur in pregnancy, and you may experience pimples, dull or blotchy skin, and pigmentation marks. Drink plenty of water to keep your skin hydrated and use a light moisturizer to keep your skin moist.

Little moles and freckles that existed prior to pregnancy may now become bigger, and brown spots or birthmarks become browner. New moles may also appear. If these moles seem particularly raised, dark, or have irregular borders, see your doctor.

Pregnancy myths

The experts don't put much stock on the many myths that surround pregnancy. However, that doesn't stop people from repeating them and believing them. Fortunately most are harmless, but do some contain a grain of truth?

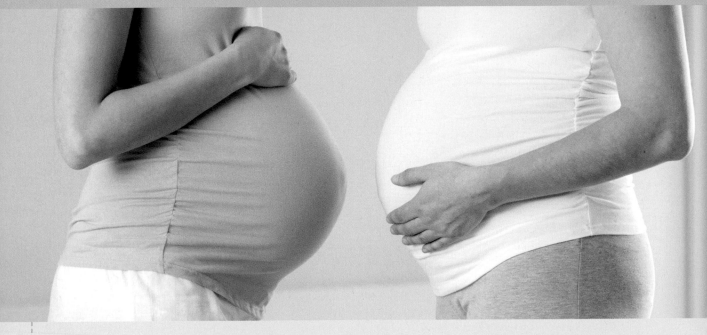

BUMP SHAPE
Many people believe that the shape of your bump can predict the baby's gender, but your shape has more to do with your baby's position in your uterus.

Many pregnancy myths can be intriguing, especially the ones guaranteed to predict the gender or personality of your baby, but some can lead you into less than healthy ways of living. In parts of Ghana, for instance, it is said that eating protein—an important part of a nutritious diet, especially during pregnancy—can cause a pregnant woman to give birth to a thief!

Myths have developed more recently in the western world that a pregnant woman can hold down a high-powered job, a whirlwind social life, have a perfect relationship and dream home, give birth to a mini Mozart, and then be back in her skinny jeans and busy office, days after the birth. Don't believe the hype! Try to enjoy the lighter side of these tales, but don't let them stop you from leading a healthy lifestyle—eating well, engaging in a little bit of gentle exercise most days, and getting plenty of rest and sleep.

Just for fun

Enjoy these myths if they make you laugh, but remember that they are mostly nonsense!

HEARTBURN MEANS HAIR
Many women have heard the myth that suffering from heartburn means you will give birth to a child with a luxuriant head of hair. Although many medical professionals don't buy it, a study at

Johns Hopkins University published in the journal *Birth* found that women who reported more heartburn tended to give birth to babies with more hair. The study's researchers put it down to high levels of estrogen and other pregnancy hormones, which influence both fetal hair growth and the opening of the sphincter at the bottom of the esophagus, which causes heartburn.

LOSE A TOOTH FOR EVERY BABY

You might think this is true if you have noticed your gums bleeding more often during pregnancy, and heard it said that if there is not enough calcium in your diet, the baby "borrows" it from your own teeth and bones. But dental health professionals say there is no truth in the notion that pregnancy leads to increased calcium deficiency or tooth loss. However, a large study of women in the United States carried out by New York University and Yale School of Medicine, published in the *American Journal of Public Health,* found a strong correlation between tooth loss and motherhood. Researchers have posited that this might be linked not just with the increased likelihood of developing gum disease during pregnancy, but also with the detrimental effects of depression and anxiety on oral health, as well as the way in which North American dentists treat pregnant women.

The best advice to counter this myth is to eat a good diet containing calcium-rich foods—cheese, milk, and yogurt—which maintain the strength of your teeth and bones, and build strong teeth and bones inside your baby. To combat the risk of developing gum disease, which is common and can be more problematic during pregnancy, visit the dentist more often while you are pregnant, brush your teeth after meals, and floss daily. If you find yourself vomiting more often than usual, rinse your mouth and brush your

teeth afterward to get rid of the enamel-attacking acid. If you find that toothpaste brings on nausea, try switching brands.

SWEET FOR A GIRL, SOUR FOR A BOY

So you crave chocolate and ice cream? The myth would suggest you are carrying a girl. Lemon and pickles? Then it must be a boy. Until a scientific study proves otherwise, there's as much truth in this myth as in the nursery rhyme, which tells us that boys are made of "slugs and snails and puppy dog tails" and girls are made of "sugar and spice and everything nice."

Cravings are thought to be a mechanism set up by the body to correct nutritional deficiencies, although no in-depth studies have been carried out to confirm this. Studies in Ethiopia do suggest, however, that women with cravings consume a more diverse range of foods, which can lead to a higher quality diet. So the best way to safeguard your health and that of your baby is to eat a well-balanced diet (see pp.48–51) and to get regular gentle exercise.

CARRY LOW FOR A BOY, HIGH FOR A GIRL

Both male and female babies can be carried high or low, and the way you carry is dependent on several factors. If you are carrying "high," it's possible that this is your first pregnancy and/or your stomach muscles are in good shape. With every subsequent pregnancy, the muscles in your abdomen become more elastic. The looser the muscles, the lower you'll carry. Similarly, if your uterus is better toned (as it tends to be in first pregnancies), your bump is more likely to be higher. The position of your baby in the womb will also affect the shape and height of your expectant belly, as will the height of your own torso. If you are tall and long-bodied, there is much more

room for your uterus to expand upward, making your bump higher. Finally, most babies eventually drop lower into your pelvis as you approach your due date, so your low-slung bump may actually be a sign of imminent labor, rather than an indication that it's time to paint the nursery blue. The truth is that the only guaranteed methods of assessing your baby's gender are CVS and amniocentesis (see pp.118–119).

AN ACTIVE BABY MEANS A HYPERACTIVE CHILD

There is little truth in this statement, since activity levels in the womb vary according to your hormones, your baby's position, how much room he has to maneuver, and your own behavior, eating patterns, and sleep/wake cycles. What we do know, however, is that personality and behavior are both established in the womb. Research has found that babies who are very active in the womb tend to be more irritable babies. The reason for this is that some hormones—particularly those that are released when we are stressed—encourage activity levels. So, highly stressed moms-to-be tend to have more active babies inside the womb, and more irritable babies outside. We also know that fetuses with high heart rates tend to become more unpredictable and active babies. Test this out yourself, but don't decide in advance what kind of baby you are likely to have, or you could create a self-fulfilling prophecy!

I AM SUPERWOMAN

This is one of the most pernicious modern myths—that life carries on as normal during pregnancy; you just gain an amazing bust and glowing skin. But it's important to get plenty of rest and sleep, taking daytime naps if you need to, and to give yourself time to reflect before your life changes dramatically.

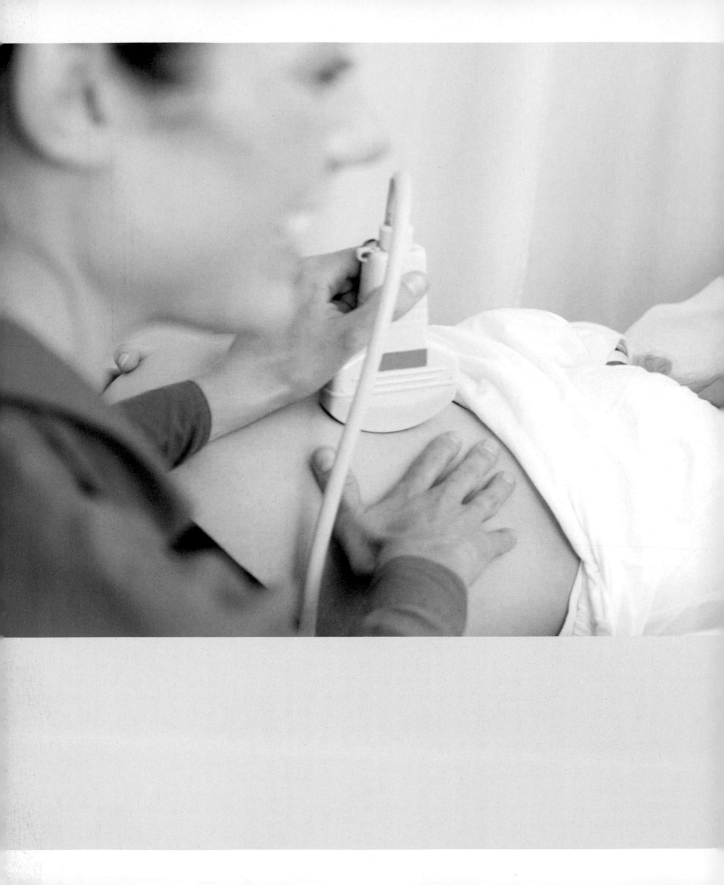

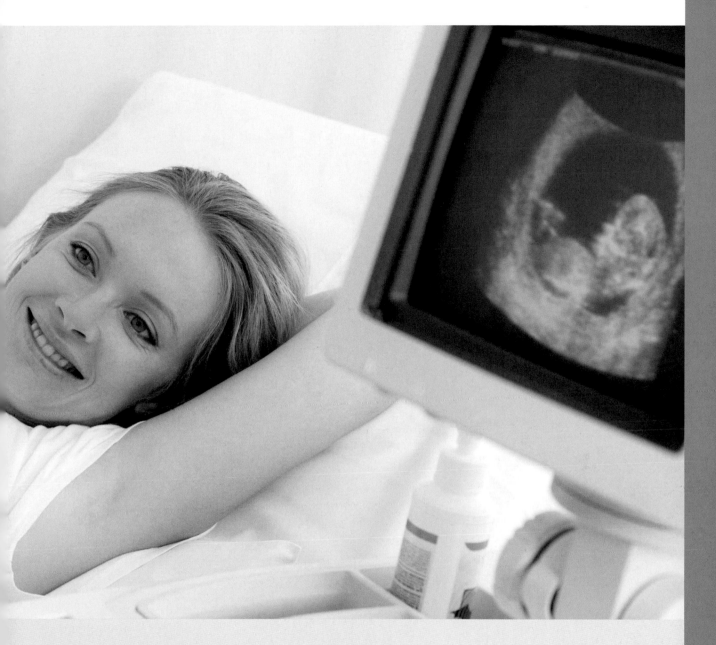

My prenatal care

A team of experts will monitor the health of you and your baby, giving reassurance, support, and the care you need throughout pregnancy.

What can I expect?

You can look forward to regular checkups, ultrasounds, and tests to confirm that your pregnancy is progressing well and identify any problems. You'll also be given information and support to help prepare you for birth and beyond.

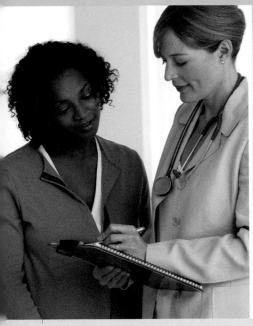

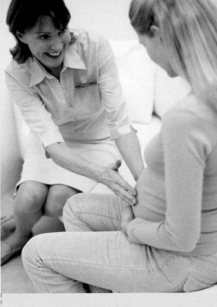

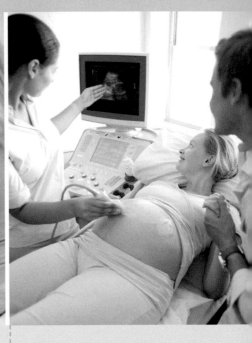

SEEING YOUR DOCTOR
Make an appointment with your GP or ob/gyn when you think you're pregnant. She'll confirm your pregnancy and continue to care for you throughout your pregnancy.

THE ROLE OF A MIDWIFE
Some women choose to see a midwife instead of an ob/gyn or family doctor throughout pregnancy, often because they plan to deliver the baby at home or a birthing center.

SEEING A SONOGRAPHER
You will normally see a sonographer for at least two ultrasound scans during pregnancy. You will be able to watch your baby on screen as each examination is carried out.

The prenatal care you receive will be the same whether this is your first pregnancy or a subsequent one, as long as you are healthy and your pregnancy is progressing normally. If, like most Canadian women, you see an ob/gyn or your family doctor during pregnancy, you will have 14 prenatal appointments over the course of 9 months (see box, opposite). In some circumstances, for example if you have an existing medical condition or are expecting twins, you may be monitored more closely.

Who you see for your prenatal care

If your ob/gyn or doctor works in an office with partners or colleagues who could be on call when you go into labor, it's a good idea to schedule some appointments with the other doctors to get to know them. Some doctors may also have nurse practitioners on staff who may handle a limited number of routine appointments.

Your choices

At your first pregnancy appointment, your doctor or midwife will give you the information you need to make informed decisions. For example, you'll learn about all of the recommended screening tests and other appointments that should be scheduled in the upcoming weeks. If the tests aren't available in her office, your doctor will be able to provide you with a list of local specialists or hospitals that offer the screenings, so you can plan ahead and decide which screening tests you'd like to have.

You can also expect your views, values, and beliefs to be taken into consideration, along with any cultural requirements or other special needs. Your doctor or midwife will be able to give you recommendations about what foods to eat and which to avoid during pregnancy, and what medications are safe to take for headaches, colds, or other common ailments. She'll also ask about your drinking and smoking habits to ensure that you aren't doing anything to harm your growing baby, and she can offer information on where to go for help if you need to cut back. And she'll be able to provide guidance about ideal exercises for pregnant women, so you can safely stay in shape, which can help prevent excess weight gain and keep your system running smoothly. Speak up if there are issues you feel strongly about, or if anything is unclear or confusing.

Types of care

Your care may be arranged in one of the following ways.

DOCTOR-LED CARE

This is the type of care that most women receive. Your ob/gyn or family doctor may have a solo practice or be a member of a group practice. If your doctor is a solo practitioner, you'll get to know her well, but she may not be on call when you go into labor, which means that another doctor she partners with could deliver your baby. If your doctor is part of a group practice, you'll have the chance to meet the other doctors who could be on call, so even if your doctor isn't working when you go into labor, a familiar face will greet you at the hospital. (Most doctors deliver babies at only one or two local hospitals, so when you choose your doctor, you'll find out where your baby will be born.)

> "Speak up if there are issues you feel strongly about, or if anything is unclear"

Your prenatal appointment schedule

As soon as you know you're pregnant, call your doctor or midwife to make an initial appointment. At around 8 weeks, your doctor or midwife will confirm your pregnancy, advise you on folic acid supplements and prenatal vitamins, lifestyle, screening tests, and scheduling upcoming appointments.

You'll see your doctor about 14 times during your pregnancy, under normal conditions. At the beginning, you'll visit the office about once a month, but the

appointments will gradually become more frequent until you're seeing your doctor weekly at the end of your pregnancy. At each appointment, you'll be measured and weighed, give a urine sample, and a nurse will listen for the fetal heartbeat. You should also have ultrasound scans at 11–14 weeks, and at 18–20 weeks.

Blood tests to look for abnormalities are normally arranged early in pregnancy: at about 12 weeks and

sometimes up to 20 weeks, depending on your doctor's practice.

Early in your pregnancy, you should be given written information on what to expect from your prenatal appointments, and the chance to discuss the schedule with your doctor.

It may seem like there are a lot of checkups, but they are important to maintain the best care for you and your baby and ensure that any problems are detected early.

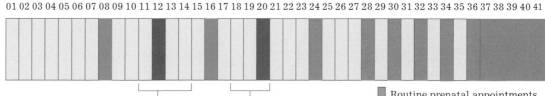

Weeks of pregnancy 01 02 03 04 05 06 07 08 09 10 11 12 13 14 15 16 17 18 19 20 21 22 23 24 25 26 27 28 29 30 31 32 33 34 35 36 37 38 39 40 41

1st scan between 11 and 14 weeks

2nd scan between 18 and 20 weeks

Routine prenatal appointments
Blood tests

SHARED CARE

Sometimes your care may be shared between an obstetrician (or group of obstetricians) and a nurse practitioner, who may handle certain routine checkups.

PERINATOLOGIST-LED CARE

If there are concerns about your health, for example if you have high blood pressure or diabetes (see p.25), you may come under the care of a maternal-fetal medicine specialist (perinatologist), an obstetrician who's specially trained to handle high-risk pregnancies. You may continue to see your usual doctor for some appointments and your perinatologist for others, or you may switch over to the perinatologist for all of your care.

MIDWIFE CARE

Some women prefer to be seen only by a midwife or team of midwives, who can see them all the way through pregnancy, labor, and delivery. If you are healthy, have a low-risk pregnancy, and prefer a less clinical approach to pregnancy and childbirth, this may be an attractive option for you.

With your midwife, you can give birth at home, in a hospital, or at a birthing center if one is available in your area; you'll want to discuss this with your midwife before signing on as a patient. For many patients, being able to labor and deliver at home, or in a homey, non-clinical birthing center, is a big reason to choose midwife care during pregnancy. For others, the allure is being able to see midwives rather than doctors for the regular pregnancy appointments, because appointments with midwives tend to be longer, giving women a chance for all of their questions or concerns to be addressed. Midwives work in collaboration with other health professionals and consult with or refer to medical specialists as needed throughout a woman's pregnancy and labor. Wherever midwives practice, they must have an obstetrician on call for assistance in case something goes wrong.

Patients of midwives often report that they don't feel as rushed as they may have felt in a doctor's office. They also prefer the strong feeling of support that they get from their midwives during labor and delivery. A midwife will stay by your side throughout your labor, helping guide you, to make the situation as pleasant as possible; a doctor, on the other hand, may be absent for most of the labor, instead focusing mainly on the actual delivery.

In Canada, most provinces and territories regulate midwifery. A registered midwife (RM) is a graduate of a university program accredited by the local College of Midwives. Public funding for midwife care varies for each province and territory—check with your local government or midwives' association for the details in your area. Also, ask to review the credentials and references of any midwife you plan to use during your pregnancy to be sure that she's qualified to care for you.

To find a qualified midwife in your area, visit the website of the Canadian Association of Midwives at www.canadianmidwives.org.

ASKING FRIENDS ABOUT THEIR PRENATAL CARE
Family members and friends who have recently had babies can be an invaluable source of information. Talk to them about their experiences and find out if they were happy with the care they received. Any lessons they learned could prove useful for you.

MAKING NOTES
You'll probably have lots of questions about your prenatal care, so it can help to jot them down as they occur to you. It's easy to forget things during a checkup.

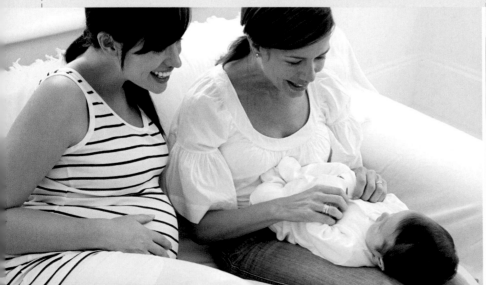

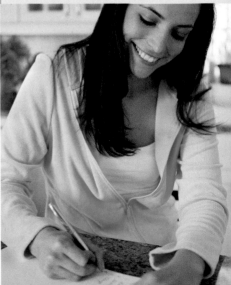

Where will you have your baby?

Where you deliver (see pp.132–135) may influence the care you receive. You can choose a hospital, your home, or, in some cases, a birthing center. Take time to visit the places where you could give birth, and ask questions. How do you feel about the environment? Will you feel safe, comfortable, and relaxed there? Talk to as many people as you can: friends, new moms, your doctor or midwife. The more you learn early on, the more confident you'll feel later in pregnancy.

OPTIONS TO CONSIDER

Most women give birth in the hospital. Hospitals offer the best medical technology, many options for pain relief, and specialists should the need arise. It is often reassuring for moms to know that there's medical backup in case anything goes wrong. However, hospital births are more likely to include interventions such as assisted birth (see pp.310–311), and busy hospitals may not have enough nurses to provide continuous support.

Birthing centers offer a cozy, informal atmosphere and homey comforts. Most are independent, but some hospitals now have birthing centers alongside their traditional maternity units. Birthing centers mostly cater to women who have low-risk pregnancies, so intervention is less likely. You are more likely to have one-on-one care from one midwife throughout your labor. Epidurals and caesareans are not available; if they are required, you will be transferred to a hospital.

For a home birth, your midwife may bring a home-birth pack before your due date, and will attend when you go into labor. If you want a water birth, you can rent or buy a pool (see pp.306–307). Be sure that your midwife is trained and experienced in water deliveries.

Home births are controversial in some medical communities because of potential for complications, but you have the right to decide where you want to deliver your baby.

> "Visit the places where you could give birth and ask questions . . . will you feel comfortable, relaxed, and safe there?"

Talking about prenatal care and choices

With so many choices out there, this can be a very confusing time—so be sure to ask questions. Take your time and don't be embarrassed. Even as an obstetrician, I had a million questions to ask, and although I probably knew the answers, just being able to ask was reassuring. MG

When choosing where to have my baby, I had a few points to consider. As a midwife, the hospital where I worked was naturally my first choice. However, it wasn't entirely straightforward because the hospital is close to a major sports arena, and the roads are either closed or grid-locked whenever there's a home game. My husband and I needed to assess how we could get to the hospital if I went into labor when the team was playing at home. Being able to get there quickly is important to factor when making choices. NK

As you set about choosing your prenatal care, take into consideration not just your physical health, but the emotional and social support you might need. The classes and activities you select need to support you in your pregnancy, but, equally importantly, they may offer up friendships that sustain you long after your baby is born. CH

It really helps to be familiar with the hospital where you'll be delivering— where to go, what is in the delivery rooms, and so on. Ask to look around and see exactly what the facilities are like before your due date so you will be more comfortable with your surroundings. LJ

I was sure that I didn't want a home birth for my first baby; I chose a hospital, in case I needed any medical assistance. Still, I was hoping for as little intervention as possible. Ideally, I planned a water birth and yoga breathing techniques and movements to help me through. But nothing went according to plan! My baby was breech and never turned, so I ended up having a C-section. My second baby was delivered naturally, but due to my previous C-section I had to be very closely monitored, so I didn't get to choose a water birth that time either. TL

My initial appointment

Once your pregnancy is confirmed, you'll schedule your first prenatal appointment. This is the time for you and your partner to ask questions and start getting a handle on what the coming months have in store.

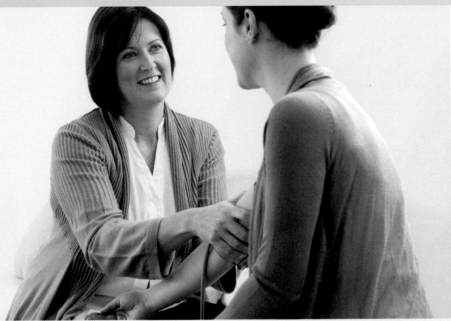

ROUTINE CHECKUPS
Your blood pressure is an important gauge of your health throughout pregnancy. For this reason, it's checked at each prenatal appointment so that variations can be picked up and investigated if necessary.

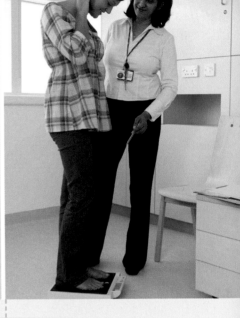

WEIGHING IN
If you're a healthy weight at the start of pregnancy, a one-time weight check at this first appointment may be all that's needed.

Your initial appointment, scheduled by your doctor or midwife at your first contact visit, should take place ideally around 8 to 10 weeks so that your health can be assessed early on and you can be given important information about upcoming screening tests for your baby.

This is your longest prenatal appointment. Your doctor or midwife will ask you about your medical history and carry out routine tests. She will use this information to compile your prenatal notes, which will be kept for use as reference in all future appointments.

Planning your care

As well as carrying out general health checks, your caregiver will discuss issues relevant to pregnancy, including folic acid, food hygiene, and birth options. She will estimate your due date, based on the date of the first day of your last menstrual period, and will plan the level of care you need during your pregnancy. Your caregiver will ask you lots of detailed questions about your health

and lifestyle. Don't be taken aback by the level of personal information you may be asked to provide—it is important that your doctor is aware of anything at all that could affect your own health or that of your baby. Typical areas for discussion include:

● Diet and exercise. Your caregiver will talk about healthy eating and foods to avoid (see pp.48–55). She will ask whether or not you exercise, and also about your alcohol intake and if you smoke or take drugs. Support will be offered if necessary, with details of the help that is available to give up smoking, or anything else that could harm your baby.

• Your medical history, including: any previous operations; sexually transmitted diseases; conditions such as asthma, high blood pressure, or a known allergy; any medication you're taking; and any mental health problems.

• Your family medical history as well as your partner's family history, including any multiple births, or inherited genetic conditions such as cystic fibrosis, or health problems such as diabetes, heart disease, and high blood pressure.

• Any previous pregnancies, including those that may have ended in miscarriage or a termination. If you have children already, your doctor will record the birth weight and sex of your previous babies.

• Screening and diagnostic tests (see pp.116–19). Your caregiver will give you information on these and discuss which you may want to consider. She'll also arrange your dating ultrasound (see pp.114–15)—or may even do this now, depending on the facilities and her expertise.

• Where you want to give birth. Your doctor or midwife will talk you through all the options available. Now is a good time to ask about hospital facilities, birthing centers, and the possibility of a home or water birth. Although it may seem early, she may ask how you plan to feed your baby and may give you literature about breastfeeding.

• Maternity rights and benefits. Your caregiver will help you assess any risks involved with your job, and how to work around them. She may also be able to help you understand your insurance benefits and leave policies.

PHYSICAL CHECKUPS

As part of her assessment of your health, your caregiver will carry out some medical checks. Some are one-time checks; others will be done at each appointment.

• You will be weighed and your height measured. Your caregiver can then assess if you are a healthy weight for your height by calculating your level of body fat, known as your body mass index, or BMI (see p.19).

• Your blood pressure will be taken, and this initial reading will be recorded as your "normal" blood pressure that later readings will be measured against.

• You will be offered routine blood and urine tests (see p.113)—your caregiver will ask for a urine sample, and will either do the blood tests now or arrange for an appointment to have them done.

ASKING QUESTIONS

You'll have plenty of opportunity to discuss any concerns you may have and to ask questions. Your doctor or midwife can inform you on most aspects of pregnancy and birth, including weight gain, nutrition, and exercise; prenatal classes; how to deal with pregnancy symptoms; how often you will be seen; and who to call if you have any pressing worries. Bring along your partner, if you wish, and take your time so you're sure to cover everything.

> "Every piece of information your doctor gathers now helps her to tailor your care to your specific needs"

How to get the most from your first visit

This is your opportunity to ask all about the care you can expect throughout your pregnancy—learning about the nature and timing of prenatal appointments, and about tests or ultrasounds can be very reassuring.

• Go armed with all the information your doctor or midwife might need, such as the date of the first day of your last period (to help establish your estimated delivery date) and any relevant details about your family's health or your partner's family's medical history. It's a good idea to talk to extended family before you go so that you can get an idea about any medical problems that run in the family.

• Ask your partner if he has any questions he would like answered. He might raise some useful issues.

• You may feel uncomfortable about disclosing certain personal information. However, although questions may seem irrelevant to you, they can be significant. Try to be as open as possible: The purpose of all this questioning is to determine if there are any risk factors that might affect your pregnancy.

• Studies show that people remember only about 70 percent of information given in medical appointments, so it's a good idea to make notes as you go.

Routine tests and checks

Testing blood and urine is a standard part of your prenatal care. These tests provide important information, such as your blood type and immunity to certain infections, and enable your doctor to keep tabs on your health.

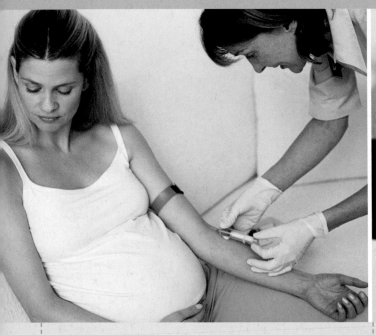

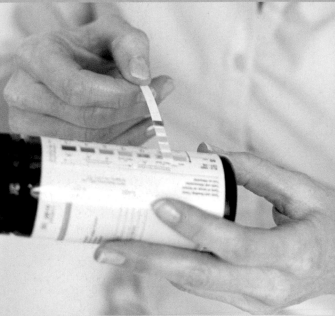

GIVING A BLOOD SAMPLE
Taking blood is a quick and painless procedure. Your doctor will explain beforehand what your blood will be tested for and will gain your consent before arranging for the tests to be carried out.

CHECKING YOUR URINE
Using a dipstick to check your urine enables your doctor to spot immediately any substances that may warrant further investigation. This quick, efficient test is an invaluable part of your prenatal care.

From your first appointment, your caregiver will record all the results of your routine checks in your prenatal notes, building up a detailed picture of your pregnancy. Having taken your blood pressure at your initial appointment (see p.111), it will probably be checked at every visit. You may be asked to bring a urine sample to each visit, too, or to provide a sample at the appointment. If you didn't have a blood sample taken at your initial visit, this should be done now, and again later in pregnancy. Your doctor or midwife will inform you of the results and will write them in your prenatal notes, and advise you if any action needs to be taken.

Monitoring blood pressure

It's important to monitor blood pressure in pregnancy because high blood pressure (hypertension) can affect your baby's growth and, later in pregnancy, could be a sign of a life-threatening condition called preeclampsia (see p.386). Your caregiver will record your blood pressure each time, compare it with the reading taken at your initial appointment, and investigate changes if necessary. Your blood pressure is written down as two numbers, one on top of the other—for example 110/70—and will be recorded in your prenatal notes.

Blood pressure often goes down at the start of pregnancy, rises in the second trimester, and returns to normal later on, so your caregiver will watch for variations beyond this norm.

> "You may feel daunted by the list of conditions being tested for, but such thorough prenatal care means that you and your baby are in safe hands"

Urine checks

Your caregiver will check your urine at each appointment to see whether it contains any of the following substances:

• Protein—this could be a sign of a urinary tract infection (UTI), in which case antibiotics will be prescribed. Protein in the urine later in pregnancy may also indicate preeclampsia.

• Sugar (or glucose)—sugar can show up in your urine if you have recently consumed a lot of sugary foods or drinks, but it can also be a sign of gestational diabetes (see p.385)

• Ketones—these are produced when your body begins to break down fat stores for energy, perhaps because it isn't getting enough fuel in the form of carbohydrates. This is more common in women who have severe nausea and vomiting in pregnancy. If both ketones and excess sugar are found, this can be a sign of gestational diabetes.

Testing blood

Your blood sample will be analyzed to determine your blood type, to screen for certain conditions, and to find out if you have immunity to certain infections.

BLOOD GROUP/RHESUS FACTOR

Your prenatal team needs to know if you are blood type A, B, O, or AB, and if you are Rhesus positive or negative. Women who are Rhesus negative develop antibodies if their babies are Rhesus positive. This isn't usually a concern in a first pregnancy, but can affect subsequent Rhesus-positive babies. The mother's antibodies attack the baby's red blood cells, seeing them as "foreign," which then causes anemia in the baby. If you are Rhesus negative, injections will be given at 28 and 34 weeks to prevent antibodies from forming.

HEMOGLOBIN

This molecule found in red blood cells carries oxygen around the body. Your body needs iron to produce hemoglobin, and even more so in pregnancy as your blood volume increases. If you're not getting sufficient iron, you could develop anemia. If your hemoglobin is low, your doctor or midwife will advise you to include more iron-rich foods in your diet (see p.49) and may prescribe iron supplements.

RUBELLA IMMUNITY

If you catch rubella (German measles) while you are pregnant, it can seriously harm your unborn baby. For this reason, your immunity needs to be tested so that if you have low or no immunity, your doctor can advise you on what steps to take. You will be offered immunization against the virus after the birth.

HIV

The HIV virus, which leads to AIDS, can be passed on to your baby in pregnancy. However, the chance of this happening can be reduced by taking medication. You will be offered an HIV test, and if it is positive, you will be offered counseling and advised on how to reduce the risk of transferring HIV to your baby.

HEPATITIS B

Hepatitis B is a virus that can cause liver disease. If undetected, it can be passed to your baby during the birth. If your blood test reveals you have this virus, your baby can be protected with medication.

SYPHILIS

A sexually transmitted infection, syphilis can cause congenital and developmental problems in your baby. However, if detected it can be treated and the risks to your baby reduced.

SICKLE CELL TRAIT AND THALASSEMIA

Sickle cell and thalassemia disorders are inherited blood conditions. They are more common in people of African and Mediterranean origin. For this reason, it's important to tell your doctor if you think you or your baby's father may have an ancestor who came from outside northern Europe (for example, someone who is Italian, Maltese, Portuguese, Spanish, Indian, Chinese, African, or Afro-Caribbean). Depending on your ethnic background and family medical history, you may be tested for one or both. If you carry a blood disorder, your partner will also be tested, and you may be offered genetic counseling.

My dating ultrasound

This is your chance to see your baby for the first time. Your first ultrasound is known as the "dating" scan because it checks your baby's measurements to confirm when your baby was conceived and give an accurate due date.

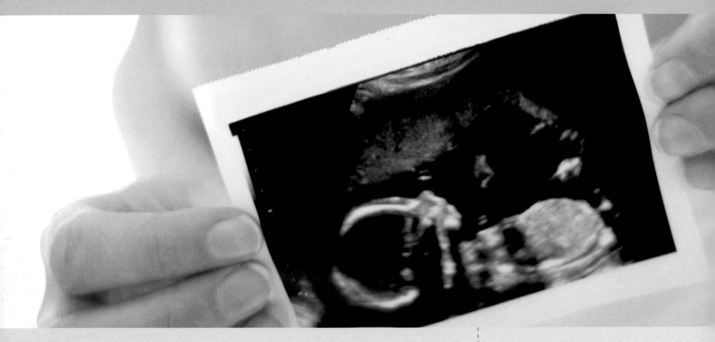

The dating scan takes place between 11 and 14 weeks. It's a memorable moment in your pregnancy, and one you may wish to share with your partner or a friend.

You may be asked to drink a lot of fluid beforehand. This is because a full bladder helps to push up the uterus to make it easier to view. The sonographer puts lubricating gel onto your abdomen, and then moves a handheld ultrasound monitor over the area.

Ultrasound uses high-frequency sound waves to build up a picture of your baby, placenta, uterus, and other pelvic organs, which can all be viewed on a screen. Scans are painless and low-risk for moms and babies. Establishing your baby's gestational age helps confirm your due date and ensures that screening tests are carried out at the correct time. If the findings differ considerably from your estimated due date based on your menstrual cycle, this original date will change. Dating scans are especially helpful if your menstrual cycle is irregular or you became pregnant right after coming off the contraceptive pill.

If your scan is done before 13 weeks, a "crown–rump" measurement (from the top of the head to the base of the spine) will be taken. If it takes place after 13 weeks, the head circumference will be measured to give the most accurate gestational age.

The dating scan provides other useful information, too. It establishes that the pregnancy is in the uterus, rather than in a fallopian tube (known as an ectopic

YOUR FIRST PICTURE
You will usually be offered a copy of your scan picture to take with you. This first grainy image of your baby is something you will undoubtedly treasure for years to come. Keep it in a dark place to prevent fading, since the paper is light-sensitive.

pregnancy, see pp.44–45), and reveals if there is more than one baby. It also confirms that the baby's heart is beating and she is developing normally, although her organs won't be looked at in detail until the 20 week ultrasound (see pp.120–123). The dating scan may be combined with a nuchal translucency scan (see p.116) to assess the risk of some chromosomal abnormalities and heart defects.

"You may feel emotional when you see your baby for the first time; for many women, this is the point when their pregnancy feels real"

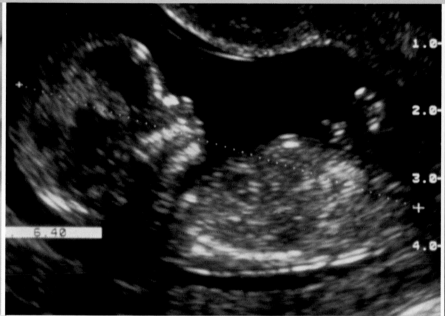

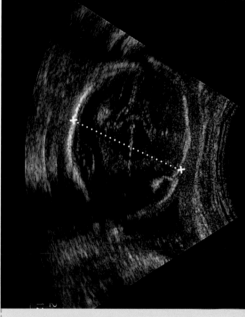

MEASURING YOUR BABY
Early in pregnancy, your baby lies in a curled position, which makes it hard to gauge the length of her limbs. The most accurate way to assess her growth now is by measuring her from the crown of her head to her bottom.

THE BIPARIETAL HEAD DIAMETER
Measuring the distance between the two bones on the head—the parietal bones (shown with crosses)—helps to assess your baby's growth.

Remembering our first ultrasounds

At our first ultrasound, I just remember feeling overwhelming amazement that this child was actually growing inside me; it seemed incredible that such a delicate creature was in there, and it brought out a very strong protective urge. CH

When I had my first ultrasound with my son, the sonographer was so quiet while she was scanning—I was sure she was finding something wrong. I was fixated on her face to see if I could pick up clues about what she was finding. Thankfully everything was normal and we picked up our conversation once she'd finished. MG

I experienced pain and bleeding at around six to eight weeks, and an ectopic pregnancy was suggested. I was referred to my local hospital for an ultrasound, which fortunately confirmed the pregnancy was in the correct place in the uterus. My husband and I were facing the screen and I immediately saw the beating heart of our baby. The bonding started from then. NK

While I had seen many, many ultrasounds during my medical training, it was entirely different when the scan was of my own baby. Seeing my daughter's flicker of a heartbeat with my own eyes made my pregnancy seem so much more real. LJ

Routine screenings

These assess the likelihood of your baby having Down syndrome or some other chromosomal disorder. In the majority of cases, parents-to-be are reassured that their baby is healthy and developing normally.

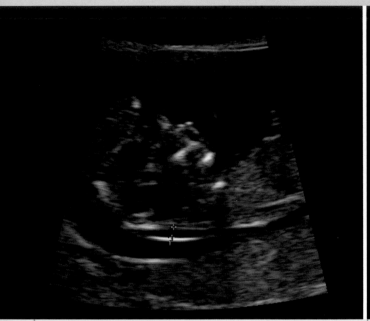

A SMALL NUCHAL FOLD
The nuchal fold is the area at the back of your baby's neck. The low depth of fluid shown here indicates that the baby has a relatively low risk of developing Down syndrome.

ADDITIONAL FLUID
This scan reveals a larger depth of fluid in the nuchal fold. This means there's a greater possibility that the baby has Down syndrome, and a diagnostic test will be suggested to confirm this.

Pregnant women are offered screening tests, which involve an ultrasound and/ or blood tests, depending on where you live. You don't have to have a test, but many women feel they would rather be prepared should a problem arise.

What's available

For most women, the first trimester screen (FTS), which combines a blood test with a nuchal scan (see right), is the preferred option because it's done reasonably early (at between 11 and 14 weeks) and is accurate. However, if you miss this window, or the FTS isn't available in your area, you will generally be offered a maternal serum screen (MSS), done in the second trimester. There is one more test, the integrated prenatal screen (IPS), which is highly accurate but not available everywhere and involves waiting until the second trimester for results. If any test results do indicate a high risk of a chromosomal disorder, you will be offered a diagnostic test to provide a definite result (see p.118).

NUCHAL TRANSLUCENCY SCAN
The NT scan is carried out between 11 and 14 weeks and is sometimes combined with the dating ultrasound (see p.114). It measures the depth of fluid at the back of your baby's neck, known as the nuchal fold, or translucency. An increase in fluid is associated with Down syndrome and other chromosomal abnormalities. A nuchal translucency (NT) measurement of up to 2mm is normal at 11 weeks, increasing to 2.8mm around 14 weeks.

The risk of having a baby with Down syndrome increases with age. This scan calculates the risk by combining your age with the results of the test. The result may revise the risk up or down, or it may remain the same for your age.

The sonographer may also check your baby's nasal bone, since a short nasal bone can indicate Down syndrome.

FIRST TRIMESTER SCREEN

The first trimester screen, which is carried out between 11 and 14 weeks, combines a maternal blood test with an NT scan. The blood test checks the levels of the pregnancy hormone hCG (human chorionic gonadotrophin) and the pregnancy protein PAPP-A. High levels of hCG combined with low levels of PAPP-A can indicate a chromosomal abnormality in your baby.

If your blood tests are done ahead of the scan, your sonographer will probably be able to combine the results and assess your overall risk on the day of the ultrasound. The FTS has a detection rate of 85 percent; there is also a 5 percent "false positive" rate, which means that sometimes it suggests a problem when there is none.

INTEGRATED PRENATAL SCREEN

This test is performed in two stages using results from screening tests carried out in both the first and second trimesters. The first test is carried out between 11 and 14 weeks, and then another blood test is done in the second trimester, between 15 and 20 weeks. The first trimester test includes a blood test to measure the level of the protein PAPP-A, and an NT scan (see opposite). In the second trimester, a further blood test is done to measure the levels of the pregnancy hormones hCG and estriol, and of the pregnancy protein alpha-fetoprotein (AFP).

The results of the blood tests and the scan are combined with your age to give a fairly clear indication of your baby's overall risk of Down syndrome. The disadvantage of the integrated test is that you have to wait until your second trimester before you get the results.

MATERNAL SERUM SCREEN

If an NT scan isn't provided routinely in your area, you will probably be offered a maternal serum screen instead to assess your baby's risk of Down syndrome, trisomy 18, and neural tube defects such as spina bifida. The maternal serum screen measures the levels of three pregnancy hormones (hCG, AFP, and estriol) from blood tests alone. The test is given between 15 and 20 weeks, and results are available in about one week.

Your results

If the ultrasound and/or blood tests show that you have a low risk of having a baby with a problem (less than 1:200), this is described as "screen negative." This means that there's a good chance that your baby is perfectly healthy. If your risk is higher than 1:200 ("screen positive"), you may be offered diagnostic tests.

Try not to panic if your results show that your risk is higher than expected. A positive test does not mean that your baby has a chromosomal abnormality. Talking to your doctor, midwife, or a genetic counselor can help you to decide whether to undergo definitive diagnostic testing (see pp.118–119).

Handling screening test results

Some women may not be sure what they should do or how they should feel if a first or second semester screening test shows that they have an increased risk for having a baby with a certain birth defect. Most importantly, you should not become convinced that a screening test result is a diagnosis for a birth defect. Screening tests only assess your risk; they aren't diagnostic tools.

In order to get definitive results, you'll need to have a diagnostic test done, such as amniocentesis or chorionic villus sampling (CVS) (see pp.118–119). Both these tests require that a doctor insert a needle through your abdomen and into your uterus to extract some cells, which are sent to a lab for processing.

(Amniocentesis samples the amniotic fluid, while CVS samples the placenta.) Both tests slightly increase a woman's risk for miscarriage, although that risk hovers around 1%.

Some women decide not to go through with diagnostic testing because they plan to have their babies no matter what, regardless of any medical conditions. Others feel that knowing definitively that their babies have a condition helps them prepare mentally for the arrival of a special-needs baby. Most of the time, however, women who go through diagnostic testing because their screening tests indicated a higher risk for a medical condition find out that their babies are healthy and doing fine.

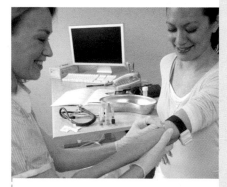

GETTING SOME PEACE OF MIND
If screening tests indicate an increased risk of Down syndrome or another condition, a diagnostic test such as amniocentesis can offer a definite answer.

Diagnostic tests

There are two main diagnostic tests—amniocentesis and chorionic villus sampling (CVS). These are offered if you had a positive result in a screening test, and give a definite diagnosis of Down syndrome and other abnormalities.

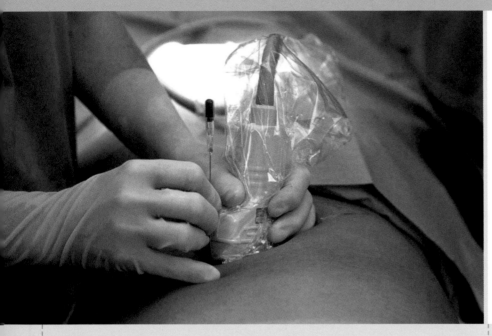

CLEAR GUIDANCE
Diagnostic tests are carried out under the guidance of ultrasound so that the doctor can view the uterus during the procedure and pinpoint exactly where to place the needle without harming your baby.

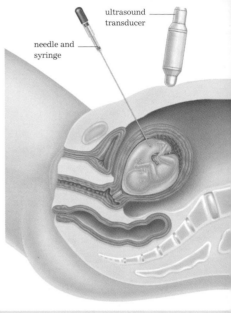

ultrasound transducer

needle and syringe

TAKING AMNIOTIC FLUID
The fluid around your baby is reached by passing a needle through your abdomen, then a sample is collected in a syringe.

A diagnostic test will be recommended if your screening test showed a high risk of a genetic or chromosomal disorder. There are two main types of test, which involve taking a sample of the amniotic fluid or placenta from inside your uterus. The samples are sent to a laboratory and tested. Chromosomes 21 (responsible for Down syndrome), 18, 13, and the sex chromosomes will be looked at. The results are 99 percent accurate.

If you don't want to know the sex of your baby, let your doctor know this before you get the results. If your baby is at risk of a specific genetic disorder such as cystic fibrosis or thalassemia major, you may also be offered a diagnostic test to detect the specific defective gene.

Your doctor will explain each procedure and help you to decide which test would be best for you. A benefit of CVS over amniocentesis is that it can be done earlier in pregnancy, which means that you can make difficult decisions sooner rather than later. However, having an invasive test earlier in pregnancy increases the risk of a miscarriage: CVS has a slightly higher risk at around 1 percent, as compared to amniocentesis, which is about 0.5 percent. The risk of pregnancy loss means that most women don't opt for diagnostic tests unless they think they would end an affected pregnancy.

Amniocentesis

This is performed between 15 and 20 weeks of pregnancy. Under the guidance of ultrasound, a thin needle attached to a syringe is inserted into your abdomen

"The majority of diagnostic tests show that babies are healthy, and women then progress normally through the rest of pregnancy"

(which may be numbed with a local anesthetic), then through your uterus and into the amniotic fluid surrounding your baby. Within this fluid are cells that contain the same chromosomes as your baby. This is called a "transabdominal" procedure and takes less than 30 minutes.

THE RESULTS

Results are usually available within 3 weeks. This can seem like a long time, so do ask for support if you have any concerns. The reason for the wait is that once the laboratory takes some of your baby's cells from the fluid, they need to be left to divide. The cells are then analyzed to check for genetic and/or chromosomal abnormalities. (See Why we decided to have amniocentesis, p.176.)

Chorionic villus sampling (CVS)

This procedure is carried out at around 11–13 weeks. Tiny samples of the chorionic villi—finger-like projections on the placenta—are extracted, and the chromosomes in the cells of this tissue are examined.

CVS is usually performed transabdominally, which involves having a needle inserted through your abdomen (the area may be numbed with local anesthetic first) and into the placenta. Sometimes, the position of the placenta can make it difficult to reach through

the abdomen, and CVS will be carried out through the cervix instead, known as a "transcervical" procedure. In this case, the placenta is reached via a small tube or forceps inserted into the cervix. Both procedures are carried out with the use of an ultrasound scan, take less than 30 minutes, and may feel a little uncomfortable.

THE RESULTS

Results should be available around seven to ten days after the procedure, although it can take up to four weeks to get the results for certain genetic disorders.

REACHING THE PLACENTA THROUGH THE ABDOMEN

As with amniocentesis, the placenta is usually reached by inserting a fine needle into the abdomen and on into the uterus. A sample of the placenta is drawn up into the attached syringe.

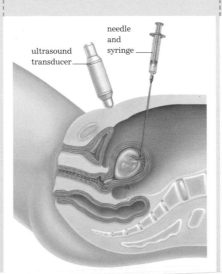

ultrasound transducer

needle and syringe

After the procedures

You may feel a bit uncomfortable and sore, and some women experience mild menstrual cramps. Contact your doctor if pain is severe, or if you have vaginal bleeding or a fever. You may be advised to avoid strenuous exercise and take it easy for a day or two afterward. If the result of a diagnostic test is positive, your doctor will explain the implications of this, and will talk to you about your options and offer support.

GETTING A SAMPLE OF THE PLACENTA THROUGH THE CERVIX

If an ultrasound shows that the position of the placenta makes it difficult to reach through the abdomen, a thin tube will be placed through your cervix and a sample of the placenta obtained in this way.

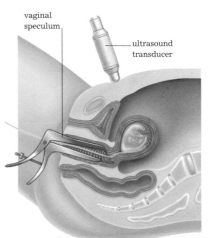

vaginal speculum

ultrasound transducer

My 20-week ultrasound

Your second ultrasound takes place at around 18–20 weeks. You'll probably feel excited and emotional when you see your baby in such detail on screen. Try not to worry as the scans are carried out—your baby is likely to be fine.

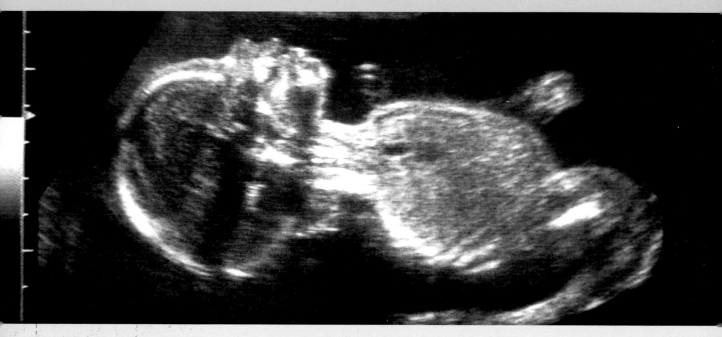

HOW YOUR BABY LOOKS NOW
Your baby will have grown considerably since you last saw her. Her position may have changed, and by now she will probably have "uncurled," making it easier to view each of her limbs on the screen. Her facial features are more pronounced, and you may marvel at the amount of detail you can see.

The second ultrasound is known as the anatomy scan because it checks all your baby's organs and body systems—which are now developed enough to be seen and assessed on screen. This may sound frightening, and indeed parents-to-be often approach the second ultrasound with a degree of trepidation because they worry it might reveal a problem. However, for the majority it is very reassuring to discover that their baby is developing normally.

The anatomy scan is usually the longest ultrasound, taking around 20 minutes; the sonographer will take plenty of time to look at each structure and organ in detail. You may be asked to have a full bladder to give the sonographer a good view of your baby.

What is checked

Your baby's major organs and body systems will be checked to ensure that they are developing normally. The position of the placenta will be assessed to confirm that it is not too low in the uterus (see p.122). The level of amniotic fluid around your baby will also be checked. Your baby's sex may also be determined at this appointment if you wish to know it before the birth.

YOUR BABY'S SIZE
Your baby is too large now to fit on the screen completely, so it's no longer possible to assess growth with a crown–rump measurement. Instead, a number of measurements will be taken to calculate

her size. The sonographer will measure her head circumference (HC), abdominal circumference (AC), and her femur, or thigh bone (FL). These measurements can confirm that she is growing normally for her gestational age. Although less accurate than a dating ultrasound, this ultrasound may also be used to confirm your baby's estimated due date.

YOUR BABY'S FACIAL FEATURES

The sonographer will check your baby's face and upper lip for a cleft lip (see pp.388–389), which occurs very rarely. While the sonographer is checking this, you will have an opportunity to see your baby's features for the first time. Many parents remark on how clearly they saw these at the 20-week ultrasound.

YOUR BABY'S SEX

By the 20th week of pregnancy, your baby's sex is easily identifiable—as long as your sonographer has a good view and sufficient time (her priority is to check for abnormalities). Many parents choose to learn the sex of their baby simply because they can't stand the wait, or

because they want to get organized in advance with the baby's name, clothing, and nursery equipment. Others prefer to wait for a surprise. The sonographer will check before starting the ultrasound whether you want to know your baby's sex. It's worth noting that the policy in some hospitals is not to reveal the sex, even if parents request it. Remember, too, that it's not 100 percent accurate.

There are circumstances when parents and doctors need to know the baby's sex because of a family history of gender-linked genetic problems. If this is the case, your doctor will talk to you about this before the ultrasound, and you will be offered advice, support, and counseling.

INSIDE YOUR BABY'S BODY

• Each of your baby's major organs and body systems will be carefully checked to ensure that they are growing and functioning normally.
• The heartbeat will be checked, and the structure and size of the heart will be looked at to ensure it is developing normally. Some problems that are

identified at this stage, such as a hole in the heart, can be treated after the birth with medication or surgery.
• Your baby's lungs will be looked at to confirm that they are beginning to develop.
• The brain will be examined—the shape of the brain will be checked and the ventricles inside it will also be looked at.
• The kidneys and bladder will be checked to confirm that both kidneys are present and that there are no blockages in the bladder.
• The stomach and bowel will be examined carefully to ensure that they are developing properly.
• The abdominal wall will be checked to ensure there are no defects and that the intestines are enclosed inside.
• The sonographer will check that the spine is properly aligned and will look at each vertebra to check for any signs of spina bifida.
• Your baby's limbs will be checked to help measure her rate of growth, and to identify any abnormalities in the hands or feet.

The latest ultrasound technology

Ultrasound technology is constantly changing. Some hospitals and private clinics now offer 3D, and sometimes 4D, ultrasounds, which provide incredibly clear images of your baby and show her movement in the uterus. These scans are normally offered from around 26 weeks onward.

3D and 4D ultrasounds provide an amazingly sophisticated, three-dimensional view of your baby and all her bones, organs, and body systems.

With a 3D ultrasound, you will be able to see the width, height, and depth of your baby in great detail. It can also provide a very accurate check for abnormalities such as cleft lip and palate, as well as congenital heart defects.

4D ultrasounds are actually moving 3D images that show your baby in action, which can be a breathtaking experience. You might see your baby yawning, sucking her fingers, or perhaps stretching her limbs and moving around.

Some hospitals use these advanced scans to encourage and promote early bonding, which is often considered particularly useful for women who have experienced difficulties in the past, perhaps with postpartum depression and bonding issues.

If you have an additional ultrasound out of curiosity rather than for any medical reason, it's worth checking what the clinic's procedure is if anything untoward is found.

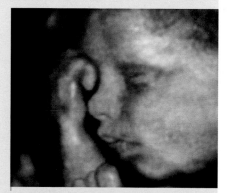

GLORIOUS DETAIL
Seeing such a clear image of your baby's face in the uterus can be incredibly moving. You may even detect some family resemblances now!

THE PLACENTA

The sonographer will check the position of the placenta, which will be either on the front wall of your uterus, referred to as an "anterior" position, or the back "posterior" wall. The placenta should be near the top of your uterus, known as the fundus. If your placenta is low-lying at this stage, which means that it reaches down toward or covers the neck of your womb (cervix), you will be offered a second scan at 32 to 34 weeks to check whether or not it has moved upward. In the majority, low-lying placentas do move up later in pregnancy. If, however, your placenta is still low and obstructing the cervix, a condition known as placenta previa (see p.386), you will need to deliver your baby by caesarean section, as the placenta will probably cover the entrance to the vagina.

AMNIOTIC FLUID

The sonographer will measure the volume of the amniotic fluid to check that there isn't too much or too little.

This is done by measuring the depth of the largest pockets of amniotic fluid found in different parts of the uterus. These measurements are then added together, and the "amniotic fluid index" (AFI) is calculated, which should be normal for your week of pregnancy.

Low amniotic fluid in the first or second trimester can occasionally be an indication of a birth defect in your baby, such as a kidney disorder, although often, a lower-than-expected level of amniotic fluid does not have any particular cause.

Too much amniotic fluid can sometimes indicate a problem such as an abnormality of your baby's intestinal tract or a congenital heart problem. If this is a concern, further ultrasounds and subsequent investigations will be recommended. It may also be a sign of gestational diabetes (see p.385).

Rest assured that amniotic fluid abnormalities aren't always concerning, but you may be offered additional monitoring just as a precaution.

THE UMBILICAL CORD

In most cases, a quick check ensures that the umbilical cord is healthy and functioning normally.

Some sonographers make sure that they are able to count the three blood vessels of the umbilical cord. If, in rare cases, there is one fewer vessel than expected, your baby's kidneys will be checked. If these are found to be normal, there is usually no need for concern, although you may have one or two additional scans later on to keep an eye on your baby's growth. However, it's unlikely that any further intervention will be needed.

ONE BABY—OR MORE?

If you didn't have an earlier dating ultrasound that confirmed whether you are having one or more babies, or, as occasionally happens, a multiple pregnancy was missed at a dating ultrasound, you will certainly find out now. There can be no mistaking more than one baby by this stage.

LOOKING AT YOUR BABY'S HEART

Even though the heart is still tiny—about the size of a peanut—at 20 weeks, it's possible to view it in detail on the ultrasound now. Its four chambers are clearly visible. The sonographer can also look at the major blood vessels of the heart to check that these are functioning properly.

YOUR BABY'S HEAD

The sonographer will check your baby's profile, the bones of the skull, and the brain. Each part of the brain will be examined in detail, including the fluid-filled spaces known as the ventricles, and the shape of the back of the brain, called the cerebellum.

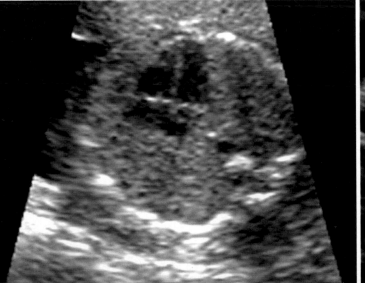

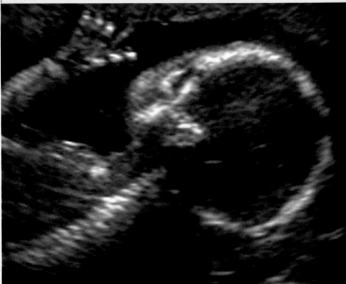

If a problem is found

Rarely, a condition in your baby may be identified at the 20-week ultrasound that requires referral to a specialist. If this is the case, you'll usually be given an appointment for a repeat ultrasound with a fetal medicine specialist within 72 hours. If a heart problem is suspected, you'll be invited for a detailed ultrasound of the heart (a fetal echo).

Further tests, such an amniocentesis (see pp.118–119) may be recommended. If a serious problem is revealed, you may be offered the option to end the pregnancy. Other problems may mean that you are referred to specialists such as cardiac or orthopedic surgeons to plan your baby's care after delivery.

Such serious problems are rare, and there will be a whole range of people to support you through any difficult times, including obstetricians, pediatricians, and physiotherapists.

Finding out our babies' sex

With my first child I had no idea of the sex, but in my second and third pregnancies I was given that information as part of additional test results during the pregnancy. I really didn't mind and had no preference about having a boy or a girl. Whether or not you want to discover the sex of your baby is a personal decision; however, if you have a very strong view about the sex you want, finding out in advance may help you adapt your thinking if your baby isn't the boy or girl you'd hoped for. CH

My husband wanted to know the sex of our baby before the birth, whereas I had always thought that I would want to wait and discover my baby's sex at the birth. However, I ended up changing my mind during the ultrasound when the sonographer asked if we wanted to know! NK

My husband and I like to plan— that's just the way we are. When asked "But don't you want to be surprised?" my husband would respond to the question by saying, "Sure, I want to be surprised . . . on the day of the ultrasound!" I personally feel there are plenty of other things to be surprised about in the delivery room—a great deal of which you have little control over. I was in the last year of my pediatric training when I was pregnant with my first child. Fully intending to find out at the ultrasound scan, my baby decided not to cooperate and the ultrasound technician was unable to say for sure if it was a boy or a girl, until we had a subsequent ultrasound! LJ

I didn't want to find out the sex of either of my children—I loved the element of surprise. Somebody said to me that there aren't many true surprises in life, but having a baby without knowing its sex was one of them that I was eager to experience. My first child was a girl and my second a boy. TL

CHECKING THE SPINE
The spine can be seen clearly now, and the individual vertebrae will be counted. The sonographer will check that the skin covers the spine and there are no signs of a neural tube defect such as spina bifida.

YOUR BABY'S LIMBS
The hands and feet will be checked and the digits examined. Your baby's limbs will be checked at this stage, and the length of the thigh bone (the femur) is a good indicator of how your baby is growing.

LOOKING AT THE UMBILICAL CORD
The umbilical cord has three blood vessels —two arteries and one large vein—which may be counted at this appointment. If there are concerns about your baby's growth, a Doppler scan may check the blood flow.

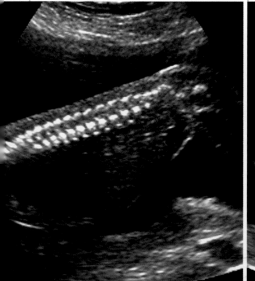
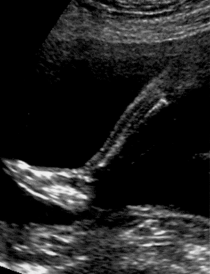
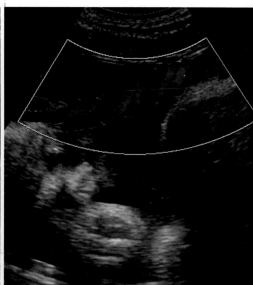

Expecting more than one?

Being pregnant with twins or more will mean that you will have a few more appointments and ultrasounds to ensure that you are all doing well. You may also be given extra support to help you care for your babies once they are born.

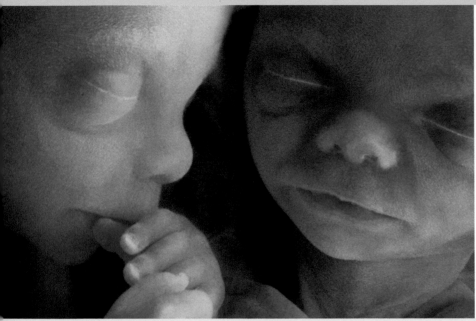

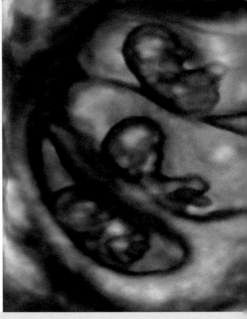

SIDE BY SIDE
Twins tend to react to each other's movements in the uterus, touching, kicking, and grabbing each other. In late pregnancy, when space in the uterus is restricted, they are less likely to turn around and change position.

CARRYING TRIPLETS
This ultrasound shows each baby developing in its own amniotic sac, safely cushioned by the surrounding fluid and membranes.

Discovering that you are expecting more than one baby can come as a shock, and you may wonder how you will cope with the pregnancy and birth—and life after the birth. Rest assured that most twin pregnancies are straightforward, but because there is a slightly higher risk of certain conditions and complications, you will be seen more often and monitored more closely than women expecting just one baby.

Your prenatal team will have plenty of experience in dealing with multiples, so you can be confident that they will be able to provide the expertise and level of care you and your babies need during the pregnancy and birth.

Regular care

Some women having twins are referred to maternal-fetal medicine specialists, who are trained to handle high-risk pregnancies, but you'll more than likely keep your usual ob/gyn. You'll also have one or more ultrasounds in your last trimester to check the growth and development of your babies and their positions in the uterus. Your level of prenatal care will be affected by whether your twins are identical or non-identical, since there tend to be more concerns with identical twins. For example, you may have an additional specialized cardiac (heart) ultrasound at 24 weeks, since identical twins tend to have a greater risk of heart problems.

Identical twins can share an amniotic sac and sometimes share a placenta, too. If the placenta is shared, there is a risk of the babies developing a condition known as twin-to-twin transfusion syndrome (TTTS). This is when, very rarely, blood from one identical twin passes to the other twin, which can cause anemia and restricted growth in the first twin). The good news is that TTTS can be diagnosed early in pregnancy, and treated while your babies are still in the uterus.

Delivering twins and multiples

Twins or more have a greater chance of being born prematurely. This is because the placenta is more likely to lose efficiency earlier, and also because the space in the uterus is more restricted.

For this reason, 37 weeks is considered full term for a twin pregnancy, and 34 weeks for triplets. Your birth options will be more limited with a multiple pregnancy. If you dreamed of a home birth before realizing that you were pregnant with twins, you'll have to come to terms with having your babies in a hospital environment. Home births in general are frowned upon by the Canadian Medical Association, and the potential for complications with twins makes such a procedure too risky.

A caesarean section is more likely with twin pregnancies and will be recommended unless the first twin is in a head-down (cephalic) position. Triplets and higher multiples will need to be delivered by caesarean.

"Joining a twins support group puts you in touch with other women with the same pregnancy issues"

Will your twins be identical?

Around one third of twins are identical. The easiest time to distinguish between identical and non-identical (fraternal) twins is within the first three months of pregnancy, when it's easier to see if the babies share a placenta and/or an amniotic sac. In most cases this is picked up during the dating scan.

Identical twins, known as monozygotic, develop from the fusion of one sperm and one egg (oocyte), which splits in two after fertilization. One third of all twins are monozygotic, and these twins are the same sex, with the same genes, blood type, and visual appearance.

Non-identical, or dizygotic, twins develop from two separate eggs and are fertilized by two different sperm. They may be different sexes and look different; they can even, in mixed race families, have a different skin color.

Dizygotic twins run in families, while monozygotic twins occur randomly. Female dizygotic twins have a one in 17 chance of giving birth to their own set of dizygotic twins.

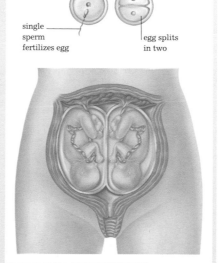

single sperm fertilizes egg

egg splits in two

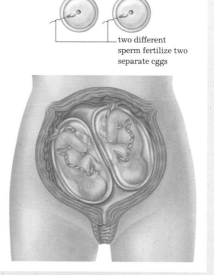

two different sperm fertilize two separate eggs

IDENTICAL TWINS
Monozygotic, or identical, twins, develop when one egg splits into two, and may share the same placenta in the uterus, as shown here. Each baby has its own umbilical cord, attached to the placenta at different points. The babies may have separate or a single amniotic sac.

NON-IDENTICAL TWINS
When two eggs develop at the same time, each baby will have its own amniotic sac and its own placenta. Not sharing a placenta means that non-identical twins have a lower chance of developing growth problems, which sometimes occurs when twins share a blood supply.

My special pregnancy

Every pregnancy is special, of course, but sometimes there are reasons to give you extra care, such as when you're an older or younger mom, overweight or underweight, or have an underlying health condition.

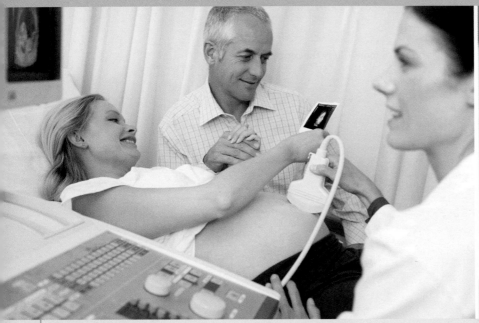

BEING AN OLDER PARENT
If you're over 35, you are considered in medical terms to be an "older mother," however young you feel. You will probably be monitored more closely, but if you're healthy, the risk of complications is low.

CHECKING YOUR SUGAR LEVELS
Easy-to-use home test kits make it easy for diabetic women to monitor blood glucose levels closely during pregnancy.

When your doctor compiles your prenatal notes early in pregnancy, she will take into account any factors that indicate you may need additional attention. You can be confident then that you will receive the best possible prenatal care throughout pregnancy.

Older moms

There has been a huge increase in recent decades in the number of women delaying parenthood until their 30s and beyond, particularly in women over 35. Being over 35 means that you are likely to see a couple of unflattering terms in your medical chart: namely "geriatric pregnancy" or "advanced maternal age." Don't be shocked by these, they are simply the medical terminology used to describe older mothers. Although being an older mom does carry some associated health risks, you are still highly likely to have a healthy, problem-free pregnancy.

However, older moms have a higher chance of miscarriage and of having a baby with an abnormality such as Down syndrome (see p.388), and are also more likely to have an underlying health problem such as diabetes (see p.128) or high blood pressure. Some problems with the placenta are more common, too, and you are more likely to develop preeclampsia (see p.386). As a result, you may have more ultrasounds to screen your baby for potential problems. You should be prepared for the possibility that you may need to stop working earlier than a younger mom-to-be, either for medical reasons or because you need to rest.

Teenage moms

If you're a young mom, you may have more stamina than an older mother. However, teenagers are still growing and developing themselves, so it's doubly important to take good care of yourself during pregnancy so you remain healthy, and your baby grows well and develops normally. Diet plays an extremely important part in a healthy pregnancy, but many teenagers may not be as concerned as older women about eating a nutritious diet. Your doctor may recommend supplements, such as iron, folic acid, and calcium.

It's important, too, that you attend all your prenatal appointments, because your doctor will give you helpful advice on leading a healthy lifestyle, and will inform you about any supplements you need to take.

HEALTH CONCERNS FOR MOM AND BABY

Due to biological immaturity or, perhaps, social circumstances, many teenagers have smaller babies. Additional ultrasounds may be required, therefore, to keep tabs on the baby's growth and development.

Teenage pregnancies are also linked to an increased risk of miscarriage, premature labor, and blood-pressure problems (including preeclampsia, see p.386), so young moms will be closely monitored to ensure that all is well.

PRENATAL SUPPORT

If you are a teenage mom, it's a good idea to attend a prenatal class with women of your own age so you can share your concerns with like-minded moms-to-be. Prenatal education is vital, as you probably won't have the life experience necessary to make confident choices for the care of both you and your baby. Classes designed for teenagers also provide a support network, advice on relationship and family issues and financial problems, and will help to set you up with the tools you need to become a confident, successful parent.

Overweight moms

If you are overweight (with a BMI of over 30, see p.19), you will be given extra attention during pregnancy, since certain complications are more likely the more weight you are carrying. You can expect your weight to be monitored throughout pregnancy, and you will be given advice on your diet and nutritional intake.

Problems include a higher risk of miscarriage, gestational diabetes (see p.385) (or a worsening of existing diabetes), high blood pressure; premature labor or a late delivery; and preeclampsia (see p.386). It may also be more difficult to detect abnormalities in your baby, because excess weight can cause technical difficulties with ultrasound.

Larger women also have an increased risk of developing blood clots in the legs or lungs and of having a longer and more complicated labor, with an increased chance of a caesarean delivery.

REVIEWING YOUR DIET AND ACTIVITY

It is very important that you don't attempt to diet during pregnancy, because you may compromise your baby's intake of the key nutrients that are required for her optimal growth and development.

Instead, you should take a look at your overall nutritional intake and, if necessary, think about changing or adapting your diet to ensure that it includes plenty of fresh, whole foods (see pp.48–51), and take steps to cut out—or at least cut back on—any refined and processed foods from your diet. If your lifestyle is sedentary, it's also important to incorporate some regular

"If you are overweight, you may need to think about changing or adapting your diet and engaging in regular exercise"

WATCHING YOUR WEIGHT
Your doctor will keep a closer eye on your weight during pregnancy if you were overweight at the outset. Taking steps to regulate your weight gain by eating sensibly and staying active will help ensure that you don't put on more weight than is healthy.

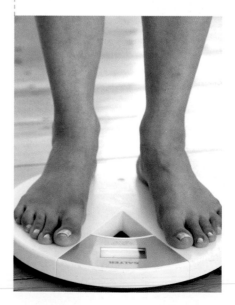

exercise into your schedule. Together, these measures can balance your weight naturally and help to ensure that you gain only the amount of weight that is healthy for you and your baby.

Underweight moms

If your BMI is lower than 19 (see p.19), you will be given expert advice from a nutritionist or an experienced doctor, and you will have extra ultrasounds to make sure that your baby is growing as expected.

You will be at increased risk of having a baby that is growth-restricted (see p.388) and that may need to be delivered early if it is not growing adequately.

CALORIES AND NUTRIENTS

You'll need to include in your diet plenty of nutrient-dense, healthy foods with good levels of healthy fats (see pp.50–51). While it can be difficult to change your eating habits, it is necessary to increase the number of calories you consume in the form of healthy fats and proteins. Not only will you need these calories to provide the resources your body requires during pregnancy, but they are also essential for your baby's healthy development.

You may need to include more nutritious snacks, such as yogurt, dried fruit, or smoothies, between meals every day, for example. Your doctor may recommend vitamin and mineral supplements to make up for any shortfalls in your diet.

The aim is not to put on excess weight, but to ensure that you get the nutrients you need to sustain a healthy pregnancy, to provide the optimal environment for your baby, and perhaps to prepare you for breastfeeding.

Conditions that need extra care

If you have a preexisting medical condition or you have suffered miscarriages, your care may need to be managed more closely during pregnancy, particularly if you take medication or if your symptoms worsen.

ASTHMA

Around one third of women find that their asthma symptoms improve in pregnancy, while one third find their symptoms remain the same and one third find their asthma gets worse.

If you suffer from a worsening of symptoms, talk to your doctor about the possibility of altering your medication: It may be that a simple change to your regular dosage will make a difference. Inhaled medication, including steroids, will not harm your baby. On the contrary, it is extremely important that your asthma is controlled; severe asthma attacks can have serious consequences for your baby.

DIABETES

This is a condition that arises if there is too much glucose (sugar) in the body. The hormone insulin, produced by the pancreas, helps glucose enter the body's cells to be metabolized. If not enough insulin is produced, glucose builds up and diabetes can develop.

There are two main types of diabetes. Type 1 is when the body produces no insulin for reasons that are unknown. This develops most commonly in childhood and needs to be treated with daily insulin injections.

Type 2 diabetes occurs later in life, usually after the age of 40. The body makes some insulin, but not enough. This type can often be controlled through diet and exercise.

Another type of diabetes, gestational diabetes, arises only in pregnancy, usually in the second and third trimesters. (For more information on this see p.385.)

The increased blood-sugar levels caused by diabetes can affect your baby's growth and make her larger than normal—a condition known as macrosomia. Having a big baby can cause complications at the birth, and increases the likelihood of an assisted delivery or an emergency caesarean, and there's a greater chance of going into premature labor.

If diabetes is not diagnosed and controlled in pregnancy, either through diet or medication, there is a slightly increased risk of stillbirth toward the end of pregnancy.

Diabetes also increases your risk of developing high blood pressure and preeclampsia (see p.386).

If you have preexisting diabetes, as well as making sure that it is well

CONTROLLING ASTHMA
During pregnancy, it's as important as ever to keep your asthma symptoms well under control. Taking your medication sensibly will prevent your symptoms from worsening, which in turn protects your baby and reduces the stress and worry you experience.

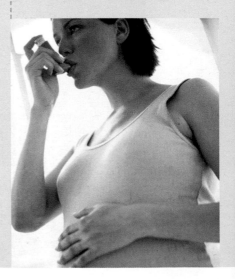

controlled before you conceive (see p.25), it is also very important to control your blood glucose throughout pregnancy. You will be referred to a team of specialist doctors who will care for you and give advice about controlling the condition, and you will also have regular ultrasounds to make sure your baby isn't getting too big.

You will also have regular blood-sugar checks, your insulin requirements will be monitored, and you may be switched to a different medication. You may need supplementary insulin to balance your sugar levels. Taking steps to eat healthily can make all the difference in how you feel and the health of your baby. You'll be given plenty of support with this.

Gestational diabetics will also have their sugar levels closely monitored. Treatment will involve diet control and sometimes pills or insulin injections.

Many diabetic moms are induced at 38 to 39 weeks to reduce the risk of complications during labor—for example if your baby is too large. Your blood-sugar levels will be monitored during labor, and you may be given intravenous insulin and glucose to help steady them.

PREVIOUS MISCARRIAGE

If you have suffered a miscarriage, there's usually no reason why you shouldn't go on to have a perfectly normal pregnancy the next time. If you feel anxious, you can request an early ultrasound to reassure you that all is well with this pregnancy.

If you've had three or more miscarriages, or a mid-term or third trimester loss, the advice and prenatal care you receive may differ. You may be seen more regularly to keep tabs on the health of you and your baby.

Additional ultrasounds may be recommended, or perhaps medication. Sometimes a stitch may be placed around the cervix if it is thought to be weak. Taking good care of yourself by eating

well, getting plenty of rest, and relaxing can all help to reduce stress and make your experience more positive.

CARDIAC CONDITIONS

If you have a known heart condition, such as an abnormal heart valve, it is likely that you will have discussed the implications of pregnancy with your cardiologist. Some women will need to have their babies delivered in a unit with special facilities. An epidural may be recommended, and the time you spend pushing may be limited.

Sometimes, minor heart murmurs are detected in pregnancy that are unlikely to cause any problems. If you have a congenital heart condition, you will be offered a detailed heart scan for your baby.

EPILEPSY

Women who have epilepsy have a higher risk of complications during pregnancy. However, it is very difficult to predict

how pregnancy will affect epilepsy. Some women see an improvement in their condition; others suffer more frequent and severe seizures, perhaps as a result of the physical and emotional stresses of pregnancy.

In women who take medication to control seizures, there is a higher risk that their babies may suffer a birth defect, such as spina bifida and cleft palate (see pp.388–389). For this reason, before you become pregnant, or as early in pregnancy as possible, you'll be referred to a specialist who will discuss and plan your care during pregnancy.

During pregnancy, you may need extra blood tests to check the levels of treatment drugs in your blood. It's also very important for you to take prenatal vitamins and folic acid.

Eating a healthy diet, making sure that you get enough sleep, and exercising regularly are other things you can do to have a safe and healthy pregnancy (see Chapter 2, pp.46–103).

Living with a special pregnancy

- Nine months can seem like a long time, but in reality, with input from different professionals, this time will go quickly and favorably. Stay calm, as this is the best way to understand and control your condition, whatever it is. Consider finding other women who have the same problem; sharing ideas and experiences can help. (See pp.391–392 for organizations and support groups.)

- Being pregnant is one of the most natural things in the world. Even if you do have health concerns during pregnancy, you can still enjoy it and find reassurance in regular monitoring. Listen to your body, stay positive, and relax whenever you can; a healthy outlook can help ensure a healthy pregnancy—and baby.

- Whatever difficulties you are experiencing in your pregnancy, don't keep them to yourself or try to do it alone. Your partner, friends, and family are probably just waiting to know how they can help, from offering practical support to a listening ear. Medical staff are on hand to assist, too. They are often able to give advice over the phone and follow up on or put to rest a concern. So don't hesitate to call if you are worried.

- Learning yoga breathing techniques can help women to remain calm in stressful situations, and practicing yoga regularly can help to bring a sense of serenity and well-being. The more relaxed and positive you feel, the better it is for your baby.

Choosing my prenatal class

The aim of classes is to prepare you for the birth and the arrival of your baby. Meeting other couples also provides a ready-made support network for after the birth. Look for classes that suit your personal approach to pregnancy and birth.

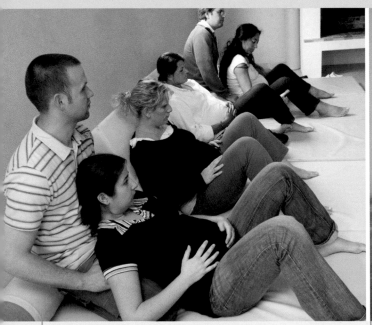

PREPARING FOR LABOR TOGETHER
Taking your partner along to some or all of your prenatal classes will ensure you both understand the birth process and encourage you to talk about how you can work together during labor.

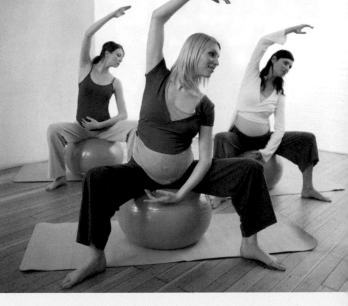

GETTING PHYSICAL
Exercise-based prenatal classes have many benefits, helping you maintain fitness levels, build stamina, and think about positions for labor. Staying fit now also ensures a swifter recovery after the birth.

Before signing up for prenatal classes, think about your approach to pregnancy and labor and what you hope to gain from the sessions. One of the main purposes of prenatal classes is to ensure that you understand the process of labor and are aware of the options you have for pain relief and intervention.

Check whether classes cover all the areas you want to know about. For example, if a course focuses primarily on natural approaches to pain relief, it might be worth finding out whether it also covers medical pain relief, or if you

will need to get this information elsewhere. Look too for classes with women who have roughly the same due date as you. This enables you to share experiences and swap advice for your stage of pregnancy. Being at a similar stage also helps to establish friendships that can prove supportive after the birth.

If you don't have time to attend a full course, which usually runs for six to eight weeks during your third trimester, you could consider a one-day workshop or weekend course, which concentrate on specific areas such as

pain-relief options and breastfeeding. Try to find a class led by a teacher in whom you have confidence and who gives you plenty of opportunity to ask questions. Also, make sure your proposed birth partner attends at least one session with you—it's important that they understand the process of labor and the best ways to cope with it.

Book classes early; the best often fill up months ahead. If you're expecting twins or more, it's recommended to start classes at around 24 weeks, because your babies are more likely to be born early.

Types of classes

There is a range of classes available, from those offered at your hospital to independently run local courses. You can look for women- or men-only classes, classes run in foreign languages, those organized for teenage moms, or couples' classes. Most have a choice of times, with many couples' classes being held in the evenings or on weekends. Often, an eight-hour course is either offered in eight one-hour chunks on weeknights or one eight-hour chunk on a weekend. Ask your doctor or midwife for information on classes in your area.

HOSPITAL-BASED

Most hospitals have their own prenatal classes, usually held within the maternity unit. You may be offered a tour of the delivery suite and find out what to expect when you arrive at the hospital. The course broadly covers what happens during labor, both medical and natural types of pain relief, and information on the kind of birth experience you can expect. It will also talk about how to care for your baby after the birth and offer advice on breastfeeding.

PRIVATE

If you'd rather take a prenatal class in the privacy of your own home, a private course might be right for you. Classes can cover all aspects of labor, newborn care, and breastfeeding. You'll be encouraged to learn natural birth techniques in the company of your birth partner, including breathing and positions during labor.

Ask your caregiver for referrals to nurses or midwives who teach private prenatal classes, and find out before booking whether its ethos matches yours.

GROUP CLASSES

There is a variety of group classes run by individuals or organizations, such as the YMCA or a community health center. Content will vary according to the instructor's philosophy, but it will generally include basic information on pregnancy and preparing you and your partner for labor and birth. Some may incorporate relaxation techniques and include yoga and meditation; others are based on hypnotherapy (see p.137), gentle stretching, or water births.

EARLY PREGNANCY

These are not a replacement for classes that take place later on in pregnancy, but are instead designed for women who would like some support and guidance in the early stages of pregnancy. You may find classes aimed at teaching the basics of a healthy lifestyle, or providing help with symptoms, tests, or emotional changes throughout pregnancy.

REFRESHER CLASSES

These are aimed at women who already have children, and offer the chance to find out the latest theories and research, refresh knowledge, and receive advice on how to do things this time around.

EXERCISE CLASSES

Many specialist classes focus on your health during pregnancy and encourage you to stay active throughout, guiding you on safe levels of exercise at each stage of pregnancy. There are classes in Pilates, aquanatal classes (water exercise), yoga, aerobics, and many more, all of which are aimed at keeping you healthy. Some exercise classes go further and teach the most effective positions for labor, as well as advising you on how to get back on your feet after the birth.

TWINS

In some areas, there are classes designed for parents expecting twins or multiples, with a focus on preparing for an earlier-than-usual delivery date, what to expect with a caesarean section or vaginal delivery, breastfeeding more than one, and life after the birth.

These classes are extremely useful for parents-to-be of twins and create an instant support network that often proves invaluable during pregnancy and after the birth.

ONLINE

If you are pressed for time or find it difficult to get out, you may wish to consider one of the various online classes available. These classes are broken down into modules that focus on the various aspects of pregnancy and birth.

While you will miss out on the social support offered in group classes—and probably the practical elements of learning labor and birth positions— you will nonetheless gain a good grounding in what you can expect during labor and in the period following the birth of your baby, including how to care for and nourish your new baby. Think about joining a group after the birth for social support.

> "Book your classes as early as possible— the best courses often fill up months in advance"

Where should I give birth?

There are many factors to consider when choosing where to have your baby. Your doctor or midwife can advise you on the options, but ultimately the choice is yours. Being informed will enable you to make a decision that's right for you.

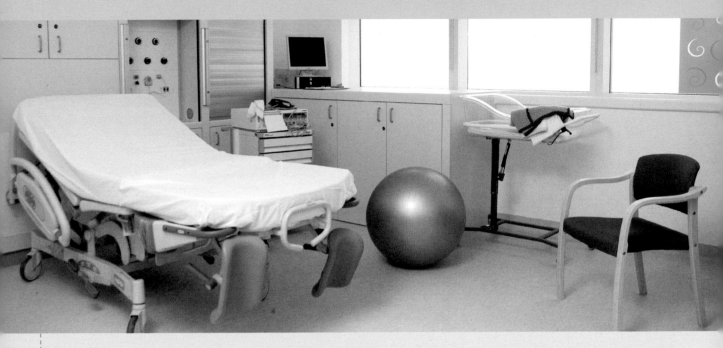

THE LABOR AND DELIVERY ROOM
Attending a tour of your hospital during pregnancy gives you the chance to view a delivery room so you know what to expect. These rooms contain delivery beds and all the necessary technical equipment, such as monitoring aids, and most have their own bathroom facilities.

When choosing where to have your baby —in a hospital, in a birthing center, or at home—your health and that of your baby will be taken into account by your doctor or midwife. Most pregnancies and births in Canada are straightforward, but sometimes there are factors that can influence your available options.

Your doctor or midwife will look at any complications during previous pregnancies. If, for example, you had a caesarean or bleeding after the birth, they may advise a hospital birth this time. They will consider your general health and whether you have a condition that needs extra care during labor. Also, the position of your baby, the number of babies you are carrying, and, of course, your personal wishes will be considered.

There are advantages and disadvantages to most birth scenarios, so think things through before you make a final decision. There's no reason you can't change your mind at a later date, but it can be reassuring to organize the birth as far as possible, so that you can get yourself in the right frame of mind and know roughly what to expect.

However, bear in mind that things do not always go according to plan, and sometimes arrangements need to be changed at a late stage. Adopting a flexible approach and treating your plans for labor and birth only as a guide can help you avoid stress and disappointment if circumstances mean that you need to change the place or manner in which you give birth.

In the hospital

Most babies are delivered in a hospital setting, under the care of a doctor or midwife. Some women like knowing that there's a range of medical pain-relief options available and high-tech equipment on site in the event of an emergency. You'll deliver at the hospital where your doctor or midwife has hospital privileges. Try to visit in advance to ask questions and view the facilities (see box, below). You may, for example, want to check the availability of tubs if you are planning to spend some of your labor in water.

Find out about hospital policies for things that matter to you, such as how many family members or friends are allowed in the labor suite; what comforts, such as music players, you can bring with you; continuity of nursing care; and what breastfeeding support is available.

The care available to you in a hospital is comprised of a team made up of an obstetrician, your midwife, a team of nurses, an anesthesiologist, and sometimes other specialists. Who actually assists your doctor during the labor and birth will depend on your health and that of your baby, and the progress of your labor.

PROS AND CONS

When deciding whether to give birth in a hospital, think about your needs as well as how you would like to handle labor.

There are circumstances when a hospital birth is necessary, for example, if you're in a high-risk category or you need to be monitored in labor, in which case hospitals provide all the staff and facilities needed. Hospital births are also appropriate if a problem with your baby is suspected, since specialist staff, including a neonatal intensive care unit, will be available right after the birth.

In a hospital, epidurals are available for pain relief, and a delivery can be assisted with forceps or a vacuum (see pp.310–311) if required. Obstetricians and anesthesiologists are readily available to perform a caesarean (see p.316–317) if necessary, and resuscitation and other equipment is on hand in an emergency.

"Try to be flexible: If things don't go according to plan, you may need to make alternative arrangements— sometimes at the last minute"

Visiting the hospital

As a part of the preparation for the delivery of your baby, you may be offered a tour of the hospital, which is worth doing. You see firsthand where you are likely to be delivering your baby, and can ask questions about hospital policies. You may want to ask about the following:

• What the admissions procedure is, what you'll need to bring with you, and what the hospital supplies.

• Visiting hours, the number of visitors allowed at any one time, and the policy on young children in the hospital.

• Maternity wards and rooms. You may want to know the number of moms per room, and whether there are private rooms available for after the birth.

• How the hospital deals with birth plans, and when they will intervene. Finding out the intervention and caesarean rates for a hospital can give you an idea of the hospital ethos.

• Who will be delivering your baby, how long the shifts are, and continuity of care.

• Natural pain relief in labor. Are there birthing pools or showers available, and will you be allowed to use natural remedies or have a complementary therapist with you?

• How long you are likely to have to wait for an anesthesiologist.

• The hospital policy on fetal monitoring during labor, and whether this might affect your ability to walk around and remain active in labor.

• What happens to you and your baby after the birth.

• What support there is for breastfeeding and whether the hospital supplies breast pumps (in case for any reason you can't breastfeed for a period of time).

• Whether the hospital has a neonatal intensive care unit—some do not have facilities for very small babies.

• Anything else that springs to mind, no matter how minor. This is your birth experience, and you have every right to know what to expect, and how you can adapt your plans accordingly.

On the downside, research indicates that there tends to be more medical intervention with hospital births. Furthermore, you aren't always guaranteed continuity of care with nurses, particularly if you have a long labor. Many women also find the environment sterile and clinical, which, in some cases, is thought to slow labor.

In a birthing center

Birthing centers are run by midwives and are either attached to a hospital or are stand-alone centers within the community. At the moment, they are not widely available in Canada

You and your partner should visit the facilities in person, and confirm that the midwives are correctly trained and registered, and that the center is regularly inspected.

These centers are best for women with a low risk of complications and who are interested in having a natural childbirth overseen by midwives in a non-medical, low-tech environment, with as little intervention as possible. Centers attached to hospitals enable women to give birth in a home-like environment, while knowing they can be quickly transferred to the hospital if medical intervention is needed.

If you're considering a birth center, make sure that you look into the facilities in different centers (if more than one is available in your area), and whether, for example, proximity to a hospital is important to you if the unit is a stand-alone one.

PROS AND CONS

At a birthing center, your care will be managed by a team of midwives with a great deal of experience, and if you organize your prenatal care through the center, you will receive continuity of care with this team through to the birth.

For some women, a main disadvantage of birthing centers is that they do not offer the full range of pain-relief options. You won't be able to have an epidural, for example. Although many centers do have some modern technology that equips them to deal with certain complications, you will need to be transferred by ambulance to your nearest hospital (unless the center is attached to a hospital) if a caesarean is required, if your labor does not progress, or if there are any concerns about your health or that of your baby during labor.

At home

Having your baby in the comfort of your own home may be an option if you are in good health and your pregnancy is problem-free. Some women think that being at home helps them to relax and makes labor run smoothly, however many medical associations frown upon home births because of the potential for complications.

You will need to organize a home birth in advance, but once it has been planned, your midwife will arrive with everything you need to have your baby at home (see pp.306–307).

DELIVERING IN A BIRTH CENTER
A low-tech, home-away-from-home environment with labor managed by midwives is a good solution for some women.

GIVING BIRTH AT HOME
Being in your own home allows you to create the perfect birthing environment, helping you to relax. Many women believe this helps labor run smoothly and makes interventions less likely.

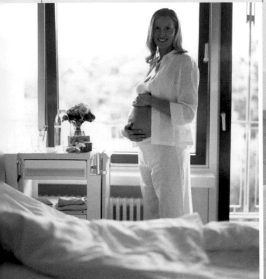

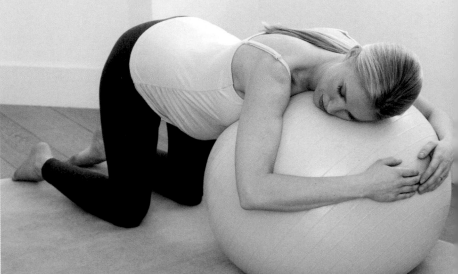

PROS AND CONS

As with a hospital birth, think carefully about your needs and preferences before deciding whether a home birth would be a suitable option for you. If your pregnancy is uncomplicated, then giving birth in a comfortable, familiar setting can help you to feel more relaxed, and you can also be more active. Feeling less tense increases your ability to manage pain, and moving around more can result in more efficient contractions and a faster labor. Statistically, at home you are more likely to have a normal vaginal birth with fewer interventions, since your pregnancy will be "low-risk." You will be guaranteed continuity of care, and you will give birth in familiar surroundings with your family around you to provide support.

Because of the potential for complications during labor and delivery, even for healthy women with low-risk pregnancies, the Canadian Medical Association and certain medical professionals oppose home births. And certain conditions, such as diabetes, high blood pressure, or being pregnant with multiples, may rule out the possibility of a home birth. Large or overdue babies may be better off being delivered in a hospital environment because of the potential for complications during a vaginal delivery.

Pain relief during a home birth is limited, and an epidural is not possible. Finally, if there are complications during or after labor, you will need to be transferred by ambulance to your nearest maternity hospital. Around one in six women who opt to labor at home will need to transfer to a hospital.

Where we had our babies

Our daughter was born at the hospital where I worked. I knew most of the nurses and the pediatric staff, so felt very comfortable being in their care. I was induced at term, because my baby was not growing and had a condition called intra-uterine growth restriction (IUGR) (see p.388). Due to my age (40) and because my baby had IUGR, both being potential risk factors for complications, we were advised to have a hospital birth. She was eventually delivered by forceps and needed admission to the neonatal intensive care unit for a short while afterward. NK

I chose a hospital to have my first child. Since I was so uncertain about how I would handle labor, I wanted all the pain-relief choices available on the spot. In reality, I got through most of labor without an epidural—but knowing I had immediate access to all the pain-management options was a comfort. CH

I had three children over the course of three-and-a-half years, and all were born in the hospital. During my first pregnancy, my husband and I were both still finishing our medical residency training. We lived near the hospital where he worked, which was 45 minutes away from the hospital where I worked, and where I hoped to deliver. Both of us worked full days prior to the start of my labor, which began five days early. Hoping to have a natural childbirth, we had decided to wait to drive the 45 minutes to the hospital (in order to remain at home for as long as possible during early labor). I continued to have contractions throughout the evening, but by 10 or 11pm, they were slowing down and less intense. We decided to take showers and get ready for bed. I went first, and quickly learned what obstetricians all seem to know: that warm water can kick labor into high gear. With much harder and more frequent contractions gripping me, I tried to get into bed while my husband showered, but found myself vomiting. After a long and very uncomfortable drive to the hospital, I was checked into a room, found to be 5cm dilated, and my water broke after a couple of contractions. My daughter was born minutes later! In the end my goal of natural childbirth was accomplished, both with my quick first labor and my subsequent deliveries. My second and third labors were equally quick—both under five hours. LJ

After a caesarean with my first baby, I was determined to try and have a vaginal birth for my second, and my obstetrician agreed to let me try. Things started very well: I was having contractions every three minutes from the start, and when I arrived at the hospital I was already about 5cm dilated. Labor accelerated rapidly and within an hour or two I was almost fully dilated. There was concern about the level of blood loss, and when my baby's heart rate suddenly dropped dramatically, I was rushed to the operating room. On examination, my obstetrician decided I was dilated enough to have the baby quickly delivered with forceps. The problem was that I'd had no pain relief, and there wasn't enough time to wait for an epidural to kick in. They therefore decided to give me a general anesthetic. They gave me just the right dose, so that after about 20 minutes I woke up to discover my husband holding our baby boy! TL

I chose to have my baby in the hospital—maybe because after working with many obstetricians, this seemed like the natural choice for me. Also, we had recently moved into a beautiful old house, but it was a bit of a building site, without any central heating—because my baby was due in November, I was worried that she wouldn't be warm enough. The hospital provided all the comfort and support we needed during those first days with our daughter. FF

How do I want to give birth?

When thinking about where you want to give birth, it's natural to consider also the type of birth you would like to have. Looking at all your options early on will make you aware of any arrangements you need to make.

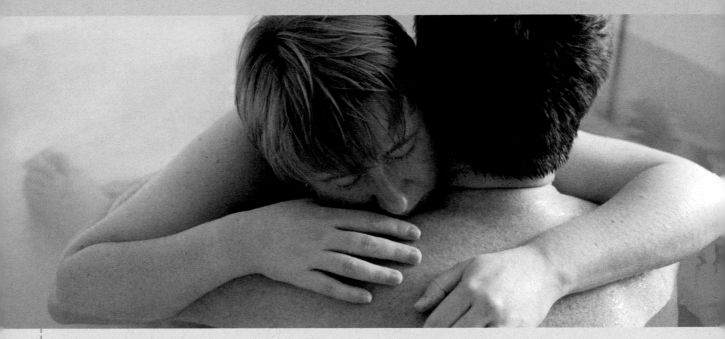

GIVING BIRTH IN WATER
Under the expertise and guidance of an appropriately trained doctor or midwife, giving birth in water can be a positive experience for both mom and baby, and can reduce the need for medical interventions.

While the birth options available to you will depend on how straightforward your pregnancy is—or whether a concern later on means you have to change your plans—there's no harm in thinking early in pregnancy about coping techniques you might like to use during labor.

You may be sure that you will want medical pain relief at some point, and your doctor and prenatal classes can inform you of the options.

Other birthing techniques, such as a water birth or giving birth using hypnosis, require a bit more planning from you, and you may have to seek out information, enroll in classes, or find out where to rent the necessary equipment. Take time to consider all the options and make the right choice for you.

Using water

Some women sit in a warm tub while laboring or giving birth, and it's a safe option for you and your baby, provided the birth is attended by a doctor or midwife trained in water births. Some hospitals and many birthing centers have birthing pools, which you may use for the labor and/or delivery of your baby, or you can rent one to use at home.

Being in warm water can be a relaxing, low-stress method of laboring and giving birth. The water provides a form of natural pain relief as it helps you to relax and reduces tension, which in turn is thought to help you to cope better with pain and encourage a more efficient labor.

"The realization that focusing on pain can increase tension may motivate you to find ways to relax during labor"

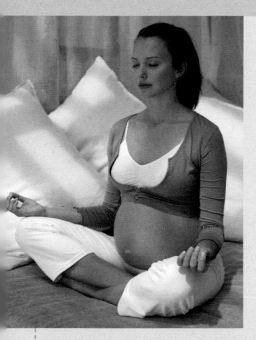

CALM FOCUS
HypnoBirthing can help you to have a natural, drug-free labor, but it requires knowledge of the techniques and practice.

Being in water also helps you to have an active birth because the buoyancy of the water supports you and allows you to move and change position with the minimum of discomfort, which can help to make labor more efficient.

Studies show that laboring in water is particularly useful for the second, pushing stage of labor (see pp.300–302). Women who labor in water also have far less chance of having an episiotomy (a surgical cut to increase the vaginal opening) or a tear to the vaginal area—so are less likely to need stitches.

There is evidence that water provides a more peaceful and calming environment for your baby's birth, since the warm water of a pool is similar to her home in the womb, and therefore makes for a less traumatic transition. For most women, laboring and giving birth in water is a positive experience.

PLANNING A WATER BIRTH

If you wish to have a water birth, or perhaps to spend most of labor in water and then get out for the actual delivery, talk to your doctor or midwife about it well in advance of your due date. She will have all the information you need about which local hospitals have water-birth facilities, or, if facilities are limited, whether you need to look into birthing centers or renting a birthing pool to use at home.

If there are birthing pools available at the hospital, ask the staff there how often it is used for pain relief, how many women give birth in the pools, who would supervise the water delivery, and what training they have.

If you are planning a water birth at home, ask your midwife for details of agencies that rent pools, or organizations that provide this information. You'll need to think about where you will set up the pool, bearing in mind that birthing pools come in various shapes and sizes. Some are inflatable, others more permanent structures. Some have built-in heaters; others have to be filled with water from your own hot-water system.

Apart from the practicalities, try to find out about other women's experiences of laboring in water. How beneficial did they find it? Was it difficult to get out of the pool during labor? How did it feel to give birth in the pool? You may also want to find a prenatal class focused on natural birthing techniques.

Using hypnosis

In the 1920s, obstetrician Dr. Grantly Dick-Reid founded the theory that panic and fear cause pain during labor. He promoted breathing and relaxation techniques to help women focus and overcome the fear of pain, in turn enabling a natural labor.

Today, women are taught to breathe rhythmically through their contractions, using deep physical and mental relaxation techniques that reduce the "fear, tension, and pain" syndrome through guided imagery and self-hypnosis. Studies show that labor time is decreased when hypnotherapy is used, there are fewer complications and interventions, and drugs are not used as frequently. Some research even suggests that 70 percent of women experience an entirely pain-free childbirth.

PREPARING FOR A HYPNOBIRTH

You can buy a CD to teach yourself the techniques, or find out about classes in your area. These are usually held from 25 weeks onward.

Choosing my birth partner

Giving birth is one of the most significant events of your life, and it is important that you surround yourself with people who will provide you with the confidence and support you need to make it a positive experience.

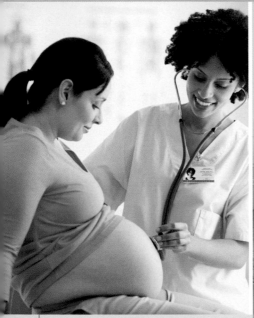

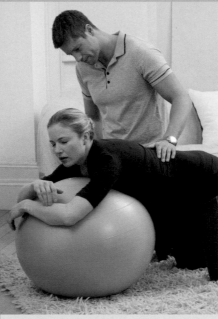

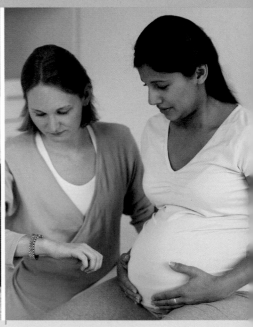

YOUR NURSE OR MIDWIFE
This is the person you will rely on first and foremost to guide you through labor and ensure that you and your baby are well.

YOUR PARTNER
If your baby's father is supportive, calm, practical, and sensitive to your needs, he'll probably make an excellent birth partner.

CHOOSING A DOULA
The support of a woman experienced in childbirth can be invaluable and help you to feel confident in your ability to give birth.

Whether your birth partner is the baby's father, a family member, a close friend, or a combination of these, you need to be confident that the person or people you choose to be with you during labor will be able to provide calm emotional and practical support throughout.

Whoever you choose to share this extraordinary event with you, their role will be to understand the birth process and to ensure that your birth plan is recognized and respected during labor, so it's important that they are well prepared in advance.

How support can help

There is plenty of evidence to show that an encouraging and supportive birth partner can have a hugely beneficial effect on how women cope with pain, and can improve the outcome of labor for both mother and baby. Studies show that women who feel well supported during labor, both emotionally and physically, manage to cope more successfully with the pain and may even have shorter

labors. The evidence reveals that they have less need for epidural pain relief and are likely to have fewer medical interventions, such as an assisted delivery or a caesarean birth.

Your primary birth partner is likely to be a hospital nurse or your midwife, who will guide and support you during labor and throughout the birth. Many women choose to have additional support during labor, since they won't know the nurse assigned to them at the hospital beforehand, they may not have the same nurse throughout (especially if there's a shift change and you haven't delivered yet) and there will be times when the nurse isn't by your side. Your doctor will also provide support, but she'll be present less often than your nurse or midwife. Having a chosen birth partner with you ensures that someone is there constantly.

When deciding who else you want to be with you during the birth, think about whether that person will remain calm and reassuring. You need someone who will allow you to focus on your labor, rather than cause you to worry about how they are dealing with the event.

YOUR PARTNER

For many women, the obvious choice of birth partner is the baby's father, and it's certainly the case that he is often the person who understands your needs best and can offer continuous support. For many men, being at the birth is a momentous occasion that they wish to participate in. They are confident of the support they can provide and wish to be by their partner's side to help her, and to witness the birth of their child.

However, the baby's father is not always the most appropriate birth partner. In fact, some men are concerned that they will find labor stressful and may not want to attend the actual birth. They may feel guilty about this and feel it is their "duty" to be there. It's important that you and your partner have an open and honest discussion about the birth. Allow your partner to express how he feels and listen to his views and concerns. If he has doubts about his ability to remain calm, he may not be the best person to have with you. Or you may both agree that he will be with you during the early stages, but not present for the actual birth, if he feels nervous about this in particular.

FAMILY AND FRIENDS

Instead of, or in addition to, your partner you may choose a friend or a family member, such as your mother or sister, to be with you. If you want more than one birth partner, check with the hospital to see whether there is a limit to how many people are allowed in the delivery room.

DOULAS

Some women decide to pay for the services of a doula to support them in labor and birth. Doula comes from the Greek word meaning "woman servant or caregiver," and in the context of childbirth refers to an experienced woman who offers emotional and practical support before, during, and after the birth. Hiring a doula may be a good choice if you feel that the baby's father won't be able to provide the right support during labor.

Doulas undertake training and have a good knowledge and awareness of female physiology and the process of childbirth. You and your partner will get to know her in advance of the birth, and she can offer support during pregnancy, for example, by advising you on how to prepare your body for labor. During labor, a doula will offer emotional and physical support. She can act as a go-between, making medical staff aware of your wishes and ensuring that, as far as possible, they are met. After the birth, she will assist you with breastfeeding, and may also provide practical support at home for the first few weeks.

It's important to feel completely comfortable with the doula you choose, that she can be on call around your due date, and that she has qualifications or references you can check.

Who makes the best birth partner?

The ideal birth partner is someone who knows you well, and who has researched labor and delivery. He or she needs to act as an advocate for you, and know you well enough to understand your capabilities. Patience is important, too. While bossy isn't ideal, neither is passive!

• You will rely on your birth partner to follow your birth plan, guide health professionals about what you need, and tune in to what you're going through. Someone you trust, who can be calming but assertive during times of need, is the ideal. You may find you need more than one person to fit this bill. If so, think carefully and choose compatible birth partners—you want harmony, not squabbles, at this time.

• Most fathers are eager to be there at the birth. Some women, though, worry about their partner being present for the actual birth because they are concerned that they may not be sexually attracted to them afterward. It's a very individual choice; only you know your partner's individual personality. Let him know about your concerns and talk about them before making any decisions.

• Sometimes a birth partner doesn't take such an active role, for example if you need a caesarean section. However, even in this case, your partner plays an important part. Provided he can stay with you, he can help you stay calm and reassure you that all is going well.

• You may find that a labor and delivery nurse is all the help you want. If you have supportive and caring medical staff, you may be unconcerned about who else is present. Some women feel they need just one person who knows what to do—and to have no other distraction.

Writing my birth plan

Creating a birth plan gives you an opportunity to communicate what you'd like to happen during your labor and birth with the specialists looking after you, so that the whole experience goes as smoothly as possible.

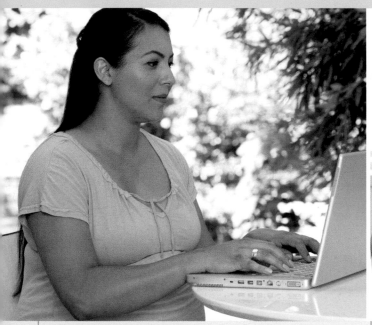

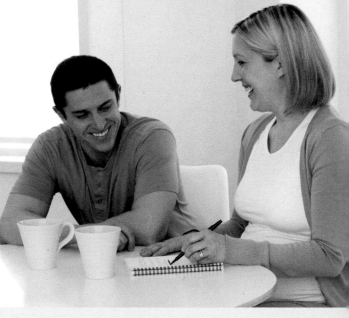

DO YOUR RESEARCH
It's a good idea to investigate the place where you'll be giving birth and to talk to other women before creating your birth plan. Online forums can be a good place to start.

INVOLVE YOUR PARTNER
Talk your birth plan through with your partner, especially if he's going to be with you at the birth. Nothing has to be set in stone, and you can keep reviewing it right up until the delivery if you wish.

You may want to write a birth plan to set out your preferences for what happens during labor and the birth of your baby. A birth plan is a useful tool to tell your doctors, nurses, or midwives how you'd like to be treated. It should be your wishes, rather than a list of demands, and it pays to be flexible, since you can't be sure what will happen on the day. Instead of saying that you absolutely don't want something to happen, it's better to state what you'd rather avoid if possible. This way, you allow your caregivers room to deliver your baby safely.

How do you get started?

Before you create your birth plan, it's a good idea to do some research. First of all, talk to your doctor or midwife to find out what is realistic for you, based on your health and that of your baby. Ask the hospital (or wherever you're giving birth) about their policies on topics such as water birth, if you'd like to have one, and their rates of interventions—how many women have episiotomies or

caesareans? Ask other women what worked for them—your family and friends will probably be a mine of information. Your prenatal teacher should also be able to guide you. And of course, your doctor or midwife will always be on hand to answer questions.

The idea is to set out the details of what you consider to be the ideal labor experience, focusing on your birth environment, pain relief, positions during labor, interventions (for example, a drip to speed up labor if it slows), natural remedies or treatments you'd like to use, who you'd like with you during labor, how you'd like your baby monitored, whether or not you'd like your partner to cut the umbilical cord, and how you'd like your baby presented to you after the delivery. You can include any aspect of labor and birth that matters to you.

WHAT TO INCLUDE

The most important things you can include are:

• Details of your chosen birth partner or partners and their role.
• The positions you'd like to try for labor and birth.
• Your choice of pain relief.
• How you'd like your baby monitored.
• Whether you want your third stage of labor (delivery of your placenta) to be natural or "managed" (see pp.304–305).
• Who should cut the umbilical cord
• Whether you'd like to have skin-to-skin contact with your baby, and how you'd like to feed her after the birth.
• Whether you'd like to use a birthing pool, and whether you want to give birth in the pool or simply use it for pain relief.
• Whether or not you are willing to have medical students in the labor room.
• How you'd like to respond to unexpected situations; for example, methods for speeding up a faltering labor, or an emergency caesarean. The unexpected is less scary if you have considered the options.

STAY OPEN TO CHANGE

It is, however, important to be flexible and to understand that things sometimes change. Every labor is different and may not always go exactly as planned. It's also perfectly possible that you'll change your mind during labor itself. Give your birth partner and the doctor or midwife overseeing your labor a copy of the plan. It's a good idea to star or highlight anything that is very important to you— for example, skin-to-skin contact with your baby as soon as she is born. It's also helpful to make a list of alternatives (for example, would you consider a spinal instead of an epidural?) so you're prepared for most situations.

"The priority is a safe delivery and a healthy mom and baby, so be prepared to be flexible and realistic"

Thinking about your birth plan

Birth plans are very useful when it comes to delivery, since you may not be in a position to explain to your doctor what preferences you have. It is important to know all the facts in order to make an informed choice, and you should be able to get most of the information you need well before the time of delivery. Many delivery units can provide you with a pre-printed questionnaire, which you can fill in to save as your birth plan.

• Creating your birth plan gives you a chance to consider carefully what you need at every stage of your labor. Bear in mind the practical aspects of labor—such as the place you will give birth, examinations, pain relief, and interventions you prefer, and how you want your baby to be handled after birth.

Consider, too, what helps you feel calm and supported—for example, what music or touch soothes you and, conversely, what does not help, so your birth partner can avoid it. Ensure that if you can't make decisions yourself, your birth plan clearly states who can act for you.

• Write out your birth plan in list form, and make sure it isn't too long, or it won't be read in its entirety. You might want to consider points such as asking for people to talk to your birth partner rather than directly to you, so that you can concentrate on what you are doing.

• Be as flexible as you can; for example, there may be situations where your doctor will ask you to get into special positions to aid the delivery of your baby.

A doctor or midwife may also advise you to have a certain type of pain relief, such as an epidural. If you have a rigid birth plan, you may be disappointed if circumstances dictate otherwise. It is therefore very important to have a realistic and safe plan, but one that you're prepared to stray from if necessary.

• While your birth plan is your ideal, don't hold onto it so tightly that it feels like failure if it must be set aside.

• After you've written your birth plan, give a copy to your doctor, midwife, or doula if you know she'll be with you for the birth, or ask to have it put in your file at the hospital or birthing center. Put another copy in the bag you're packing for the day you give birth.

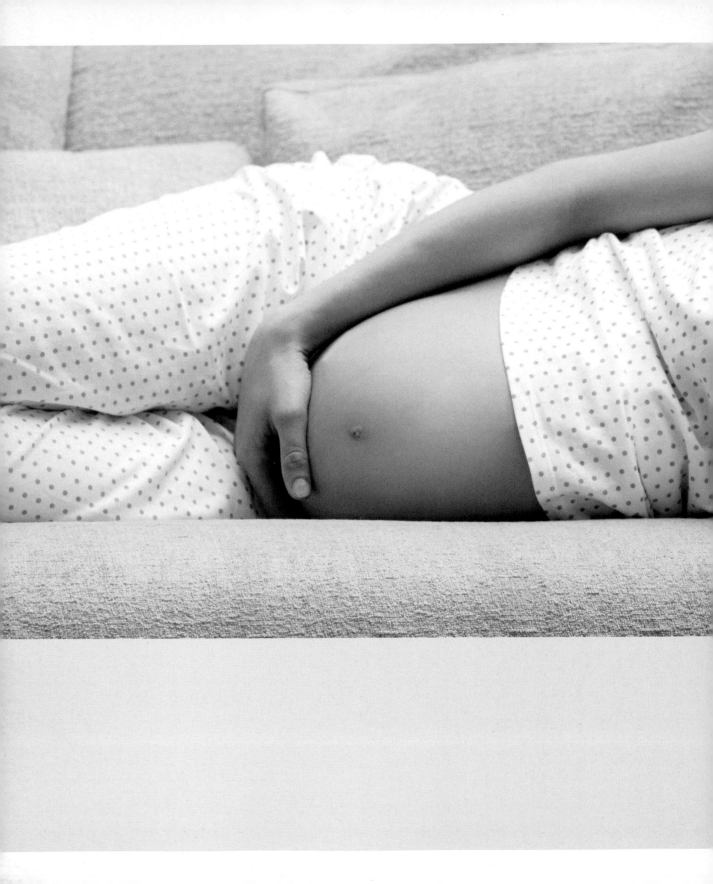

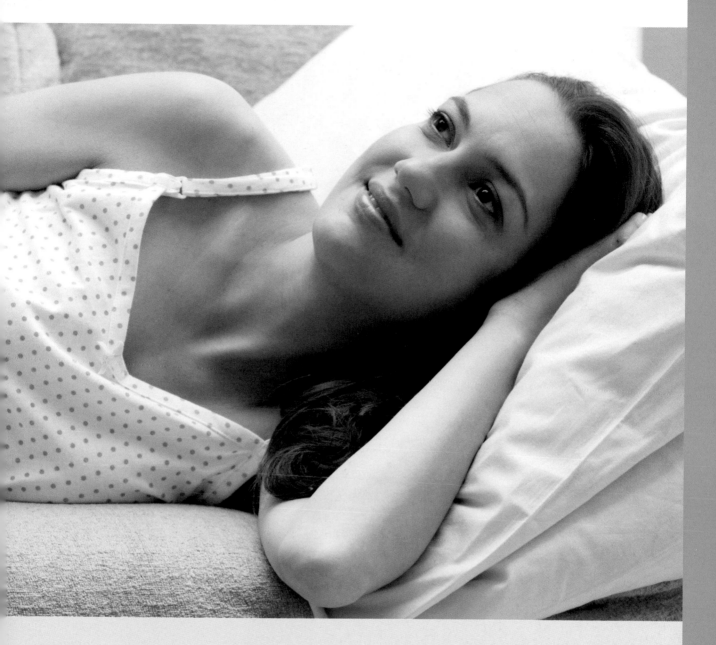

My pregnancy calendar

It is fascinating to see your baby's growth and development and how your body changes during every week of your pregnancy.

The first trimester

From that first exciting moment when you unveil your positive pregnancy test up to 13 weeks of pregnancy, your first trimester is a period of rapid physical and emotional change.

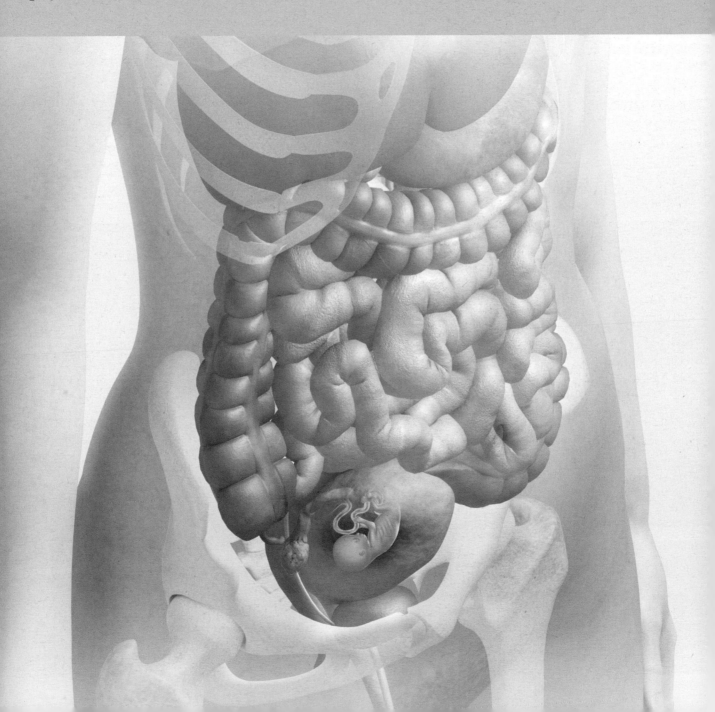

"Your baby will grow from a single cell to a tiny human being, as your body changes to accommodate his needs and nurture his development"

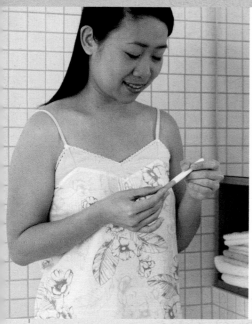

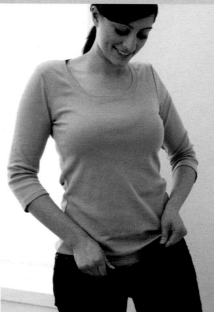

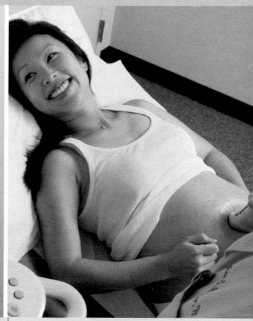

IT'S POSITIVE!
It's normal to have mixed feelings about a positive test result, even if you planned your pregnancy.

A TIGHTER FIT
One of the early symptoms of pregnancy is abdominal bloating—a sign that your body is preparing for the next nine months.

I CAN SEE HIM!
During this trimester you'll get your first chance to see your baby live on screen, at your dating scan.

MIRACULOUS CHANGE
You may not begin to show for several months, but deep inside your pelvis your baby will be growing and developing at an astonishing rate during the first trimester.

The first trimester marks the beginning of your pregnancy experience. Over the next 40 weeks an astonishing series of changes will take place, as the miracle within you grows and develops from a microscopic cluster of cells to a bouncing new baby. You, too, will experience a profound transformation as your body prepares your unborn baby for life.

Smaller than a poppy seed at the outset of pregnancy, your baby will develop all of his major organs within the first trimester and, by 13 weeks, will weigh around 0.5oz (12.5g) and measure

2in (5.5cm) from the top of his head to his bottom. He'll have toothbuds and fingernails, and his heart will be beating.

Your body and emotions will change dramatically, too, as hormones begin to surge in preparation for the creation of a new life. Excitement may alternate with anxiety, and you may experience some uncomfortable pregnancy symptoms, such as nausea, sore breasts, and fatigue, as your baby undergoes this period of rigorous development. The good news is that by the end of the first trimester, an equilibrium will likely be restored.

3 weeks

Early symptoms, some much like PMS, may lead you to suspect that you are pregnant. These indicate that hormonal changes necessary to support your baby are taking place.

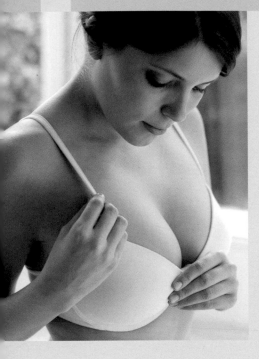

Tender breasts

Even before you have an opportunity to take a pregnancy test, you may be aware of changes already occurring in your body. You may feel a little unsettled emotionally—more tearful, anxious, or excited than usual—and your breasts may tingle and feel fuller than normal. It's not unusual to experience a little nausea, headaches, and even unusual food cravings well before you've even missed a period. Some women also experience a strange sensation known as "air hunger," which causes you to feel short of breath. You may also experience a feeling of complete exhaustion.

Soon after your egg is fertilized, the part of the embryo that will develop into the placenta begins to release the pregnancy hormone hCG (human chorionic gonadotrophin), which prevents the release of further eggs from your ovaries and encourages the production of estrogen and progesterone. Estrogen works to boost the blood flow to your organs and promotes the dramatic growth and development of your uterus and breasts. Progesterone is essential to prepare your uterus for the embryo. It is these hormones that will kick-start the very first symptoms of pregnancy.

You may experience a small amount of bleeding and possibly some mild cramping, which occurs when your baby implants in the lining of your uterus (see below), and you may feel slightly bloated.

What happens at implantation?

When your egg is fertilized, it becomes a "blastocyst," or a tiny ball of cells that will multiply at a rapid rate while moving down the fallopian tube (see pp.30–31) to your uterus, where it will implant in the lining. Once in the uterus, the cells become known as an embryo, which burrows into the wall of your uterus and connects to your circulatory system.

SIGNS OF IMPLANTATION
Implantation usually occurs between six and twelve days after ovulation. There are typical signs, including implantation

spotting (light, brief bleeding), mild cramping, and a drop in your body temperature for about a day. This is followed by an increase in temperature that will remain until your pregnancy has been established. Some women do not experience any tangible symptoms of implantation, so don't be alarmed if there is nothing to suggest that implantation has taken place.

Once the process of implantation has occurred, amniotic fluid begins to collect around your baby; this will become the amniotic sac, in which your baby will be protected and nurtured until he is born.

The placenta (see p.158) will also begin to develop, supplying the oxygen and nutrients that will sustain him inside the womb.

In certain rare cases, the fertilized egg develops and implants outside your womb, either in your fallopian tube or, more rarely, in your abdominal cavity. In the tube, the embryo soon outgrows the narrow space. The tube may begin to rupture and there may be bleeding, which can cause severe abdominal pain and irregular vaginal bleeding. This condition is referred to as an ectopic pregnancy (see pp.44–45) and requires immediate medical attention.

3 weeks

Your baby is still a microscopic collection of cells, but exciting developments are taking place—all his organs, including his brain, spinal cord, and heart, will soon begin to form.

MY BABY

From egg to blastocyst

During ovulation, an egg will be released from an area on your ovary known as the "follicle." Once the egg is released, this area is called a "corpus luteum" (which literally means "yellow body"). This small, fluid-filled sac becomes increasingly "vascular," developing blood vessels and starting to produce progesterone—which is required to prevent the lining of your womb from shedding and helps your fertilized egg to survive in your uterus.

As your egg travels down your fallopian tube and is met by a healthy sperm, fertilization takes place. Your fertilized egg, now known as a "zygote," is propelled by tiny hairs ("cilia") toward your uterus. As the zygote travels, the cells divide repeatedly—from two, to four, to eight, and then sixteen cells, and so on—until it enters the uterus three to five days later. Every time the cells divide, they become smaller and smaller, in a process called "cleavage." The cells remain inside the original egg cell, which continues its journey toward your uterus.

This solid cluster of cells enters your uterus and remains there, unattached, for about three days, after which it develops a fluid-filled center. When this cavity appears, the hollow ball of cells is known as a "blastocyst," which is the basis of the cell mass that will eventually become your baby. The blastocyst moves toward your uterus lining, where it implants itself to receive a rich supply of nutrients and oxygen from your blood. Here, it splits into two sets of cells; one set becomes the placenta and the other will develop to become your baby. At this early stage of embryonic development, the blastocyst's needs are met by a balloon-like structure called the yolk sac, which will continue to provide its sustenance until the placenta is fully developed.

At this point, your baby is known as an embryo, and is already starting to form the neural tube—a pipe-like collection of cells, from which his brain and spinal cord will develop—that will eventually become his nervous system (see p.151).

> "As your egg travels down your fallopian tube and meets a healthy sperm, fertilization takes place"

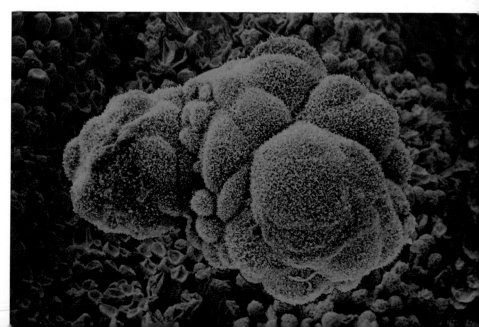

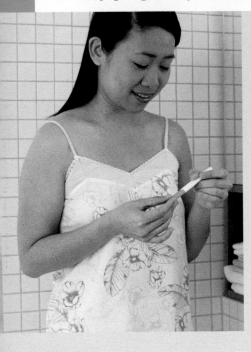

Confirming pregnancy

Many women wait for a missed period before taking a pregnancy test, but it's worth noting that many of these tests are so sensitive that you can get a positive result a few days or even a week before your period is expected. Pregnancy tests measure levels of the hormone hCG (human chorionic gonadotrophin), which is secreted once your fertilized egg (blastocyst) implants itself in the wall of your uterus (see p.147). There are normally enough hormones in your urine to measure about two weeks after you conceive, but some women have high enough levels for a positive result just a week later. Don't panic if your first pregnancy test is negative; test again in a day or so, urinating first thing in the morning. When you sleep, you release a chemical that concentrates your urine so that you do not have to get up repeatedly to empty your bladder. Therefore, your first urine of the day will be much more likely to have the highest concentration of hCG.

It's highly unlikely that if you get a positive test result it will be wrong, but a negative test may not be a firm indication that you *aren't* pregnant. Occasionally, implantation and the subsequent release of hCG can take longer in some women. By the end of four weeks, you should have a firm result. Congratulations!

How we felt when we found out we were pregnant

I felt very short of breath and had some nausea; I also noticed some breast changes—in particular, nipple soreness and tingling. In hindsight, these symptoms were pretty mild compared to a few weeks down the line. MG

I experienced a sense of relief and excitement. Having wondered if it would ever happen, I don't know how I didn't blurt it to the whole world the moment I found out. Sharing the news with my husband, I had a real sense that we were in something important together. CH

I was astonished to discover I was pregnant, as I didn't plan either of my pregnancies. However, I was delighted! FF

I was very excited to find out I was pregnant with each of my three children and, being an impatient person, couldn't wait for them to be born! LJ

Extreme tiredness hit me the most in the first trimester—before I even knew I was pregnant—and it continued for 12 weeks. Although the pregnancy was not planned, it was a wonderful surprise—despite having just started a new job, and just moved into a new home! NK

I noticed that I was going to the bathroom more a week after I conceived, so I wasn't surprised that my test was positive a week later. I was still pretty overwhelmed by what lay ahead! VB

I was really nauseated and extremely tired in the first 12 weeks or so of pregnancy. I could hardly move from the sofa most afternoons and evenings. TL

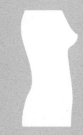

4 weeks

Critical organs are already developing in your baby, so it is important to eat a well-balanced diet, including plenty of folic acid, even if you aren't feeling particularly hungry.

Early embryonic development

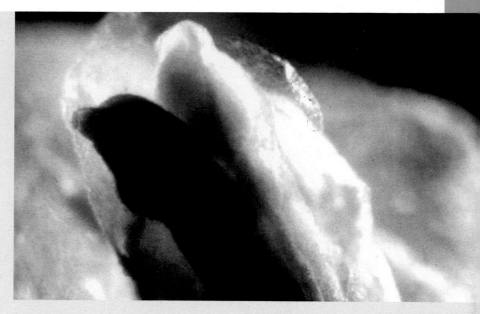

Once the ball of cells implants in the wall of your uterus and becomes an "embryo," some time around three or four weeks of pregnancy, the embryonic period begins. This is when your baby's brain, spinal cord, heart, and other organs begin to form. At about three or four weeks, the embryo is divided into two layers called the "epiblast" and the "hypoblast." All your baby's body parts will be formed from these layers.

At around four or five weeks, your baby's embryo will form three layers. The uppermost layer, known as the "ectoderm," will become your baby's top layer of skin, his central and peripheral nervous systems, his eyes, inner ears, sweat glands, and tooth enamel.

It is in the ectoderm that your baby's neural tube also develops, beginning first as a flat region that rolls into a tube about 28 days after your baby is conceived. Your baby's brain, backbone, spinal cord (the long bundle of nerves that runs inside the backbone to connect the brain with the rest of the body), and nerves are formed from the neural tube, which continues to develop until it closes in a week or so (see p.151).

In the middle layer, known as the "mesoderm," your baby's heart and a very basic circulatory system will form.

The cells in your baby's mesoderm layer will also form the basis of his bones, muscles, cartilage, kidneys, and even his reproductive system.

The innermost layer of the embryo— the "endoderm"—will become a simple tube lined with mucus membranes. This is where your baby's lungs, intestines, and bladder will develop, as well as his thyroid gland, liver, and pancreas.

By the beginning of five weeks, the embryo is visible as a tiny nubbin of tissue on the ultrasound scan. Even though it is just barely recognizable, all the building blocks for your baby's vital organs are already in place.

The period from four weeks to ten weeks of pregnancy is an exceptionally important time for your baby's development, and he will be very vulnerable to the effects of drugs, alcohol, smoking, radiation, and viruses. By 10 weeks, almost all of his organs will be formed—and some will have begun to function—although his brain and spinal cord will continue to develop throughout pregnancy.

Your placenta is not yet in place to offer some protection from toxins and pathogens (including viruses and germs), so special care should be taken to avoid anything that could harm him.

Your diet is also crucial during this time, and key nutrients, such as essential fatty acids (EFAs; see p.51) and folic acid (see p.19), are required for the growth and development of your baby's brain, nervous system, and other organs.

4 weeks

Your baby is now about the size of a poppy seed, and by the end of this week, a rudimentary placenta and umbilical cord will form, to keep the embryo nourished and well oxygenated.

MY BABY

Feeling bloated

It's not unusual to feel puffy and bloated during the first weeks of pregnancy—and well before you begin to "show." There are two main reasons for this. The first is that the hormone progesterone can cause excessive gas during the first trimester, as it works to relax the smooth muscles in your abdomen to allow room for your baby to grow. This extends to the digestive tract and intestines, slowing the passage of food through the gut and often leading to constipation. You can ease this by drinking warm peppermint tea or hot water and lemon before breakfast, to help move things through your gut and stimulate digestion.

It can also help to eat a good, healthy breakfast with plenty of fiber (see p.51), which will encourage the action of your intestines. Swapping out soda for plenty of water and eating little and often can also ease symptoms of constipation.

The second common cause of bloating is water retention—much like the edema experienced in PMS. Hormonal changes are the main cause of this type of bloating, but reducing the amount of salt you eat and increasing your water intake can help prevent discomfort.

There are, of course, a multitude of other reasons why your tummy may appear bloated, including the growing size of your uterus and the increased blood and tissue in your abdominal area.

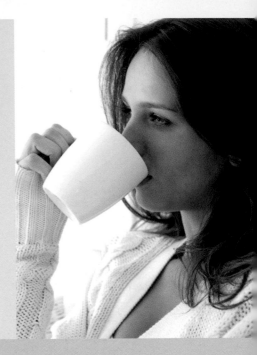

ME AND MY BODY

5 weeks

Some women experience few symptoms of pregnancy at five weeks, while others are already feeling nauseated and extremely tired. Each of these scenarios is normal.

Early pregnancy symptoms

My breasts felt much bigger and very tender early on, and I was very tired. TL

I wasn't a coffee drinker before becoming pregnant, but I definitely drank a fair bit of Diet Coke. I can still remember the day—sometime just before six weeks—when I completely lost my taste for diet soda, and for the remainder of my pregnancy I steered clear of it. LJ

Morning sickness took me by surprise. Somehow I thought it would only be mornings—that's what the name implied! Feeling sick for large parts of the day seemed unfair, not to mention the constant need for a supply of dry crackers and ginger ale. CH

Tiredness and headaches were my main early-pregnancy symptoms. I wanted to sleep wherever I could lay my head. My headaches were quite debilitating, and I was reluctant to take any medication. Undergoing a course of acupressure proved to be very effective. NK

I was extremely tired at times, sometimes nodding off midway through sentences after a day at work. VB

The first symptom I experienced in both my pregnancies was "air hunger." I could not take a deep breath and felt short of breath at the slightest exertion. This was how I discovered I was pregnant with my daughter. Nausea came next, and I could not stand the smell or taste of coffee. I also felt extremely tired in the mornings. These symptoms soon resolved after 12 weeks. MG

Heart formation

In the week to come, your baby's heart will be formed from the middle layer of cells in the embryo, known as the "mesoderm." Beginning as a simple tube, the heart undergoes a process called "looping," and then begins to divide into four separate chambers that are capable of pumping blood around his body. There is an opening in your baby's heart and a special valve that diverts the blood away from his lungs; he doesn't need to breathe to get oxygen while you are pregnant, since he receives everything he needs from your placenta or, at this stage, your own blood. This opening will close around the time of his birth.

These amazing developments take place across just one week, as your baby requires blood to grow and develop. By the end of the week, your baby's heart will begin to beat, and this can be detected during an ultrasound scan. Next week his heartbeat will be regular, and by eight weeks his heart will be fully developed, beating 150 times per minute—about twice the rate of an adult. This rate slows down as your baby grows in the womb.

During the first few weeks in the womb, your baby's heart takes up most of his midsection; in comparison to the size of his body, his heart is nine times larger when he is an embryo than it will be when he is born.

> "By the end of the week, your baby's heart will begin to beat, and can be detected during an ultrasound"

5 weeks

Growth is rapid, and by the end of this week, your baby will be 4–6mm long—or roughly the size of a small apple seed. He'll resemble a tadpole more than a baby at this point.

MY BABY

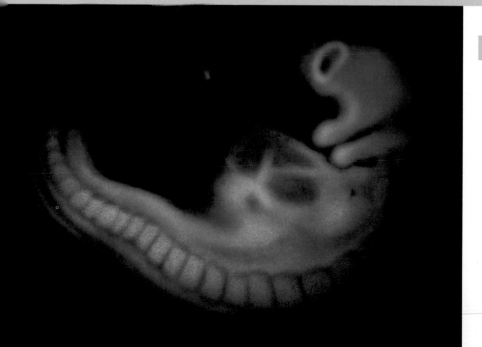

The neural tube

Around this time, your baby's neural tube, which will form the basis of his spinal cord and brain, closes. When the tube is formed, there are pores (openings) present that will begin to close during six weeks of pregnancy. One end of the neural tube (at your baby's head) will become his brain, while the remainder will form his spinal cord. If these pores do not close properly, abnormalities called neural tube defects (NTDs), such as spina bifida, can occur. These defects are rare, but they account for most abnormalities of the brain and spinal cord. Taking folic acid (see p.19) is essential for your baby's neural tube.

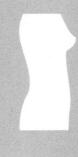

6 weeks

Pregnancy symptoms, such as nausea, vomiting, mood swings, and fatigue, may be much more noticeable now, as your hormone levels continue to increase.

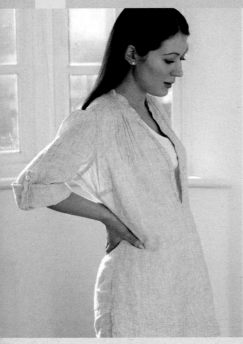

Backache

One of the earliest pregnancy symptoms, which can continue in various degrees to your final months, is back pain. All through your pregnancy, a hormone called "relaxin" is released, in order to loosen your joints to allow your baby to pass through the pelvis. What's more, your growing uterus will apply pressure to the lower part of the spine, which can cause discomfort. You may also experience sciatica (inflammation of the sciatic nerve, which runs through your buttocks and the sides of your legs). This feels like a sharp, needle-like pain through your bottom and into your thigh. It can occur on one side, or both. Finally, the increased blood supply to your pelvis can cause you to feel "congested" and achy in your lower back.

Maintaining good posture and avoiding any sudden movements can help relieve pressure on your back. It's a good idea to take stock of your work station at this stage (see pp.60–61), and ensure that you feel comfortable and have plenty of lower-back support when seated. Get used to wearing flat, comfortable shoes, too; high heels can make the ligaments in your back even more uncomfortable. Although it may seem very early in your pregnancy, it's a good idea to avoid lifting anything heavy, and to put your feet up and rest whenever you can. Regular, moderate exercise is a good way to keep your muscles toned and supple.

Pregnancy hormones and what they do

Hormones are chemical substances that are carried throughout your bloodstream to stimulate various activities in your body. During pregnancy, you'll experience a number of hormonal changes, which are responsible for the symptoms you'll experience as your body prepares to create and then deliver a baby.

Some of the hormones at play include hCG (human chorionic gonadotrophin), which stimulates your ovaries to produce more progesterone, stopping your periods. Progesterone maintains almost every aspect of your pregnancy, including relaxing the muscles of your uterus as it grows, maintaining your placenta, stimulating the growth of breast tissue, and strengthening your pelvic walls. Later on in your pregnancy, it will cause your blood vessels to relax and soften.

Estrogen helps prepare your breasts and encourages milk production; it also regulates the production of progesterone, maintains the lining of your womb during pregnancy, and promotes healthy blood flow. In addition, it regulates the density of your baby's bones, among many other functions. Oxytocin stimulates your milk glands to prepare for breastfeeding and triggers contractions during labor; endorphins help to deal with stress and pain; relaxin softens tissues and ligaments to make your lower back and pelvis more flexible for labor; and thyroxine develops your baby's central nervous system and ensures that he gets enough oxygen.

There are many more hormones involved, which play a dual role of preparing your body for pregnancy and birth, as well as helping your new baby adapt for life outside the womb.

6 weeks

Dark spots will be forming where your baby's nostrils and eyes will develop, and he is looking more recognizably human. He's about the size of a lentil or a kernel of corn now.

My baby's eyes

Just two weeks after conception your baby's eyes will begin to develop, and over the next four weeks all his major eye structures will form. At around five weeks, a pair of eye buds will appear on the sides of his head, and eye sockets will be formed.

His eyes are made up of three types of tissue: the neural tube (which creates his retina, and the color of his eyes); the mesoderm, which is responsible for his cornea (the white of his eyes); and the ectoderm, which will create the lens.

By six or seven weeks, the lens, the cornea, and the retina begin to develop. On an ultrasound, you can often see a black circle on each side of your baby's head. This is his retina, which can be seen through the lens of his eye. About a week later, skin begins to fold over his eyes, creating lids. These will fuse closed while his eye development continues over the coming months (see p.197). Your baby's optic nerve forms during the last seven months of pregnancy.

Your baby's basic eye development occurs quickly, and early in pregnancy, and it is particularly vulnerable to injury during this time. Alcohol, tobacco, drugs, and some viruses, such as rubella (German measles), can cause the eye to become malformed or damaged. This is one good reason that a healthy diet and lifestyle are essential from the moment you decide to have a baby.

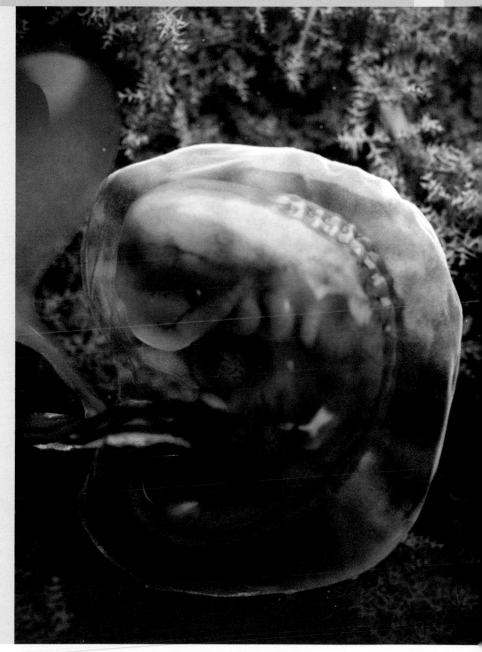

Nausea and vomiting

Sometimes referred to as "morning sickness"—a misnomer, since pregnancy sickness or nausea can occur at any time—this symptom usually abates around the beginning of your second trimester (14 weeks). The cause of nausea and vomiting isn't entirely clear, but it is believed to be due to increasing levels of estrogen and progesterone, an enhanced sense of smell, and excess stomach acid. Blood-sugar swings, stress, and fatigue can also play a role. Another theory is that it is caused by the buildup of hCG (see p.152), which is produced after

implantation and increases until about 12 weeks of pregnancy. The good news is that research has found that women who suffer from nausea and vomiting are much less likely to have a miscarriage.

Although you can't do much about your hormones, it can help to eat little and often—both to mop up excess stomach acid and to help balance your blood sugar. Whole-grain carbohydrates and a little protein are your best bets; fat can sometimes exacerbate symptoms. Try to eat something before you get out of bed in the morning. Ginger is a traditional remedy to settle your stomach, so ginger cookies or ginger ale may help you to keep things down. Yoga for relaxation and plenty of sleep may also help.

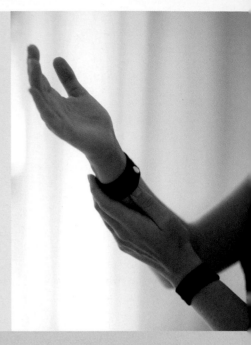

ME AND MY BODY

7 weeks

Your uterus will now be the size of a small grapefruit, and you may experience some mild cramping as it expands. It's normal to gain around 4lb 5oz (2kg) in the first trimester.

How we coped with nausea

I was lucky enough not to suffer from pregnancy sickness, but I followed my own advice from an early stage, and that may have helped. I always carried crackers to snack on—every two to three hours, even if I wasn't hungry—and would have a small carbohydrate snack before bed to prevent my blood-sugar levels from dropping in the night. I also tried to sit upright for an hour or so after eating, since digestion is slower due to pregnancy hormones. NK

I suffered from nausea on and off, throughout the day, until 12 weeks with

my first baby, and until about 14 weeks with my second. I craved carbohydrates, such as bread, potatoes, and pizza! TL

Morning, noon, and night sickness affected me for the first three months, and it was only made better by regularly nibbling on crackers. It was definitely worse when I went too long between meals. With each pregnancy the morning sickness got worse, with greater nausea and symptoms lasting longer through the day. Luckily though, no matter which pregnancy, it did ease off at the three-month milestone. CH

One of my moms suffered terribly from pregnancy sickness, which finally abated around 15 weeks. She said what worked best for her was acupressure bands—wristbands that stimulate an acupuncture point (see image, above). You put them on first thing in the morning, then when you experience a wave of nausea during the day, press on the button, first on one wrist then the other, about 20 or 30 times at one-second intervals. MG

I was very lucky to never feel sick in either pregnancy. VB

Budding arms and legs

When you are about four weeks pregnant, your baby's limbs will start to appear as small bulges or "buds"; arm buds appear first on either side of his body, followed by leg buds a few days later. As they grow longer in the coming week, nascent feet and hands can be seen. At first, they look like paddles, but the fingers and toes will soon take shape.

By seven weeks, your baby's arms are clearly divided into hand, arm, and shoulder segments, while his legs will have upper and lower leg, knee, and foot segments. Toe buds will appear at the end of his legs, and will seem very small and thin, as will his legs. There will be a light webbing between his fingers and toes, giving your baby an almost amphibian-like appearance. His elbows will become visible around this time. By eight weeks, your baby's elbows will be well formed, allowing his arms to curve around his chest throughout his development in the womb. His arms can be raised and bent at the elbow, and his hands will be by his face (or nose) for much of your pregnancy.

As your pregnancy progresses, his legs and arms will continue to become longer. The webbing will disappear, leaving distinguishable fingers and toes that will curl open and shut as he stretches and moves. His muscle tissue and bones develop over the coming weeks and months, and by 18 weeks, he'll have a good covering of muscle and his bones will start to become harder. By 20 weeks, he'll have fingernails and toenails, which will continue to grow until he is born. At around 26 weeks, your baby will begin to develop recognizable fingerprints and footprints.

Throughout your third trimester, muscle and cartilage will continue to develop on your baby's arms and legs, and his bones will become harder. Calcium is very important for bone development and for hardening of the bones; make sure to get plenty of it in your diet (see p.51), as well as vitamin D.

7 weeks

Your baby will still have a small tail, which will disappear over the coming weeks, and now he has fingers and toes with webbing between them. His little tooth buds are also forming.

MY BABY

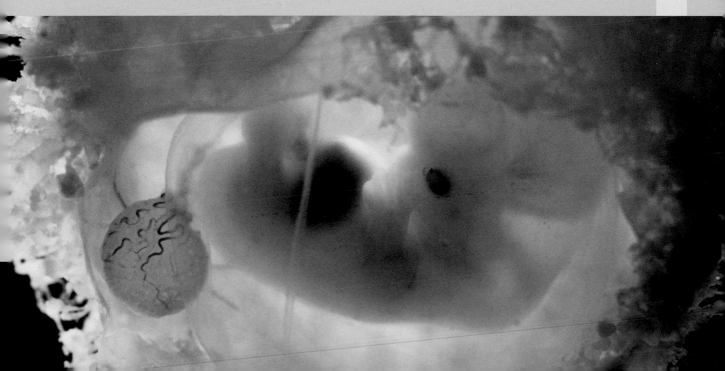

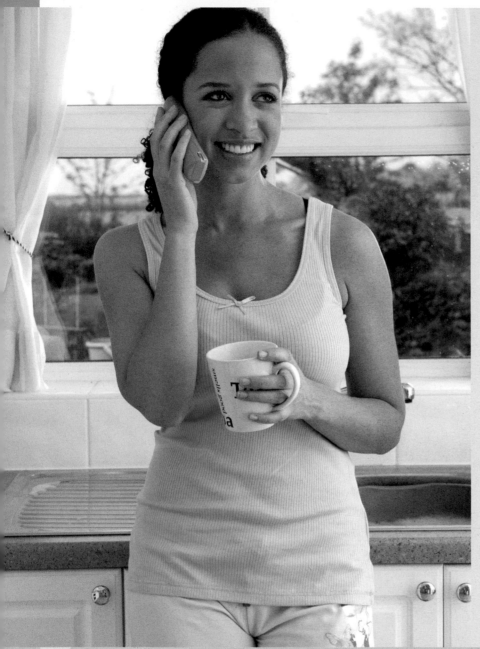

Mood swings

Pregnancy is a period of dramatic change—not just physical, but also emotional. Your moods may swing from elation and happiness to tears and feelings of depression in a short space of time, and you may find that you are snappier and more irritable than usual.

While it is easy to blame these dramatic emotional changes on hormones, it can be difficult to feel in control. Mood swings are a feature of PMS as well as pregnancy, and if you suffered from PMS before you became pregnant, chances are you'll experience more severe mood swings now.

Talk to your partner and your co-workers and explain that you are presently at the mercy of your hormones, so to excuse unusual flights of emotion. Remove yourself from the scene when you feel like you are going to burst into tears or snap; a good long walk or calling a friend can help you relax and let off a little steam. Try to eat regularly, since fluctuations in your blood sugar can make you feel even more unstable. Similarly, avoid stimulants such as caffeine. Most of all, get plenty of sleep, and reassure yourself that what you are feeling is very normal. By your second trimester, you'll feel more like yourself again. However, if you do experience periods of depression that don't seem to shift, see your doctor, who can assess the situation (see p.91).

8 weeks

You may be frustrated by unremitting symptoms, such as breast tenderness, mood swings, and nausea—or you may be one of the lucky women who has virtually no symptoms.

How the facial features develop

At about six weeks, your baby already has basic facial features, and arches where his jaws will develop. A week or so later, his mouth and tongue are evident, and his eyes have a retina and a lens. His nose and ears will begin to take form, too. By eight weeks, your baby will have tiny nostrils and a defined nose tip, as well as a distinct upper lip. His chin will show some definition, too, and tooth buds for his future baby teeth will be forming within his developing jawbones.

At this point, his ears will start developing rapidly. By eight weeks, the external part of his ear (the "pinna") will also start to develop low down on his head. The part of the middle ear that is responsible for both balancing and hearing will form by 10 weeks.

At the end of the first trimester, your baby's eyes will have moved from the side of his head to the front, but will still be set wide apart. His eyelids are closed and will remain so until about 30 weeks. His skin will be transparent, and it will be possible to see a network of veins across his face. By 20 weeks, he will have eyebrows and eyelashes, and begin to look very much like the baby you will meet in a few months. Look closely at your anatomy scan (done at around 18 to 20 weeks); his profile may fill out a little, but you'll get the first real opportunity to see what your baby will look like.

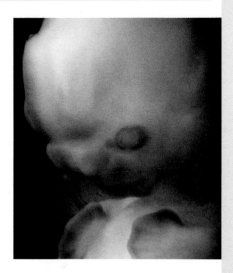

Basic perceptions

At eight weeks, your baby looks like a small human, with distinct limbs, hands and feet, fingers and toes, and more refined facial features. He has also lost his tail. This is the point at which your baby's brain, although still very simply formed, begins to grow and develop, and his nerves will be functioning to the degree that he is capable of some movement. Nerve cells in his brain are branching out in a network that will become the pathways for nerve transmission later on. By now, he has developed some very basic sensory perceptions. He can respond to touch, although it is still too early for you to be able to feel your baby's movements. Research suggests that he will also develop pain sensors, and soon be able to experience pain himself. Almost all your baby's organs are in place, and they will continue to mature and become more complex throughout your pregnancy.

MY BABY'S TAIL IS GONE

Until about eight weeks, your baby will have a tail that is about one sixth of his length. Between four and eight weeks, this tail will recede, and its tissues will form what is commonly known as the tailbone, the final segment of the spinal column (the coccyx). The reason for this tail is unclear, but it is believed to be "vestigial," which means that in the process of evolution, it has become unnecessary and is no longer formed in humans. However, the tailbone still serves as an attachment point for certain muscles and ligaments, and provides support when sitting down.

Very rarely, babies are born with a bit of a tail, containing some muscle tissue, sometimes a little cartilage, and some nerves; this can be surgically removed and poses no risk to their health.

8 weeks

Your baby is now about 0.6in (1.6cm) in length, and his organs, nerves, and muscles are beginning to function. Eyelids cover more of his eyes, and he has early tastebuds on his tongue.

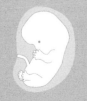

MY BABY

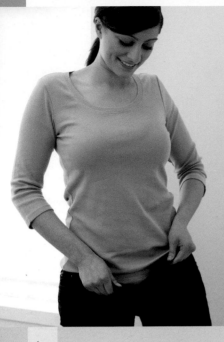

My expanding waistline

As your baby grows, your uterus expands to accommodate him, the placenta, the umbilical cord, 500 to 1,000ml of amniotic fluid, and the fetal membranes. At this stage, your uterus will be the size of a small melon, fitting neatly within your pelvic cavity. Slim moms-to-be and those who have had previous pregnancies may well begin to see the first signs of swelling in the abdomen, as the uterus begins to protrude.

Many women are surprised to find that they feel and look larger well before their uterus has begun to expand outward, and feel that they look chubby rather than pregnant! This is caused by bloated bowels and surrounding tissues (see p.150), as well as the slight weight gain that is normal early on. Putting on weight is a necessary part of pregnancy, and you can expect to gain an average of 27lb 10oz (12.5kg), although this varies a great deal between women. You'll be weighed at every prenatal appointment to make sure that you stay within the proper weight-gain range.

As your waistband tightens, you will need to make adjustments to your clothing—and your attitude! Coming to grips with looking (and feeling) larger can take time, but it's all part of accepting and embracing your pregnant body.

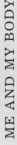

ME AND MY BODY

9 weeks

Your pregnancy hormones will continue to rage, and you may experience headaches and back problems, as well as increased vaginal discharge that can encourage yeast infections.

The role of the placenta

The placenta is an organ attached to the lining of your womb during pregnancy, which provides your baby with oxygen and nutrients via the umbilical cord. Waste products from your baby also pass back along the umbilical cord to the placenta, and then into your bloodstream for disposal. It keeps your unborn baby's blood supply separate from your own, as well as providing a link between the two.

Your placenta also produces hormones that encourage the growth and development of your baby. It is responsible for protecting your baby against some types of infections while he is in the womb. Most bacteria will not cross the placenta to your baby, but the placenta will not protect him from viruses, such as rubella (German measles; see p.21). Alcohol, nicotine, and other drugs can also cross the placenta. Toward the end of your pregnancy, the placenta passes antibodies from you to your baby, which provides him with your own immunities for about three months.

HOW THE PLACENTA IS FORMED
Your placenta is developed from layers of cells that are created when your embryo implants in the wall of your uterus. As it develops, it extends tiny hair-like projections (chorionic villi) into the wall of your uterus. These projections branch out in a complicated tree-like arrangement, which increases the area of contact so that more nutrients and waste materials can be exchanged. The placenta is fully functioning by about 18 to 20 weeks, but continues to grow throughout pregnancy. At delivery, it weighs about 1lb (400g) and is around 9in (22cm) long.

It is believed that abnormalities in this development are responsible for complications such as preeclampsia (see p.386), which can occur later in pregnancy.

Internal organs are forming

When your baby becomes an embryo, after implanting in the womb, his internal organs will begin to be formed. This formation begins around three weeks after fertilization of the egg, when your embryo elongates and develops a more human shape. The area that will become the brain and the spinal cord (the neural tube) is the first to form, while your baby's heart and major blood vessels begin to develop by around four weeks. Just a few days later, his heart will begin to pump fluid through his blood vessels, which will continue to develop in both the embryo and in your placenta.

By the time you are nine weeks pregnant, almost all your baby's internal organs—including his kidneys, liver, pancreas, intestines, gall bladder, and reproductive organs—are formed, although they will continue to mature as your baby grows and develops, and many will not be fully functional until your baby is ready to be born.

This is a critical period of structural development during which your baby is highly susceptible to the damaging effects of a variety of drugs, viruses, and other environmental factors. It is extremely rare for congenital fetal abnormalities to develop after this.

By three months, many of your baby's organs will begin working on a very basic level. Some, such as the heart (see p.151), will be in working order, and his brain will be growing rapidly. It takes until the end of the fifth month for most of his internal organs to work efficiently, and they will become larger and more effective as your baby grows. There are, however, a few exceptions to this. Your baby's kidneys will not be fully developed until your eighth month, and his lungs will not be mature until he is full term (around 37 weeks). Although his reproductive organs will be in place, it won't be possible to recognize them until around 20 weeks, when the differences are finally noticeable.

9 weeks

Already about an inch (2.5cm) in length and growing steadily, your baby's features—including his nose, mouth, fingers, and toes—are very distinct and clearly visible on an ultrasound.

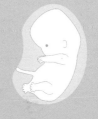

MY BABY

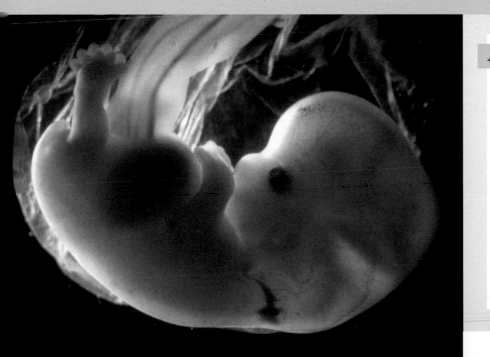

A tiny human being

Although there will be plenty of fine-tuning in the months to come and a great deal of growth, at this stage your baby has all of his essential body parts, including fingers and toes, wrists and ankles, and even tiny earlobes. His organs are in place and many will soon become functional. His head is half the size of his body, and his chin is tucked against his chest.

He'll remain in this position for many weeks. However, he'll take advantage of the space in your uterus to move freely in the amniotic fluid.

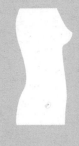

ME AND MY BODY

10 weeks

Your uterus is the size of a large grapefruit, and you may be able to feel it above your pubic bone. You now have the first wonderful opportunity to hear your baby's heartbeat.

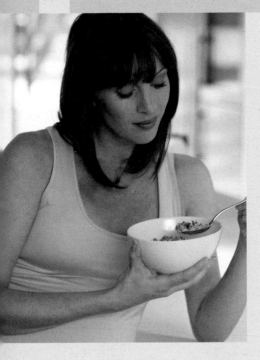

I'm constipated!

One of the unfortunate side effects of the extra progesterone is the slowing down of your digestive system. This can lead to constipation, bloating, gas, and a feeling of fullness. It's important to try to rectify this early on, because it is not uncommon for hemorrhoids (caused by straining; see p.101) to crop up at this stage, and they can become worse as your pregnancy progresses.

It is important to eat plenty of fiber-rich foods, such as fresh fruits and vegetables, whole grains, legumes, seeds, and brown rice, to bulk up your stool so it is easy to pass. Fiber does, however, require plenty of liquid to work efficiently, so you'll need to drink lots

of fluid—ideally about six large glasses of water each day. Exercise—about 20 to 30 minutes, three times a week—will also gently stimulate your bowels.

Iron supplements can often encourage constipation, so if you are taking them, it may be worth talking to your doctor to see if the dosage can be changed, or you can take a break from them for a while. If you are uncomfortable, and your bowel movements have become hard or impacted, visit your doctor, who can recommend a good, gentle laxative that is safe during pregnancy. It may be that simply adding prunes and prune juice to your diet will do the trick. Don't experiment with laxatives on your own, because some can encourage early contractions.

What's the best thing to eat now?

A healthy, well-balanced diet is essential during the first trimester. At this stage you should have a daily intake of protein, carbohydrates, and dairy products. Try following these suggestions:

● As your baby's brain, eyes, and nervous system continue to develop, it's important to include plenty of EFAs (essential fatty acids) in your daily diet. Nuts, seeds and their oils, leafy green vegetables, and limited portions of oily fish such as salmon or mackerel will provide you with everything you need.

● Iron is important: Your baby's liver is beginning to produce red blood cells, which require this mineral. Find it in lean red meat, fish, fortified bread and cereals, and beans and lentils. Folic acid, a B vitamin, is also particularly important during the first trimester. You can get it through supplements, as well as eating foods such as lentils, chickpeas, brown rice, wheatgerm, citrus fruits, and papaya.

● Foods to avoid include those high in vitamin A (such as liver), which can cause birth defects if eaten in large quantities.

Also avoid unpasteurized milk and cheeses, which present a risk of listeria.

● You don't need to "eat for two"—contrary to popular belief, you only need about an extra 350 calories a day when you're pregnant, and less in your first trimester.

● Try to commit to eating well, with a variety of foods providing key nutrients. Avoid justifying extra chocolate bars and other foods that are not "nutrient-dense" —they'll cause unhealthy weight gain and do nothing for your health.

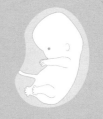

10 weeks

Your baby is now 1.2in (3.1cm) from crown to rump (the top of his head to the base of his spine), and he is becoming increasingly active. His size will triple in the next few weeks!

Now a fetus—and less vulnerable

Throughout your pregnancy, your baby will receive his nutrition and oxygen from your bloodstream, filtered through your placenta. Although the placenta is a wonderful screening device, things such as viruses and toxins in tobacco, alcohol, and drugs can pass through the barrier and affect your baby's health and development. This is of particular concern in the period before your placenta is fully functional (around 17 or 18 weeks); however, it is most important in the early stages of development, which occur between conception and 10 weeks. This is the time when your baby's organs, including his brain, heart, and nervous system, are developing, and the foundation for his growth is being laid down.

This week marks the point at which the first series of important developments in your baby ends, leaving him less vulnerable to environmental toxins that may harm him and lead to congenital defects. For many women it is an enormous relief to know that their babies are less susceptible now. That's not to say that exposure to toxins both now and throughout your pregnancy can't be harmful to your baby, but serious malformations are far less likely. This week, your baby becomes known as a "fetus" rather than an embryo. He will be known as a fetus until he is born.

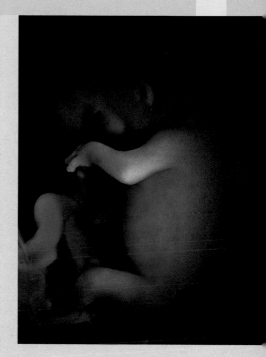

Early brain development

From just a few weeks after conception, your baby's brain will begin to grow and develop. This starts during the first three weeks, when the neural tube begins to form (see p.151), after which his three brain sections are formed: the forebrain, the middle brain, and the hind brain. By five weeks, his brain's "hemispheres" are formed and there is, unbelievably, some brain-wave activity. Just a week later, his brain formation is nearing completion.

By seven weeks, your baby's "hind brain," which is responsible for regulating his heartbeat, breathing, and muscle movements, starts up. At nine weeks, your baby's brain will be forming 250,000 neurons per minute!

By 18 or 19 weeks, your baby's brain forms millions of motor neurons, enabling him to develop and make voluntary muscle movements. The forebrain develops into the left and right hemispheres of the brain, and the nerve cells that he'll need for processing all of his senses are developing rapidly. Your baby's brain is capable of understanding complex sensory perceptions and distinguishing between different sounds just a few weeks later.

Around 24 weeks, your baby's brain can regulate all body functions. His spinal cord begins to harden and straighten, and his nervous system is more developed. By 28 to 29 weeks, your baby's brain can monitor breathing and regulate his body temperature, and it develops creases and fissures. As you enter the third trimester, your baby's brain will continue to develop, while establishing connections between the nerves. When your baby is born, his brain is only about a quarter of the size of an adult's, but perfectly formed and capable of life—and learning.

First ultrasound

Around this time you can expect to have your first ultrasound, which will offer you a priceless glimpse of your new baby. Known as your "dating ultrasound" or "dating scan" (see pp.114–115), it is designed to confirm your baby's expected delivery date, based on measurements taken by a sonographer. You should be able to see your baby's heartbeat, and his head, limbs, hands, feet, and some organs.

You may want to encourage your partner to accompany you to your first ultrasound; many couples find that it offers an invaluable opportunity for early bonding, as you see your baby for the first time. It also seems to make your pregnancy seem more real for both of you, and offers reassurance that all is progressing as it should.

You may also be offered a nuchal translucency screening (see p.116) to assess the risk of Down syndrome and other chromosomal abnormalities. Your doctor or midwife will fully explain this in advance, and you can choose not to have it done, if you wish.

Don't hesitate to go to your ultrasound appointment armed with questions; your sonographer will be in a good position to tell you how your baby is growing and developing. If anything you see on the monitor raises questions, ask. It's normal to feel nervous and anxious before your appointment, and emotional afterward.

INCREASED BLOOD VOLUME

From about six or eight weeks of pregnancy, the amount of blood in your circulatory system will increase dramatically. By 32 to 34 weeks, you will have some 50 percent more blood than you did before you were pregnant. The greatest increase is in the second trimester (see p.170); however, you will be creating more blood now, and there are two reasons for this. The first is that more blood is necessary for you to provide your baby with oxygen and nutrients, and to dispose of any waste products, such as carbon dioxide, that he produces. Secondly, it protects you if you lose a lot of blood during labor and delivery.

ME AND MY BODY

11 weeks

As a result of changing hormones, some women find that their hair and nails look stronger and healthier, while others experience a little hair loss around this time.

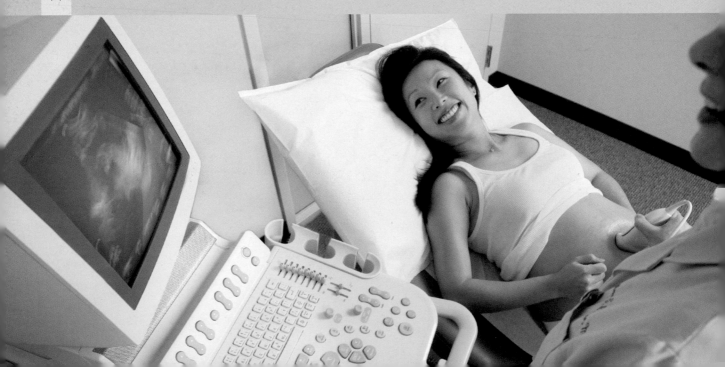

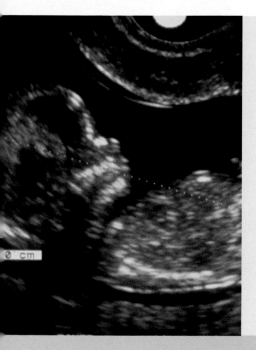

Early movements

Although it is too soon for you to feel his movements, your baby will be kicking, stretching, and moving comfortably in your uterus. He's surrounded and cushioned by amniotic fluid, so his movements are slow and gentle. At seven or eight weeks he will have started to bend sideways, and he will startle. A week or so later, he can hiccup, move his arms and legs on his own, and begin to suck and swallow. At 10 weeks, he'll begin to raise his arms, touch his face, and rotate his head. Some of his bones are beginning to harden, but this process won't be complete until much later in your pregnancy.

This week, your baby can begin to yawn, and you may be lucky enough to see this during your first ultrasound. In fact, ultrasound can show the range of your baby's movements, which are nothing short of miraculous. By just 10 weeks, he'll be capable of plenty of voluntary movements, including opening his jaw and moving his tongue, stretching, and reaching up with his hands. He'll have little spurts of exercise for several minutes, followed by periods of rest. No matter how active he is, he is buried far too deeply in your womb for you to feel anything yet, so try not to worry. Most women do not feel the first flutterings until after 16 weeks, and sometimes much later.

11 weeks

From the top of his head to the base of his spine, your baby is now around 1.6in (4cm) long, about the length of your thumb. He has toenails, fingernails, and 20 tooth buds in place.

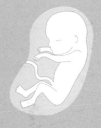

MY BABY

The umbilical cord

Your baby is attached to you via your umbilical cord, which runs from an opening in your baby's belly (known as the "umbilicus") to the placenta. It is about 20in (50cm) in length, and its main job is to transfer oxygen and food from your bloodstream, via the placenta, to your baby. It pulses with every beat of your baby's heart.

There are three channels in the umbilical cord. A vein carries oxygen-rich blood and nutrients from you to your baby, while two arteries return deoxygenated blood and waste products (such as carbon dioxide) from your baby back to your

placenta. The blood vessels are enclosed and protected by a sticky substance called "Wharton's jelly," and then a membrane known as "the amnion." As the pregnancy progresses, antibodies are also passed through the umbilical cord to your baby.

The umbilical cord is coiled like a spring, so your baby is free to move around. By nine weeks, the cord's pattern is usually established, and it coils in a counterclockwise direction. However, the cord can coil later, and sometimes isn't established until 20 weeks. Your baby's movements seem to encourage the umbilical cord to coil.

CLAMPING THE CORD
Your baby will remain attached to your umbilical cord until he draws his first breath, and the fetal blood it contains returns to his body. At this point, the cord will stop pulsating, and can be cut. There are no nerves within the cord, so cutting it after delivery is painless. There is some debate about whether to cut the cord very soon—one minute or so—after delivery, or whether to wait for up to 20 minutes. Some experts believe that delaying the cord cutting may be beneficial to your baby, because the blood that returns to him contains more red blood cells.

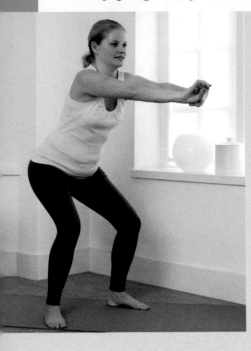

Getting more oxygen

During pregnancy, more oxygen is required in order to meet both your needs and those of your baby. In order to accommodate this, the hormone progesterone directly affects your lungs to encourage faster and deeper breathing, to exhale more, and keep carbon-dioxide levels low. Early in pregnancy, your chest will begin to expand, allowing an increase in your lung capacity (the amount of air your lungs can take in with each breath). However, as your uterus grows it pushes up against your diaphragm—the broad, flat muscle that lies under your lungs—which slowly decreases lung capacity. This may seem alarming, but progesterone ensures that you are breathing deeply enough to take in more air. Both you and your baby will be getting plenty of oxygen through your enhanced circulatory system, which carries more oxygen-rich blood.

You may, however, experience some breathlessness and lightheadedness. Gentle aerobic exercise can help; it will lower your pulse rate, which means your heart doesn't have to work as hard to pump the extra blood. Good posture will also help you breathe better. In the final weeks of the third trimester, your baby will "drop" down into your pelvis in preparation for labor, and you will find it easier to breathe.

How your uterus changes during pregnancy

The uterus is created from smooth muscle, lined with glands, and designed both to stretch to accommodate your growing baby, and to contract during labor to deliver her. At the time of conception, your uterus will be the size of a plum, but by 12 weeks will expand above your pubic bone, where you may be able to feel it. Your uterus begins to soften around six weeks, changing position, increasing in size, and ascending into your abdomen by your fourth month. As your baby grows, it will move upward and outward, so that by the time you reach the end of the second trimester (about 27 weeks), the top of your uterus will be near your ribcage. At full term, your uterus will have expanded well into your ribcage—about 5-7in (13-18cm) above your belly button. It's now 1,000 times its initial capacity, and 20 times its original weight, with more muscle, connective and elastic tissue, blood vessels, and nerves.

The shape of your uterus will also change, moving from elongated to oval by the second month, creating a gentle protrusion. By mid-pregnancy, it will become round and then back through oval to elongated at 38 weeks, which is when growth tends to peak. As your baby's birth approaches, your uterus will drop a little into the pelvic cavity, in a process known as "lightening."

As it expands, your uterus walls become thinner and, from the end of the second trimester, begin to contract—known as "Braxton Hicks" contractions. You won't actually feel them until much later in your pregnancy (see p.216). Your doctor will use the height of your uterus to check your baby's growth (see p.200); this is known as the "fundal height."

(see p.216) ... (see p.200)

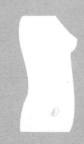

ME AND MY BODY

12 weeks

The risk of miscarriage reduces dramatically this week. If you haven't done so already, now is a good time to share your news. In most cases, nausea and fatigue will begin to wane.

Ear development

Your baby's ears begin forming as early as six weeks after conception, with the development of a few small bulges known as "bronchial arches" and passageways that will eventually form the inner ear. By the second month of pregnancy, your baby's ears will be developing in the correct position on the side of his head, and appear as little folds of skin. His inner ear will still be developing.

At 19 weeks, your baby's ears will begin to stand out on the sides of his head, and the bones within the inner ear are completely formed. The nerve endings from your baby's brain are effectively "wired" to his ears, and he will be able to hear your heart beating, your tummy rumbling, and blood moving through your umbilical cord. Some experts believe he may be able to hear earlier than this, possibly from 16 weeks. There is plenty of research to suggest that he will even startle when he hears loud noises outside the womb, although he is still heavily cushioned in amniotic fluid and many of the sounds outside your body will elude him.

Between 26 and 28 weeks, the nerves in your baby's ears are almost fully developed, and he will react to familiar voices outside the womb. He may react to sounds he recognizes, including the theme song from your favorite TV show. A little fine-tuning will continue until he is born, but the vast majority of babies are born with full hearing.

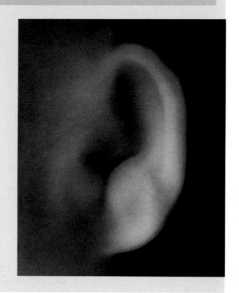

Head start

The size of your baby's head may surprise you when you see it for the first time on your ultrasound. At about 13 weeks, your baby's head is very large in comparison to his body; in fact, it is half the size of his body, when measured from the top of his head to his buttocks. At this stage, his brain is still rapidly developing its various functions that will soon be directing his body's activities.

By around 20 to 21 weeks, his head will be about one third of the size of his body, which is swiftly catching up with the growth of his head. When your baby is born, his head will be about a quarter of the size of his body, which is still large in relation to his body when we consider it in adult terms. A baby's brain will continue to grow and develop into late childhood.

The size of your baby's head is only relevant when it falls outside the norm (which can indicate problems with his development) or when it is very large in relation to the size of your pelvis (which can make a vaginal birth difficult). Your baby's head will be measured during your dating scan, and later on in your anatomy scan, and any concerns will be addressed at that time.

> "At about 13 weeks, your baby's head is very large in comparison to his body"

12 weeks

Your baby is continuing to grow, and will now weigh more than half an ounce (around 14g)! His reflexes are developing, and he may respond when you press firmly on your tummy.

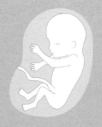

MY BABY

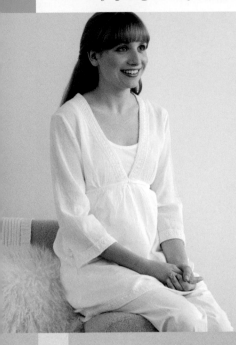

Feeling great

The end of the first trimester marks a distinct turning point as your hormones begin to settle down (in particular, hCG, which appears to be responsible for the most unpleasant symptoms, such as nausea and vomiting) and your energy levels improve. This is a perfect time to re-introduce or start a regular exercise routine, to prepare your body for labor and birth, and to encourage overall good health and well-being throughout the remainder of your pregnancy. In fact, some experts suggest that anything other than very gentle exercise should be avoided for the first trimester, as energy is better off being diverted to the important early developmental stages of your baby. So if you have been too exhausted to get going before now, you are off the hook.

You are likely to feel much more positive emotionally, since the risk of complications and miscarriage are significantly reduced and you can now begin to enjoy the prospect of becoming a mom. You may even find that your libido improves (see p.180), and that you feel more confident about your changing body. Many women begin to show around this time and will enjoy exhibiting their new bump. While it is important to make the most of your new energy, you'll also need to take time to rest and adapt to your body's demands.

ME AND MY BODY

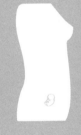

13 weeks

Progesterone may have a positive impact on your skin and hair, and you may be developing a pregnancy "glow." Your breasts may even begin making colostrum, or "early milk."

How amniotic fluid nurtures your baby

The liquid that surrounds your baby is known as "amniotic fluid," which is clear and yellowish. As your pregnancy progresses, more fluid is created—first by tissues in your uterus, and then, from about 12 weeks, your baby's urine. Amniotic fluid levels increase steadily throughout most of your pregnancy, slowing down in the final 10 weeks before birth, peaking at about 34 to 36 weeks, and then declining until the birth.

At its peak, there is roughly 27-34 fl oz (800-1,000ml) of amniotic fluid surrounding your baby. This fluid (also known as your "water") circulates constantly. Until about 14 weeks, the amniotic fluid is absorbed through your baby's skin. After this, as the kidneys start to work, he swallows the fluid and then releases it in his urine, encouraging gut development.

Amniotic fluid plays a number of roles, including helping your baby to move in the womb, which encourages optimal bone growth and muscle development; developing your baby's lungs as he "practice breathes" the fluid; keeping his temperature constant, as if he were in a custom-built incubator; and protecting him from outside injury. At each stage of pregnancy, there is a range of volumes that are considered "normal." Too much amniotic fluid is known as "polyhydramnios." This is common in cases of multiple pregnancy, gestational diabetes, and the presence of congenital defects.

Very low levels of amniotic fluid are known as "oligohydramnios," which can occur in late pregnancy, when membranes rupture or your placenta malfunctions, and also in the case of fetal abnormalities. Fluid levels can be detected mainly through ultrasound, and if there is any suggestion of a problem, you will be carefully monitored.

Using hands

By 13 weeks, your baby will have learned to use his hands, reaching up to put them by his face and possibly even managing to get his thumb into his mouth. He's too young for sucking, though. Although it isn't clear when the sucking reflex develops—some babies begin around 14 or 15 weeks, while others are much later—there are a number of studies showing that babies do find comfort sucking their thumbs in the womb from around four months.

At around 25 or 26 weeks, your baby's hands will be fully developed, although some of the nerve connections that allow him to have full control of them will continue to mature for many weeks to come. By this stage, however, he will have impressive dexterity—making a fist and clasping objects in his palms. He will use his hands to explore his environment, not only entertaining himself, but also stimulating his tactile development. Twins will begin to touch one another and begin the process of early bonding, reaching out to stroke one another's faces, and grabbing at the other's hands and feet.

Your baby has fingernails in place, and his own unique set of fingerprints are being laid down. By 20 weeks, his skin will develop four layers that contain the ridges for his fingerprints and the lines on his palms and the soles of his feet.

> "Studies show that babies find comfort sucking their thumbs in the womb from around four months"

13 weeks

Curled up in the womb, your baby is the size of a peach, and covered with fine fuzz, too. His sucking reflexes are not yet fully developed, but he may get his thumb in his mouth.

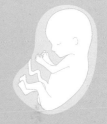

MY BABY

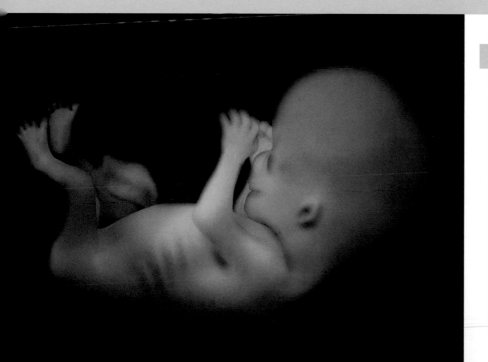

Ready to reproduce

Although your baby is still tiny—just 2in (5.5cm) from crown to rump— his or her reproductive organs are already in place. Baby girls will already have nearly two million eggs in their ovaries, and this number will increase to six or seven million by the time you are 20 weeks pregnant. After this, the eggs gradually waste away, leaving about one to two million eggs in her ovaries at birth. When she hits puberty, she will have about 300,000 eggs, which is more than enough for a lifetime of fertility. The external genitalia of both boys and girls are developing at this time, and will be complete around 20 weeks.

The second trimester

The second trimester is often called the "planning trimester," and for good reason. You may experience a period of renewed energy and greater comfort, allowing you to get on with the business of preparing for your new arrival.

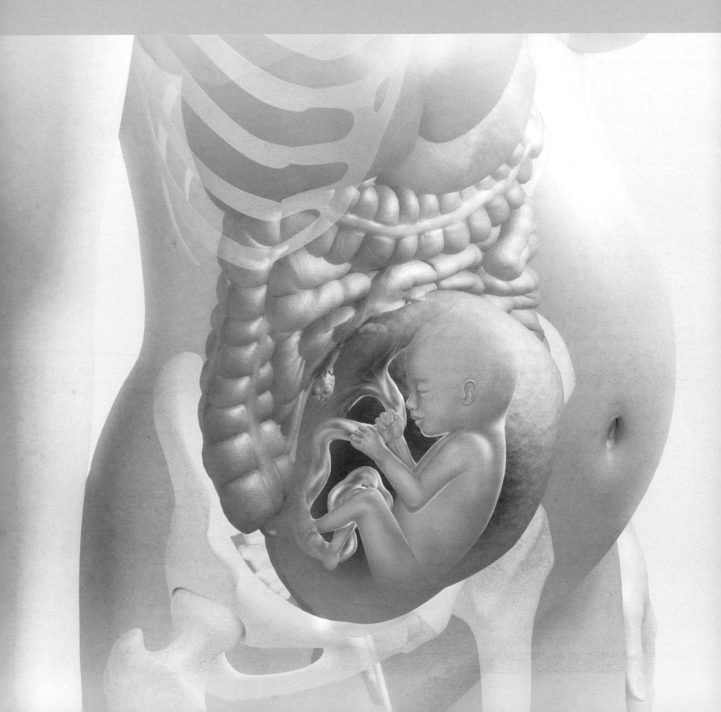

"With much of her development complete, your baby will grow at a tremendous rate, and it won't be long before you feel those first flutterings"

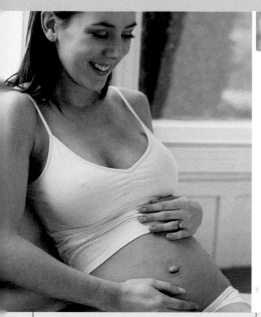

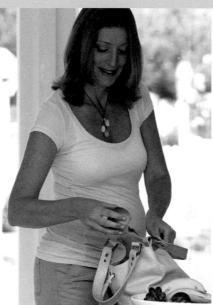

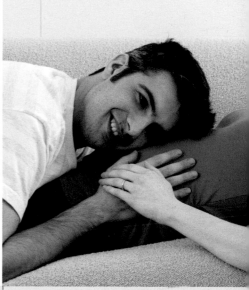

EARLY BONDING
As you begin to feel your baby's movements, you can begin the process of bonding, talking to her and stroking your belly.

KEEP YOUR ENERGY UP
Your baby's dramatic growth can make you hungrier than usual. Choose healthy snacks to keep your blood-sugar levels stable.

PARENTS-TO-BE
Sharing the excitement of those first movements with your partner will help him feel involved.

BEGINNING TO SHOW
As your baby grows, your uterus will enlarge and move up and outward. Combined with normal pregnancy weight gain, you will undoubtedly look pregnant.

Your second trimester of pregnancy runs between 14 and 27 weeks, and often coincides with the relief of pregnancy symptoms as your hormones begin to settle down. Take advantage of this time to get organized for the birth, and to be as active as you can. Not only will regular exercise release hormones that encourage a sense of well-being, but you'll also be better prepared for the birth itself.

Your baby will have been busy growing, developing, and, amazingly, playing in the womb for some time now, but her tiny size means that you are unlikely to have felt her. All this is about to change, and you can expect to feel those first movements somewhere between 16 and 20 weeks. Your baby may begin to seem more "real" to you during this trimester as she makes her presence known, and you will get a glimpse of her during your ultrasound around 20 weeks.

You may experience that famous pregnancy "glow" due to the increase in blood supply to your skin and hair. As your baby grows, your uterus expands from just below your hip bones to about 2.8in (7cm) above your belly button.

ME AND MY BODY

14 weeks

Some women find this the easiest stage of pregnancy. You may sleep more soundly, feel far less nausea, have more energy, and experience a deeper emotional connection with your baby.

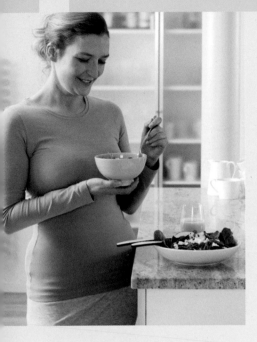

Increasing your iron intake

As your body continues to produce more blood to provide your baby (and you) with the oxygen and nutrients you need, your iron intake has to increase dramatically. Some experts suggest that pregnant women require almost double the iron they needed before they were pregnant, which means ensuring that your diet is high in iron-rich foods. Good sources include meat, leafy green vegetables, whole grains, and fortified cereals and drinks. Your body will absorb the iron in these foods more efficiently if they are eaten in conjunction with a little vitamin C. You can take this in the form of a supplement, or have some fresh fruit with your meals. It's also a good idea to avoid drinking tea at mealtimes because it contains tannin, a substance that inhibits the uptake of iron in the body.

If you don't have more energy now, and still feel unusually tired, it's worth discussing this with your doctor, who can arrange to have your blood tested for anemia (see p.113). Along with fatigue, you may notice that the red tissue around the insides of your eyelids is paler than usual—as are you. A supplement can be prescribed, if necessary, although these can have side effects, such as constipation.

How your skin may change during pregnancy

As your hormones shift throughout pregnancy, you can experience changes in the pigmentation of your skin. In particular, an increase in estrogen and melanocyte-stimulating hormone (MSH) can cause your skin to darken and make your veins more prominent. What's more, as your skin stretches across your growing bump and enlarging breasts, the tissue becomes stretched or "striated," leading to red, welt-like stripes that will eventually fade to silver. These stretch marks seem to be partly genetic and partly to do with how quickly you gain weight, but 75 to 90 percent of pregnant women will be affected. Minimize them by eating a diet rich in vitamins B and C, zinc, and silica to keep your skin healthy.

COMMON CHANGES
Different women experience different degrees of changes, but the following are normal: darkening of moles, nipples, and the pubic area; a linea nigra (a dark line on the abdomen, running down from the belly button); stretch marks on your abdomen, breasts, and even upper thighs, hips, and lower back; spider veins on your face; brown patches on your face (known as melasma); skin tags (harmless little growths of skin); varicose veins; and a worsening of acne or rosacea. It's also normal to experience mild rashes and itching; however, if itching is intense (particularly if there is no rash), or symptoms are uncomfortable or worrying, see your doctor.

The good news is that the hormones causing many of the oddities also give you that dewy, fresh appearance thanks to the increase in blood supply during pregnancy. However, remember that your skin is more sensitive during pregnancy, so take care of it (see pp.76-78).

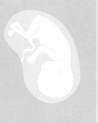

14 weeks

From crown to rump, your baby is now about 3in (8cm) long and 1.4oz (40g). Her eyes are closer together, and her reflexes are starting to develop, preparing her for life outside the womb.

Reacting to light

One of the most dramatic developments around this week is your baby's new ability to sense light. Although her eyes are still fused shut—and will remain so until as late as 30 weeks—she will react to bright light held close to your abdomen. One study found that at 16 weeks, when a blinking light was shone on the abdomens of pregnant women, the heartbeats of their babies responded.

While your baby is still very small and well cushioned deep in your uterus, she is unlikely to respond to many changes in light outside the womb. However, as she grows and your uterine walls become thinner, light will penetrate and she will respond increasingly. Some women report that their babies wriggle and kick more frequently when they sunbathe in later pregnancy.

A SENSE OF TASTE

Your baby starts to develop a sense of taste at around seven weeks when her taste buds begin to form. Between 13 and 15 weeks, your baby's taste buds are almost as mature as an adult's. Research has found that your amniotic fluid can smell strongly of foods that you commonly eat—in particular, strong spices, onions, and garlic. While we do not know whether babies can actually taste these flavors while in the womb, there is some evidence that they will prefer those flavors they have been exposed to after they are born. Many of the same flavors will also come through in your breast milk, making them instantly familiar to your newborn; what's more, when weaning time comes around, they may enjoy more tastes than you expect.

After birth, your baby will show an initial preference for sweet flavors, which is nature's way of priming her to enjoy the sweet taste of breast milk. As for other tastes, newborns typically dislike sour tastes and salty flavors until around four months of age.

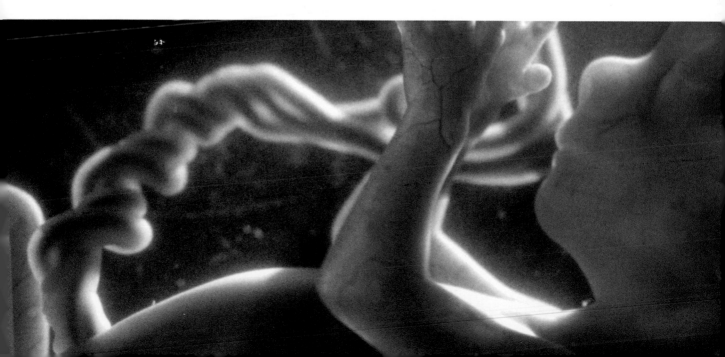

Exercise with care

One of the hormones released during pregnancy is known as "relaxin," which helps the birth process by softening and lengthening the cervix and pubic symphysis (the point at which the pubic bones meet).

Relaxin inhibits uterus contractions, and is believed to play a role in the process that kick-starts labor. It works by cutting down the production of collagen (the main component of connective tissue found in cartilage, tendons, and ligaments) and increasing its water content, which makes its fibers bigger and more elastic.

Relaxin is produced in the early stages of pregnancy by the corpus luteum (see p.30), and then, from around 12 weeks, the placenta. It is released in large quantities in your first trimester, after which it reduces a little and continues to be produced until your baby's birth.

When the ligaments become more elastic, they feel looser and they are more prone to damage. In particular, the ligaments in the groin, holding together the pubic symphysis, can widen and cause enormous discomfort. For this reason, it is very important that women exercise carefully during pregnancy—taking care not to push themselves too far when stretching or performing maneuvers that push the legs too far apart, such as lunges. It's equally important to avoid activities that put pressure on your lower back and pelvis, such as walking very long distances, climbing stairs, and standing for extended periods of time.

Although the joints most affected are those in your pelvic area and lower back, your entire body is subject to the effects of relaxin, which results in abnormal motion that can lead to pain and inflammation. Strengthening your back muscles can help prevent injury and discomfort by providing more support for the ligaments around the joints, but you'll need to exercise with the help of a professional who is accustomed to working with pregnant women. Resting frequently throughout the day and adopting good posture can also help.

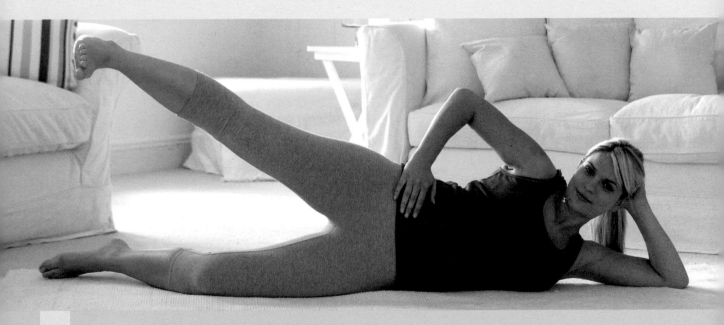

15 weeks

If you haven't yet begun to show, it's very likely to happen in the next week or so. Your uterus will have risen to just below the height of your hipbones, and is expanding outward.

Phase of rapid growth

Your baby is due for a growth spurt over the next few weeks, in which she will literally double in weight, and become centimeters longer. In turn, you may notice that your abdomen will expand quite dramatically as your uterus stretches upward and outward to accommodate her. Her sudden growth will require a surge of blood supply to your uterus, which, by the end of your pregnancy, will be receiving about one-fifth of your pre-pregnancy supply. Your baby will need extra oxygen and nutrients over this period of growth, and you may find that you are more tired than usual as your body struggles to keep up with the demand. Now, more than ever, it is important to ensure that you are getting plenty of iron-rich foods (see p.49), and lots of fluids.

WHERE DOES THE BLOOD GO?

Your blood will enter your baby's body through the vein in her umbilical cord. It travels to her liver and then splits into three branches, where it reaches a major vein connected to her heart. From here, it travels to your baby's head and upper extremities, and after circulating there, returns to the right atrium of her heart.

The moment your baby begins to breathe, her circulation changes completely, and blood is sent to her lungs to pick up oxygen.

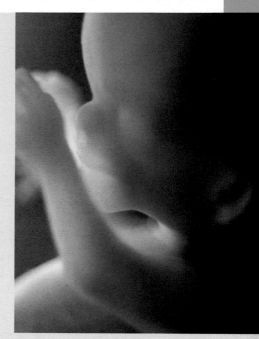

How my baby's bones develop

Early in pregnancy, the basic structure for your baby's bones is laid down as cartilage (a fibrous, somewhat rubbery substance) and connective tissue. The development of your baby's rudimentary skeleton is complete at around 14 or 15 weeks, after which the process of "ossification" begins. This literally means the gradual transition of your baby's skeletal bones from cartilage to hard bone. This process is normally complete by about 31 or 32 weeks of pregnancy, but her bones will continue to grow for the remainder of your pregnancy—and until she reaches adulthood. These bones are visible during ultrasounds, so skeletal-system problems can often be determined before birth.

STAYING FLEXIBLE

At birth, your baby has approximately 300 bones, which will eventually fuse and grow together to create 206 bones. Some of these early bones remain largely cartilage, which is flexible and protects her from fractures as she crawls and walks. The bones in your baby's skull contain soft spots, or "fontanelles," in two places, to allow the soft plates of her head to flex in the birth canal. The fontanelle at the rear of her head closes around four months; the one on the top of her head closes between nine and eighteen months. Space in her skull also allows for brain growth in the third trimester and infancy.

For ossification to be effective, you'll need plenty of calcium-rich foods in your diet (see p.49), as well as vitamin D. Getting plenty of sunshine can help with the latter; one study found that expectant moms who spent plenty of time outdoors had babies with stronger bones.

15 weeks

Your baby will begin to produce lanugo, a fine hair that will cover her body until just before birth. She may also begin to practice breathing, which can also involve getting the hiccups!

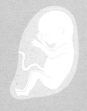

MY BABY

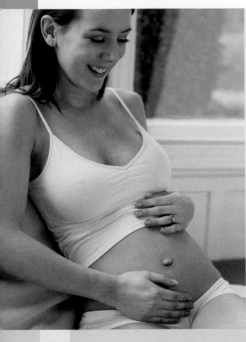

Feeling my baby move

Your baby has been active for several weeks now, but as she continues to grow during your pregnancy she will begin to take up more space in your uterus, the walls of which become increasingly thinner. Around this time, it is possible to feel her first movements, known as "quickening." Seasoned moms may recognize these flutterings earlier, while first-time mothers may dismiss them as gas or one of the other mysterious sensations that pregnancy can bring. Some women don't feel them until around 26 weeks of pregnancy.

The sensation differs between women; some moms report feeling something like a goldfish flipping around inside, while others feel a gentle fluttering or a tapping sensation. There may be bursts of activity followed by long periods when you'll feel nothing. You may also experience the sensation erratically, depending upon your baby's position in the womb. It's possible to go several days without feeling anything, but there are ways to stir her into action (see pp.208–209).

It won't be possible for your partner to experience these movements yet, even with his ear to your tummy, but it won't be long before she is kicking, punching, and pressing her elbows outward—all of which can be both felt and seen.

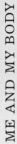

16 weeks

You will probably be feeling uncomfortable in fitted clothing, and need to start thinking about maternity wear. Your enlarged uterus may put some strain on your lower back.

Bonding with my unborn baby

Every time you think or talk about your baby, you are increasing your bond; whether you are discussing baby names or listing questions to ask your doctor, you are bringing your baby to mind.

There are direct ways to increase your connection with your baby: When you rub your bump or sing and speak to her, for example, you are soothing her and letting her know you are there. Your baby can communicate with you, too, once her kicks are strong enough for you to feel.

We know that babies respond to their mother's anxiety, stress, and anger with an increased heartbeat, and that they relax when mom is calm. Actively taking time to create a peaceful environment in which you can communicate with your baby can not only help to nurture her emotionally, but bring you closer.

MORE WAYS TO BOND
Tune into your baby's patterns of stillness and movement to intensify your bond; speak softly when she is quiet, and sing lively songs when she is more alert. If you have a picture from your first ultrasound, keep it posted somewhere to remind you of the little person growing inside you. Write her a letter; sometimes putting feelings into words can help make them more vivid. You'll also have a special document to present to her when she is a little older. Most importantly, enjoy your baby! You are planting the seeds of a relationship that will blossom throughout your lifetime.

Research suggests that bonding during pregnancy can help prevent postpartum depression, and encourage a strong, early relationship with your baby. Your partner can also begin bonding with your baby by talking to her—as close to your tummy as possible at this stage—and by stroking your bump.

How much can she hear?

There is still considerable debate about when your baby will be able to hear sounds from outside the womb. Many parents and experts report that babies not only hear loud sounds, such as music and shouting, but even respond to them with distinct movements. We do know that the tiny bones in your baby's ears are in place this week, and that she is capable of hearing sounds within the womb, which is alive with the sound of your heartbeat, blood flow, and digestion. This is one reason that babies are soothed by "white noise" during infancy;

it mimics the sounds they lived with during their cozy confinement in the womb. Various studies have found that it's not only newborns who enjoy this noise; in fact, people of all ages experience white noise as stress-reducing and find it can help them sleep. You can buy recordings of white noise if you'd like to use this to calm your baby after birth.

A study in Ireland, using ultrasound observation and measured pulses of sound, revealed that babies with normal hearing start moving in reaction to sound at around 16 weeks. This was earlier than previous estimates and occurs about two months before completion of the ear (around 24 to

26 weeks). Babies seem to respond particularly to their parents' voices—so it is very likely that your baby can hear your voice, and possibly that of anyone pressed close to your abdomen. You may notice that she startles (with a series of flutters) when there is a loud noise. Some babies may also be more sensitive to loud noises than others. It's worth remembering that at this point your baby is surrounded by fluid, and her ears are often full of the protective greasy coating that covers her skin (vernix), so even very loud noises would be muffled by the time they reach her ears.

Start singing and talking to your baby now, and see how she responds. You may be surprised!

16 weeks

Your baby's backbone and back muscles are strong enough for her to straighten her neck and lift her head even farther. She weighs 3.5oz (100g) and is about the size of a large avocado.

MY BABY

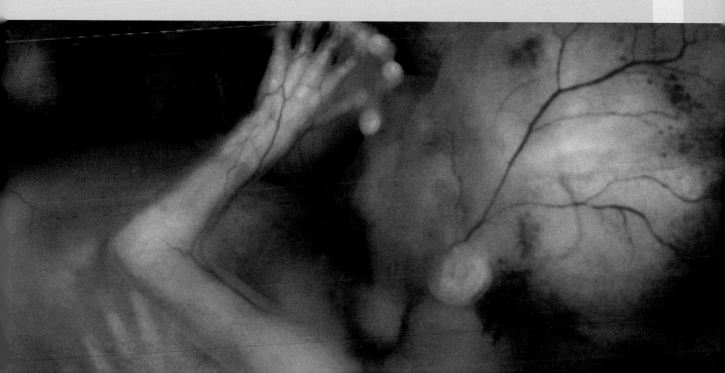

ME AND MY BODY

17 weeks

Your veins will be more prominent because of the extra blood in your body, and this may also cause nosebleeds. A nice side effect of this extra blood is glowing skin and lustrous hair.

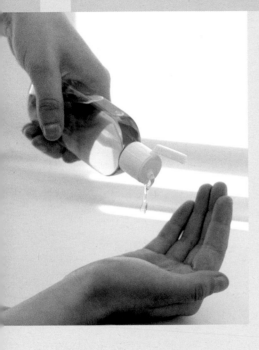

Prone to illness

One effect of pregnancy is reduced immunity, which can leave you susceptible to viruses and bacteria. The changes to your immune system are, in fact, designed to protect you and your baby. Some parts of your immune system are enhanced; others are suppressed. This creates a balance that prevents your body from building up antibodies against your baby (your body could perceive her as a foreign body), while preventing infection in her, without compromising the defenses. This does, however, leave you open to opportunistic infections and viruses, and you may find that you suffer from a series of colds.

Hormonal changes can also leave you open to infections—particularly in the urinary tract, which is relaxed by progesterone then compressed by your enlarging uterus, increasing the risk of urinary tract infection. Yeast infection can also be a result of increased estrogen in your reproductive tract.

The best advice is to get plenty of rest and eat healthy foods—particularly those rich in vitamin C, which is known to build immunity. Washing your hands religiously, including before and after you use the bathroom, and using anti-bacterial gel can help keep germs at bay.

If you are having amniocentesis, this test will take place between now and 20 weeks (see pp.118–119 for information).

Why we decided to have amniocentesis

My first son has a disability, so it was recommended that I have amniocentesis with my second child. It was a difficult decision given the risk of losing the baby, but I felt I needed to have all the information I could about what might lie ahead. CH

One of my moms took up the offer of amniocentesis when she was pregnant with her third baby. She was 40, and just wanted to rule out the risk of abnormalities. As it turned out, her baby was diagnosed with Down syndrome. She and her husband were both very shocked;

they had genuinely not anticipated the result; however, they were able to get plenty of counseling in order to make the decision that was right for them. NK

I had amniocentesis during my third pregnancy, after I received abnormal results on a screening test. While there was still a very good chance that my baby would be normal, the test put him at a greater-than-usual risk of a serious chromosomal abnormality. Given my medical background—and belief that it's much better (and safer) to know about any potential problems with the fetus

(regardless of your personal beliefs as to what to do about it)—my husband and I decided to have the amnio. The procedure itself wasn't fun, partly because I wasn't numbed where the needle went in and partly because I took the "full bladder" directive so seriously that I was pretty uncomfortable. Neither was waiting more than a week to get the results back. Most parents don't realize that results from an amnio involve a cell culture, which takes a long time to grow! Fortunately, in the end, the amnio came back normal and, on the upside, we found out definitively that we were having a boy. LJ

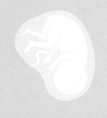

17 weeks

Your baby's size is now about the width of your outstretched hand. Fat is beginning to form across her body, which helps keep your baby warm, and encourages her metabolism.

Boy or girl?

Wondering about the sex of your baby is probably a regular pastime, and all is about to be revealed, if you wish! From around 16 weeks and depending on your baby's position, a very experienced sonographer may be able to determine your baby's gender; final changes to her external genitalia are nearly complete.

At about six or seven weeks, the site of your baby's genitals is a small bud, known as the "genital tubercle." Until nine or ten weeks, reproductive structures are the same for both boys and girls. Male genitalia are dependent upon a chemical produced in the testes, which causes the tubercle to elongate and grow to form a

penis. At this stage of development, a baby boy's testicles are located in his abdomen, and will not descend until the seventh or eighth month of pregnancy.

The development of a baby girl's genitals is promoted by estrogen and other hormones. This time, the tubercle grows to become the clitoris, with folds around it forming the labia. It is possible to determine sex between 13 and 16 weeks, but often the genitals are too small to be seen; by 20 weeks, your baby's size should allow identification. 3D scans can make this process easier.

Your baby's sweat glands are now developing, as well as her fingerprints, and her eyes are now in a more forward-facing position.

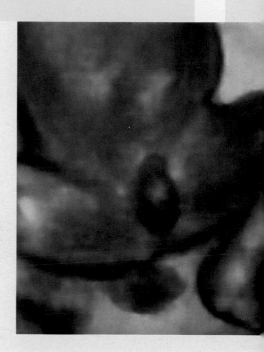

The process of myelination

Myelin is a white, fatty protective coating, made of elements of proteins and fats that coat your baby's nerves, rather like the insulation on an electrical cord. Around 16 weeks, the process of "myelination" begins, as the nerve fibers around your baby's nervous system are lined with a coating of myelin to protect and insulate the neurons they contain.

Myelin helps to encourage the transmission of nerve impulses, which carry information from one nerve cell to the next. The brain is made up of gray matter (neurons) and white matter (nerve fibers and their insulating material).

Researchers have found that the process of myelination (in the white matter) may play a role in the development of talent! When we use our brains, the connections between nerves are established. Using these connections repeatedly (by thinking, reading, adding, and using our motor skills, for example) triggers special cells that wrap layer upon layer of myelin around them—optimizing their efficiency.

STRONG CONNECTIONS
Our ability to grow stronger and newer connections takes place in early life, which is one reason why it is important to

stimulate your baby and encourage her to practice and develop new skills in the early years. While myelination begins in the womb, it continues throughout life in a "use it or lose it" capacity.

A healthy diet helps to ensure that your body has the nutrients it needs for myelination. Smoking during pregnancy can affect the formation and action of myelin, causing problems such as attention deficit hyperactivity disorder (ADHD), depression, and autism. When myelin is damaged, a variety of health problems can result, including multiple sclerosis (an auto-immune condition).

I'm showing!

Although some women—particularly those who are pregnant with their second or third baby, or carrying twins or other multiples—begin to "show" as early as 10 to 12 weeks, the majority of first-time moms do not look obviously pregnant until they are into the second trimester. By now, however, you will have noticed that your "bump" is not just obvious, but definitely protruding.

At this stage, your uterus is about the size of a large cantaloupe, and it has expanded up to just below your belly button, and will be nicely rounded out in front. In the coming weeks, your belly button is likely to "pop" or stick out a bit; it will return to its usual shape within a few weeks of your baby's birth.

As well as a growing baby—and uterus—it is normal to be very hungry, and to put on some weight. By now, you may have gained about 9lbs (4kg) or even a little more, which is considered to be a healthy level to sustain your baby's growth. If you are concerned about your weight, don't attempt to diet. Choosing fresh, healthy foods and giving up any junk food (no matter what your cravings) and refined or processed foods may be all it takes to keep your weight in check. Pregnancy places enormous demands upon every system in your body, and you will need all the good, nutritious foods you can eat for a healthy pregnancy.

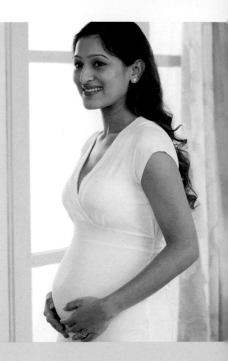

ME AND MY BODY

18 weeks

Your heart is working about 50 percent harder than it did before you were pregnant, to cope with the extra blood in your system. A little regular exercise can make it stronger.

Reactions to our growing bumps

By this stage I had a very obvious bump. I did have some suspicious looks—my colleagues were interested and desperate to ask, but did not dare in case I had just put on weight! There was lots of mumbling, and then obvious relief when I disclosed the truth. I felt I did get much more care and attention, which sometimes was a bit patronizing. I did not want to be treated as someone with an illness. It's important to let others know how you feel; it can be intimidating for people who are not familiar with pregnancy to try and behave normally toward a pregnant woman. MG

Once my bump showed, people were much more attentive and considerate. Also, there were constantly people wanting to touch or pat my bump, which I found surprising at first. CH

I barely looked pregnant until my third trimester—especially during my first pregnancy—and even then I could hide it with a big sweatshirt. So unless I told them, most people didn't know. This was frustrating, as I was excited to be pregnant and most people didn't notice! On the other hand, some family members treated me differently, and wanted me to

be excessively and unnecessarily careful as I went about my normal life. LJ

I don't think people treated me differently until my pregnancy was very obvious, around 34 weeks. I didn't enjoy strangers talking to me about my pregnancy—I found it very intrusive. FF

A very senior midwife at work looked at me intensely when I was about seven weeks and said, "You're pregnant, aren't you?" That's experience for you! She looked out for me when I was on duty, and it was our secret for a while. VB

Accumulating essential fat

Although you are nearly halfway through your pregnancy, your baby is still only a fraction of her birthweight and will look very thin when seen on an ultrasound. This is all about to change! From around 18 weeks, your baby will begin to gain about 1 to 2oz (50–60g) per week, as she lays down muscle, ligament, and fat in preparation for life in the outside world. The fat that begins to cover her body will account for much of her weight gain from this point onward, particularly during the third trimester.

Fat is actually very important for your baby, not just because it keeps her warm and provides a protective covering between her muscles and her skin, but because fat stores will provide her with the energy she needs to sustain her growth until she is born. It's worth noting that your own weight gain serves a similar purpose; laying down fat at this stage of your pregnancy will give you the reserves of energy you need to provide your baby with what she needs. Fat is initially laid down around the nape of her neck and her breastbone, before spreading downward across her torso, and then her limbs. Fat is also important for the development of your baby's nerves and brain. Every nerve cell

in your baby's body is covered with a layer of fat and protein (myelin, which is approximately 80 percent fat and 20 percent protein; see p.177) that serves to insulate it from nearby nerves and improve the connection between the different nerve cells.

It is important to ensure that you have adequate levels of healthy fats in your diet. A little saturated fat is fine (see pp.50–51), but go for healthier options, such as nuts, seeds, avocados, olives, high-quality dairy products, and lean meats and poultry. Boost your intake of essential fatty acids (EFAs; see p.51), by eating one or two portions of oily fish, such as salmon and mackerel, or a couple of handfuls of nuts and seeds, each week.

18 weeks

For the very first time, your baby is now a little larger than her placenta, and she will continue to outgrow it as she moves toward her birth. She is now the size of a medium carrot!

MY BABY

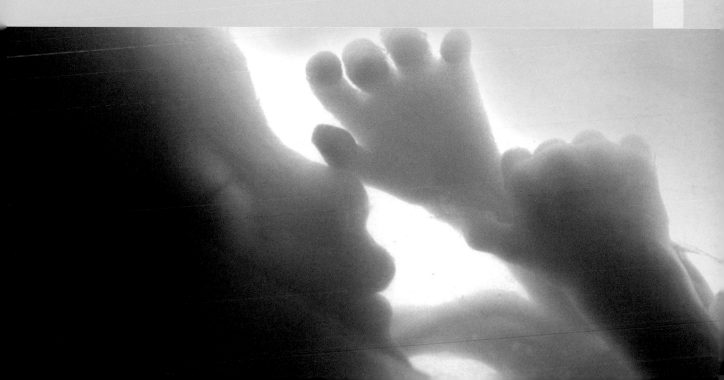

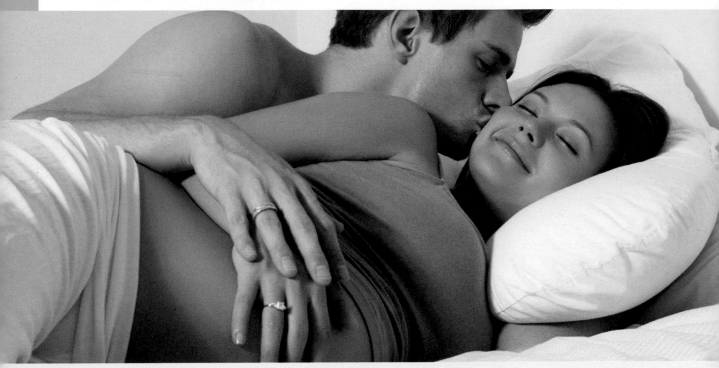

More energy— and libido!

Many women report feeling much more energetic by 19 weeks, as many early pregnancy symptoms have abated, and you are likely to be getting more sleep. Take advantage of your heightened energy levels to get organized for the birth. Your second trimester is a great time to start making extra meals that can be frozen for use when your baby is born. You may be able to fit in some more exercise, such as yoga or swimming, which will prepare you for the birth and increase your chances of a shorter labor.

It's not uncommon to experience a renewed interest in sex around this time. Higher levels of estrogen and progesterone can make you want to be intimate, while increased vaginal lubrication and blood flow to the pelvic area and greater sensitivity in your breasts can send your sex drive soaring.

You may need to prepare your partner for your heightened libido, since he may be nervous of making love when you are pregnant. Reassure him that sex will not hurt your baby, and that you can adopt a number of comfortable positions. Some pregnant women experience no sexual desire at all, and this, too, is normal. Being close, hugging, and cuddling may be enough for both of you.

Do check with your doctor if you have experienced late miscarriages in the past, have a history of cervical weakness, or are experiencing "placenta previa" (see p.386). Sometimes penetrative lovemaking needs to be avoided. Don't be surprised if your baby moves around a lot after orgasm; it's simply due to the increased blood supply to your pelvis, and your higher heart rate.

ME AND MY BODY

19 weeks

Your belly will continue to expand, shifting your center of gravity and making you feel clumsier than usual. It's normal to have gained up to 15lbs (7kg) or even more at this point.

From buds to lungs

At about four or five weeks of pregnancy, tiny buds appear in your baby's chest, and quickly develop airways known as "bronchi." Two air sacs form at the end of the bronchi, which eventually become complete lungs. Your baby's lungs will continue to develop, preparing him for his first breath, and will remain full of fluid until he is born. A substance called "surfactant" will eventually form, which prevents his lungs from sticking together, and helps him to breathe after birth (see p.203). By 19 weeks, it is possible to see (via ultrasound) your baby's chest rise and fall as he starts to inhale amniotic fluid. These rehearsals, known as "practice breathing," will continue throughout pregnancy.

Your baby will not actually "breathe" air while he is in the womb; he will get all the oxygen he needs from the blood in your placenta, via his umbilical cord. Until about 25 weeks, his nostrils will also remain plugged. If you go into labor prematurely (see pp.314-315), you are likely to be given a steroid injection (usually betamethasone or dexamethasone) to help your baby's lungs develop sufficiently to allow him to breathe.

Some research suggests that a baby girl's lungs mature more quickly than a boy's. And it does seem that premature girls typically have less breathing trouble than boys of the same gestational age.

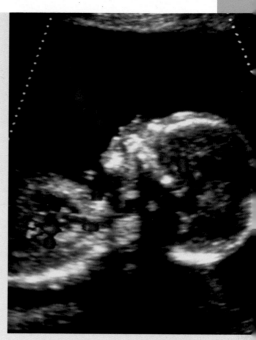

My baby's liver and kidneys

Your baby's liver develops throughout pregnancy, but its role is different from the one that it will have once she is born. Instead of performing digestive processes (which are unnecessary, because your baby gets her nourishment from the placenta, instead of food or milk) and filtering the blood, your baby's liver releases special blood stem cells that travel around her body—for example, to parts of her immune system, to stimulate its work. From about nine weeks, her liver will work to produce her own red blood cells, and by twenty-two weeks, with a little help from you, her liver is starting to break down bilirubin, a substance that is produced by red blood cells (see p.389). Her liver will be fully mature by the end of your pregnancy, but it may need a little more practice before being able to cope with the early demands placed upon it, which can sometimes lead to jaundice (see pp.389–390).

HOW THE KIDNEYS DEVELOP
Your baby's kidneys begin as buds early in pregnancy, and are in the correct place in her body and ready for development by the second month. By about 14 weeks, her kidneys start to function. From 14 weeks, the kidneys begin to produce urine. Your placenta will continue to do most of the work until the last few weeks of pregnancy.

Until she is born, waste and excess fluid are removed from your baby's body via her umbilical cord, which eventually reaches your own blood for disposal. Her urine is released into the amniotic sac and forms amniotic fluid, which plays a strong role in your baby's lung and gut development (see p.166).

19 weeks

Your baby's brain is rapidly developing the neural connections that will enable her to hear, see, touch, smell, and taste at birth. In fact, this sensory development reaches its peak this week.

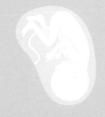

MY BABY

My anatomy scan

The time has arrived for your second ultrasound, which will offer a wonderful opportunity to see your baby's growth and development. You may be surprised to see how much she's changed, and how her facial features have developed. She really does look like a little person now, and she may exhibit a personality of her own as she performs acrobatics, waves, or sucks her thumb on screen.

It's natural to be nervous before this ultrasound, which is intended to pick up any anomalies, or aberrations, in your baby's growth and development, the health and position of your placenta, and the amount of amniotic fluid that surrounds your baby. Try to remember that the purpose of this exercise is to pick up any abnormalities that can be addressed now or shortly after your baby's birth, to ensure that both you and she are healthy.

It's a good idea to bring along your partner or a friend, to offer support and share your excitement. Ask the sonographer to explain what she is doing as she goes, and ask questions about what you are seeing on the screen. Also, decide in advance whether you wish to know the gender of your baby—you may have the chance to find out now. If you don't want to know, tell the sonographer and ask when you should look away so you won't spoil the surprise!

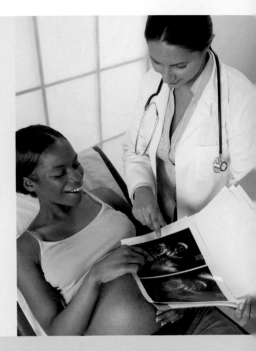

ME AND MY BODY

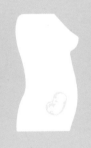

20 weeks

Congratulations! You've hit the halfway point in your pregnancy, and will now look truly pregnant. You can expect to put on about a pound (500g) per week from now until delivery.

Remembering our anatomy scans

In all three pregnancies I was very relieved after my ultrasounds. At this stage of pregnancy they have the potential to reveal a lot of abnormalities, so seeing that everything looked well and measured normally was a big relief. LJ

I recognized that an all-clear on the anatomy scan did not guarantee a "perfect" baby, but it did set my mind at ease to know that no major health issues were found. CH

My husband and I had made the decision not to tell anyone—not even family—until after the anatomy scan. Luckily my baby obliged and remained well hidden until then, as a nice, neat bump. We were obviously relieved with the all-clear, and started to relax and enjoy the pregnancy. NK

Although I was relieved after the ultrasound, there is always a small worry that something was missed, and concern over whether my baby would be OK when she was born. TL

My anatomy scan was not completed at the first visit, because my son was in an awkward position, and his heart and face couldn't be seen in detail. I scheduled another appointment to complete the ultrasound. I was convinced that there was something wrong and that the sonographer was hiding it from me. The week went by very slowly, with every possible thought going through my head. My worries were in vain, and the second ultrasound was completely normal. I think it is important to remember that whenever you have any test, there is a small chance it could show something wrong, but the likelihood of all being normal is much, much higher. MG

Organs are maturing

During the first trimester, your baby's organs were formed and systems were set up for them to work. The second trimester is very much a time for continued refinement and growth, as the connections between her brain and her organs become more capable and sophisticated. Her growth rate will slow a little, allowing energy to be diverted to the maturation of her organs and body systems, such as her immune and digestive systems and lungs.

By 20 weeks, your baby's organs are all present and continuing to mature.

In fact, some may be working efficiently already. Her kidneys are now capable of producing urine, which is discharged into the amniotic fluid. Her lungs are continuing to develop (see p.181), and although they won't be mature for a few more months, she will soon start to practice breathing.

Your baby's reproductive organs and genitals are now fully developed, and her nervous system is beginning to function. Digestion also begins a few weeks into the second trimester, and meconium (your baby's first bowel movement), begins to collect in her colon. Her brain will continue to develop rapidly over the next weeks, and start to direct bodily functions and her responses to stimuli.

This is an important time for the development of your baby's senses—her taste, smell, hearing, sight, and touch. She can hear your voice and probably that of your partner, and recognize them, too. Your baby's liver and pancreas are working hard to function properly, and will now be capable of making their own secretions.

While there are still many environmental toxins that can cross the placenta and damage your baby's growth and development (such as nicotine, drugs, alcohol, and some viruses), her organs are now much more developed and capable of better protecting themselves. For many women, this is a time to breathe a huge sigh of relief.

20 weeks

Your baby will be very active in the womb as she begins to fully explore her environment. Some of her movements will be obvious, and may startle you; she will, however, still sleep a lot.

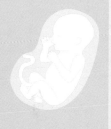

MY BABY

Growing more slowly

Your baby now measures about 6.5in (16.5cm) from crown to rump, and as she starts to unfurl it will be possible to measure her from crown to heel for the very first time. She would fit comfortably in the palm of your hand, and weighs about 10.6oz (300g). From now on, her amazing growth rate will slow a little, allowing energy to be diverted to the maturation of her organs and body systems, such as her immune and digestive systems and lungs. In particular, her skin—which is the largest "organ" in her body—is becoming more complex now.

ME AND MY BODY

21 weeks

As your bump grows, you may find that you are easily thrown off balance and much more clumsy than usual. You are also more likely to experience breathlessness, so take things slowly.

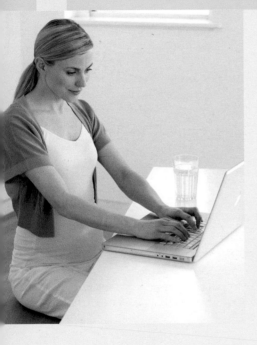

Feeling forgetful?

Are you more forgetful than usual? Do you pause mid-sentence, unable to remember what you were going to say? Do you regularly misplace your car keys, or lose track of the time? Recent research shows that this absent-mindedness, often called "pregnancy brain," is very common in the last six months of pregnancy. Fortunately, it doesn't last: Your faculties should return to normal about three months after giving birth.

Pregnancy brain may be caused by increased levels of the hormone progesterone. Progesterone often causes headaches, mood swings, and fatigue, and may also affect the way your brain operates. There's also a theory that because labor and birth are guided by the right side of our brains, our bodies encourage us to be more "right-brained" during pregnancy. It is equally likely that a change of routine, worrying, lack of sleep, and increased introspection can contribute to a slight memory loss.

Whatever the case, the best advice is to get plenty of sleep and eat a good, balanced diet. Gentle, regular exercise will improve circulation to all parts of your body, including your brain, and reduce fatigue. Finally, dehydration can disrupt the balance of your electrolytes (substances that aid in a number of body functions), so get as much fluid as you can throughout the day.

Pregnancy and memory loss

I was definitely more forgetful—I would fail to remember important things that I would never usually forget. For example, I went out of town and forgot to arrange for someone to teach my yoga class. The students all turned up, and there was no one to teach them. TL

I could not remember where I left things, or recall phone numbers and other minor facts. Of course, once you have a baby, you become so busy multitasking that your memory never truly recovers! MG

During pregnancy my memory seemed fine but, afterward, once our baby was born, I felt my brain had turned into forgetful mush. On one occasion I got the baby into the car after going shopping, then left the empty stroller on the sidewalk and drove all the way home. CH

I was working full-time as a pediatric resident at the hospital and as far as I know, was still functioning just fine. I still managed to take overnight calls at the hospital throughout my pregnancy. But then, every woman is different. LJ

My memory was undoubtedly worse during pregnancy. I found making lists of what to do and who to call was a great help (as long as I remembered to bring along my phone to make the calls). The list habit has continued post-pregnancy, too, which seems to help. NK

I managed well at work, but at home I became pretty forgetful. I agree that lists become very important—but they are even more so now, juggling work and children! VB

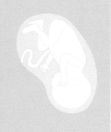

21 weeks

Your baby is now a fully formed little human, floating calmly in a pool of warm water. Her movements are more obvious, and she may have periods of intense activity.

Skin begins to thicken

Your baby's skin is the largest organ in her body, and it starts to grow early on, gradually becoming thicker and more complex as she gets older. At around five weeks, there is just one layer, which will later form the epidermis (the top layer). By around eight weeks, this layer is developing well, with tiny hair follicles beginning to form.

Between 17 and 20 weeks, your baby's eyelashes, eyebrows, and fingernails will be visible, as will the patterns of the hair follicles on her scalp. Her skin will be very transparent, appearing dark red and/or very venous, as you see the blood coursing through the veins under the surface. The absence of a good fat covering makes your baby's skin seem even thinner.

Between 20 and 24 weeks, your baby's sweat and sebaceous oil glands develop, and the top layer of her skin will turn more opaque. Her skin is becoming thicker during this period, as the epidermis develops three intermediate layers. Her skin will continue to mature between 31 and 33 weeks, when it is thick and strong enough to provide an effective barrier.

In her final month, fat will be rapidly laid down under her skin, reducing the appearance of wrinkles and making her look plumper, smoother, and less venous.

In the womb, your baby is protected by a substance known as "vernix" (see p.187), which remains in place until after the birth. Around 21 weeks, your baby will also develop a dark layer of fine, downy hair known as "lanugo"—Latin for "wool." Lanugo provides an insulating layer to help regulate your baby's temperature, and also holds the vernix in place, preventing her skin from being waterlogged. Most babies shed this hair in the week before delivery, but some are born with it. If this is the case, rest assured that it will fall out in a few days, and be replaced by a lovely peachy fuzz, known as "vellus hair."

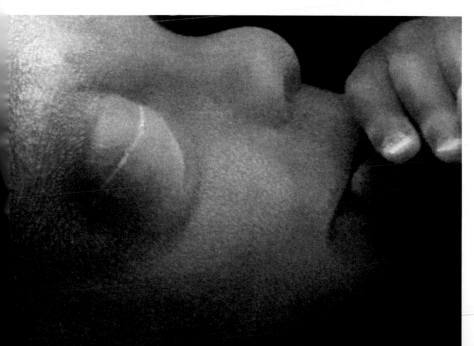

"Your baby's skin will be very transparent, appearing dark red and/or very venous"

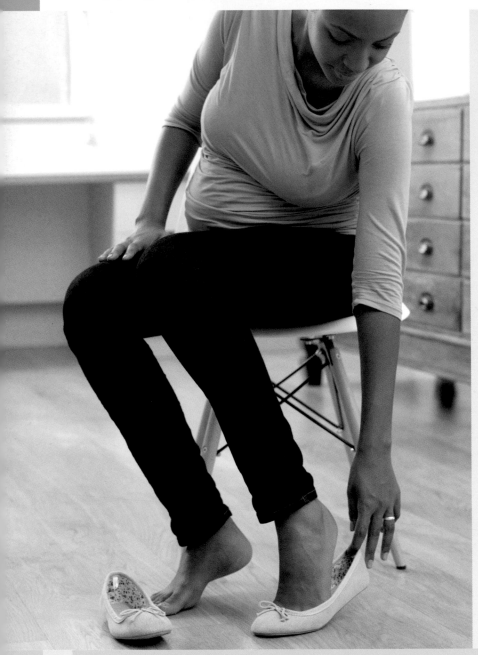

Feeling off balance

As your pregnancy progresses, your center of gravity continues to change, moving forward with the increased weight of your baby and uterus. To compensate, most women tilt their pelvises forward, to increase the curve at the base of the spine—sometimes by as much as 28 degrees. Not surprisingly, this affects posture and balance, and you may notice that you feel less coordinated as your pregnancy goes on.

Although mother nature (or perhaps evolution) has ensured that we don't topple over when pregnant, it helps to accommodate your changing center of gravity by moving a little more slowly and avoiding quick changes in direction. Watch out for uneven surfaces too.

Interestingly, practicing yoga appears to help with both posture and balance; it shifts the center of gravity very gradually, allowing you to adapt more naturally. Good posture is essential—not only to compensate for the pressure on your back and other joints, but because the effects of relaxin (see p.152) can cause you to adopt all sorts of odd stances as you struggle to stay upright! The best advice is to wear flat shoes, which encourage good posture and help to prevent accidents. The bigger your bump, the more necessary it will become to sit down when you put your shoes on.

22 weeks

If it hasn't already done so, your belly button may start to protrude. You may find yourself leaning backward on your heels when you stand, as your center of gravity shifts.

Beginning to swallow

Early in the second trimester, your baby starts to swallow her amniotic fluid, pass it through her kidneys, and excrete it as urine. She then keeps swallowing it, effectively recycling all her amniotic fluid every few hours. Researchers believe that taking in amniotic fluid may help the development of your baby's digestive system, and condition it to function after her birth.

Your baby's digestive system has been functioning in a basic way since early pregnancy. By 11 weeks, her small intestine begins to contract and relax, which pushes substances through it. It is also capable of passing sugar from inside the small intestine into her body. By 21 to 22 weeks, her digestive system is able to absorb water from the amniotic fluid she swallows, and to pass unabsorbed matter as far as her large intestine.

This unabsorbed matter is known as "meconium," a greenish-black, sticky substance that babies pass from their bowels, usually after the birth, but sometimes in labor or even before (see p.215). Amniotic fluid is normally clear, often with flecks of white vernix. If it is colored, then meconium has been passed. If your baby breathes meconium into her lungs, she may require special treatment after the birth, including being placed on a ventilator and possibly being given antibiotics to prevent infection.

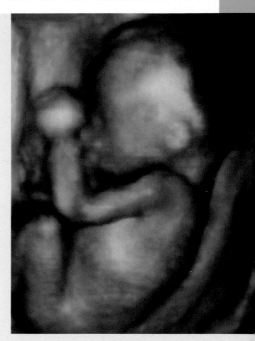

Why your baby is covered in vernix

At around 19 weeks, your baby will start to produce a white, waxy substance known as "vernix." This mainly comprises sebum—a complex oily substance—and is produced by her sebaceous glands (microscopic glands in your baby's skin). Vernix covers the entire surface of your baby's skin, protecting it and keeping it smooth and supple, while she is immersed in amniotic fluid. It also encourages the formation of the various layers of your baby's skin while she is in the womb. Vernix helps your baby to travel more easily down the birth canal, and it is believed to contain an antibacterial agent that may provide a physical barrier to infection. Furthermore, it helps to conserve heat, keeping your baby warm until she develops an adequate level of fat. Finally, vernix is thought to encourage the colonization of the skin with micro-organisms (healthy bacteria that form part of her immune system) after birth.

Most babies are born with a covering of vernix—particularly if they are born prior to full gestation at 37 to 40 weeks—and it will usually come off when your baby has her first bath.

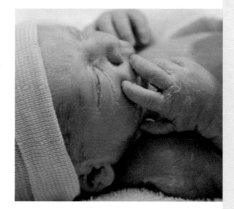

22 weeks

Your baby has room to stretch her arms, and even cross and uncross her legs. The nerve endings in her fingers are more finely tuned—she may touch her face, and perhaps suck her thumb.

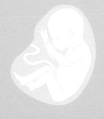

MY BABY

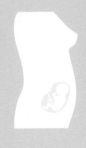

23 weeks

You may be surprised to find that the increased growth of thicker, healthier-looking hair isn't limited to your head! It can sprout in unusual places—your face, back, and neck.

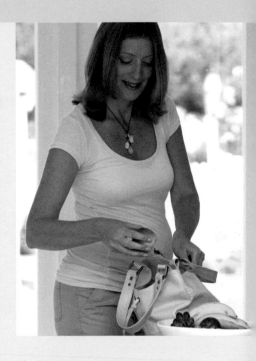

Gaining weight steadily

Many women are alarmed by the sudden increase in weight that is a feature of the second trimester, as your baby continues to grow and develop and your womb expands. Most women put on around 4lb (1.8kg) in the first 12 weeks, then about 1lb (500g) a week for the next three months (which is around 12-14lb or 5.5-6.4kg in total), and then usually only 10lb (4.6kg) over the last 12 weeks and beyond. These figures can differ between women; however, research suggests that the weight you gain should relate to your weight before pregnancy: If you begin pregnancy at a normal weight, a healthy weight gain during pregnancy is 15–25lbs (6.8–11.3kg). If you start out underweight, you should gain about 28–40lbs (12.7–18kg). If you begin overweight, aim for 5–15lbs (2.3–6.8kg).

Diet and exercise are also important to keep your weight gain steady. About 30 minutes of gentle exercise (such as yoga, walking, or swimming), three times a week, can help to encourage your metabolism and burn off calories faster. As a bonus, research has shown that women who exercise regularly are more likely to deliver a healthier baby with a stronger fetal heart rate; what's more, time spent in labor is likely to be about 30 percent shorter.

Weird and wonderful cravings

During my first trimester, I craved carbohydrates, which I did indulge to some degree. After that, I had my usual appetite for a variety of foods and was able to eat healthily again. I tried to follow an expert's gentle birth method program, which involved restricting wheat and sugar. This was fine for my first pregnancy, but I didn't manage so well in my second, when I had my toddler's leftovers in front of me every day. TL

I didn't have any particular cravings, but I did develop some aversions—and a healthy appetite! I couldn't stand the smell or taste of coffee, which made me feel nauseated. I also felt very hungry in the early afternoon and would stop and have a whole sandwich between lunch and dinner. It helped to prevent me from feeling tired and sick. MG

I craved milk, banana milkshakes, and satsumas—not too unhealthy, but an indication of something! NK

I'm not sure if this counts, but I devoured cheddar and cranberry-sauce sandwiches during pregnancy. CH

Strangely, I had a craving for carrots. I would only let myself buy a pound of carrots and the odd turnip each day, to limit my intake. My babies were not born orange, or with exceptional night vision either! FF

I didn't have much of an appetite and had to make myself eat. Having had 19 weeks of "morning" sickness, there were definitely foods that I was able to tolerate and therefore craved—especially cheddar cheese melted on a bagel. LJ

In my first pregnancy, I devoured ice in the third trimester, crunching away all day! I now realize that this is a common craving. VB

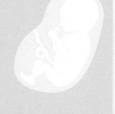

23 weeks

Although it is becoming more opaque, your baby's skin is still red and wrinkled. Her skin is being produced quicker than her new layers of fat, so it may hang somewhat loosely.

Patterns of activity

Although this may be the first time you've experienced your baby's kicks, they are now becoming more rhythmic and slower, as her room in your womb begins to decrease. Whether you feel it or not, she'll be kicking strongly by now, as she flexes and practices using her muscles. Her brain is wired sufficiently to encourage less-random movements, and she will be purposefully reaching out and kicking.

Some moms worry that their babies are "too" active, possibly subscribing to the myth that a busy baby will be a hyperactive child. There is no evidence that this is the case, nor can you predict your baby's gender from her movements in the womb (see p.103). Equally, a quieter baby will not necessarily be an angelic child! Every baby has her own pattern of activity, and as long as it remains consistent, you need not worry.

Around now your baby is developing a little cycle of sleeping and waking (see p.195), and may be determinedly active and awake when you are sleeping, while your movements throughout the day lull her to sleep. Later on, you'll be able to stimulate your baby's movements by tapping your belly or drinking a cold drink (see p.208), but it may not be until about 28 to 32 weeks that others will be able to feel her from the outside.

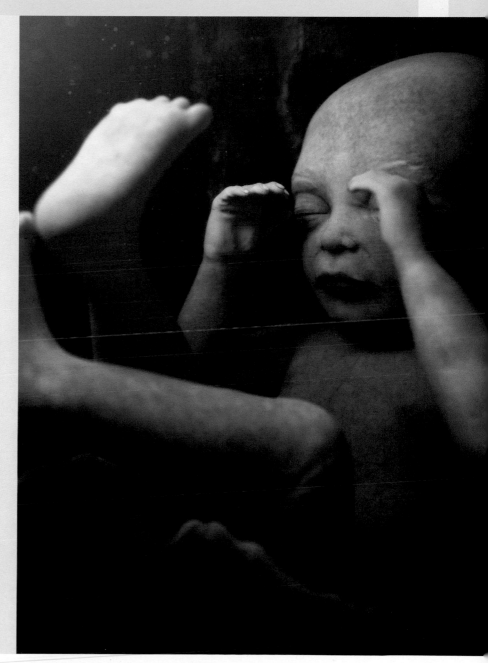

Feeling kicks

By 24 weeks, your baby is making herself at home in your uterus, and there can be little doubt that the prodding and nudging you feel comes from her. She's much larger now, having put on a layer of fat, and is continuing to grow, so she doesn't have the same amount of room to perform her acrobatics. Now, when she moves, you'll likely feel harder kicks and even rolls or twists, and you may even be able to see your abdomen move subtly as she does so.

If you haven't been pregnant before, this may be the first time you experience your baby's movements, as the tough muscles of your uterus stretch enough for them to become evident. What does it feel like? The sensation has been likened to popcorn popping, fluttering, a tickling feeling, or bubbles. Those first feelings are known as "quickening."

You may be surprised to find that you haven't felt your baby until now—some women report the first flutters around 16 weeks—however, it can depend on your weight, the position of your baby, and the location of your placenta. A lot also depends on how quickly your baby grows; to make you aware of her presence, she needs to be big enough to nudge and poke at your insides.

When you do feel her move, you're not actually feeling it on the lining of your uterus, because the uterus doesn't contain the necessary sensory receptors. But when your baby kicks, the uterus is knocked against muscles or organs such as the abdominal wall or bladder, and this is what provides the sensation of movement.

Try not to worry if your baby doesn't seem to be particularly active; after the joy of those first kicks or bubbles, you may expect to feel her constantly, which simply may not happen. It isn't until about 26 to 28 weeks that you should feel her kicks regularly.

If you don't feel her at all, do mention this to your doctor or midwife; however, if her heartbeat is strong and her other vital signs are stable, it is most likely that all is well.

ME AND MY BODY

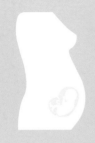

24 weeks

Your partner should be able to feel your baby's acrobatics inside the womb by now, and you may even see your stomach changing shape as she moves around.

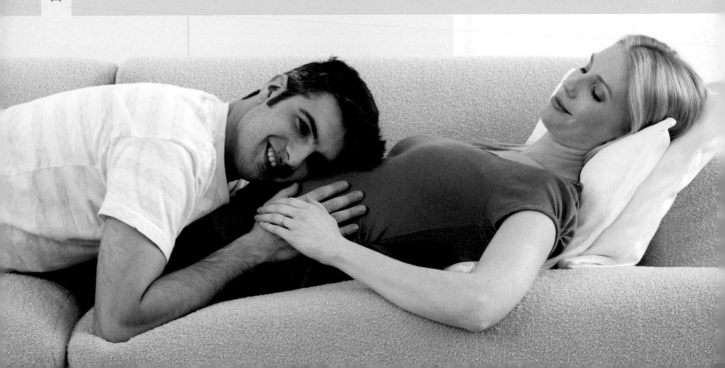

Becoming viable

It may seem impossible to believe that just over halfway through your pregnancy your baby could survive outside the womb, but this is the case. While babies born prematurely at 23 weeks face tremendous challenges to survive and then to thrive, this does mark the approximate age at which your baby can be born and still survive outside your body. Her lower airways will still be developing—babies do not yet make surfactant, which is necessary to keep the tiniest airways open and allow for oxygen to cross from your baby's lungs to her blood. However, if doctors can delay your labor long enough to provide you with steroid injections to help her lungs mature (see p.181), she has somewhere between a 10 and 70 percent chance of survival.

Viability depends on the weight of your baby when she is born—with 1lb (500g) believed to be an important threshold. If she's heavier than this, she stands a better chance. It's important to remember that this is still very early to deliver a baby, and it is probable that she will require prolonged intensive care. However, it is good to know that even if things don't go according to plan, your baby is capable of life outside you. Every day that your baby remains in the womb between 23 and 26 weeks, she has an increased survival rate of about three percent; although until about 30 weeks, there is still a high chance of her suffering from a mental or physical disability. After 26 weeks, her chances of survival jump to 80 to 90 percent; her lungs are more mature now, and there is less risk of her suffering from other problems, too.

There are many things that can affect your baby's viability, apart from her weight. For example, if your amniotic sac remains intact past 24 weeks, your baby has a better chance than if your water breaks before then. On the other hand, diabetes and high blood pressure can place your baby under stress during delivery, which increases the chances of complications.

24 weeks

Your baby's face is almost complete, with her eyes close together at the front, and her ears in their final position on the side. Her hair is growing but will appear white until pigment develops.

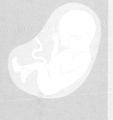

MY BABY

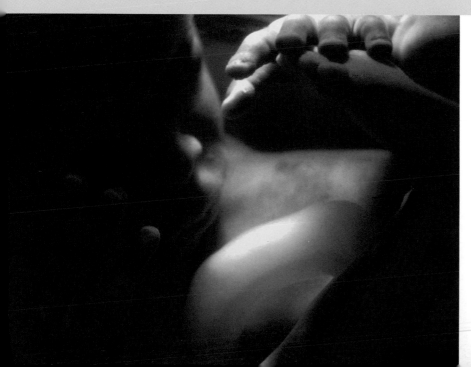

"Viability depends on your baby's weight when she is born"

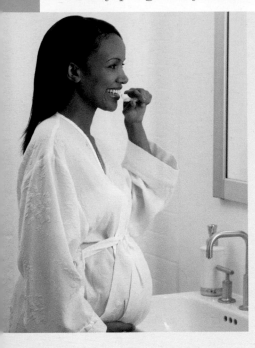

Gums and dental hygiene

While brushing your teeth, you may notice that your gums are a little sore and possibly swollen and bleeding. Not only do pregnancy hormones encourage swelling of the gums, which causes inflammation, but they also leave your mouth more vulnerable to bacteria and plaque, making them more sensitive. There is an old adage that you "lose a tooth for every baby"; however, with improvements in dental care and hygiene, this is, thankfully, no longer the case.

Choose a softer toothbrush and gently brush the area between your gums and your teeth. Floss between them at least twice a day, but try not to be too aggressive, since you may inflame your gums further. You may find it useful to use a gentle fluoride mouthwash, which will attack bacteria and help prevent plaque buildup. If you find that your gums are bleeding regularly, you may be suffering from "gingivitis," a mild gum disease. Talk to your dentist about the best ways to manage this, and increase your intake of vitamin-C rich foods (see p.49), which encourage the health of your gums. It is important to keep tabs on your oral health—gingivitis can lead to a more serious condition known as "periodontitis," which has been shown to increase your risk of having a premature or low-birthweight baby, and even preeclampsia (see pp.386–387).

Why it's important to exercise your pelvic floor muscles

Your pelvic floor muscles support your bladder, uterus, and intestines. During pregnancy, your baby's weight—and the fluid and tissue surrounding her—can stretch this floor, causing your bladder to drop down, and leading to temporary incontinence (see p.218).

The ligaments between these muscles are also softened during this time by the hormone "relaxin" (see p.152). You may find that you "leak" a little urine when you cough, laugh, or sneeze, or when you jump or run, which is a sign that your pelvic floor muscles need some work.

Exercising your pelvic floor muscles for just five minutes, three times a day, can make a big difference to your bladder control, and also help to encourage a shorter second stage of labor, when you push your baby out. Regular pelvic floor exercises (known as Kegels) encourage the health of your perineum (the area between the anus and vagina), making tearing less likely in labor, and help healing after the birth by increasing the circulation of blood to the area.

To practice Kegels, you first have to identify the pelvic floor muscles (these are the ones you use to hold the flow of urine and to hold in gas). Tighten these muscles, hold for a count of five, then slowly release them. Repeat the exercise several times a day. Think of a trigger to remind you: when the phone rings, or when you stop at a traffic light, for example. You can do them pretty much anywhere—sitting for meals, lying down, standing in the elevator.

You can also build stronger pelvic floor muscles by squeezing them tightly when you sneeze, lift, or jump; this also prevents additional damage to the area.

25 weeks

The top of your uterus will rest between your belly button and your sternum (breastbone), and is about the size of a soccer ball. This can cause breathlessness and digestive discomfort.

Developing nervous system

Your baby's nervous system is comprised of a network of specialized cells known as "neurons," which coordinate her actions and transmit signals between different parts of her body. There are two main parts: the central nervous system, which contains the brain, spinal cord, and retina; and the peripheral nervous system, which consists of sensory neurons and little clusters of neurons known as "ganglia," which provide connections between the two nervous systems and other nerves.

The foundation for your baby's nervous system is the neural tube (see p.151), which begins to develop around three weeks of pregnancy. Within just a week or two, a rudimentary brain and nervous system are in place, and by 24 weeks, brain waves can be detected.

Around 12 weeks, your baby's brain and nervous system experience rapid development, with the right and left hemispheres of your baby's brain beginning to connect, and motor fibers, which control movement, developing first. This allows your baby to move her limbs in an increasingly complex manner. At about 16 weeks, a coating known as "myelin" begins to develop on your baby's brain and nerves (see p.177), which insulates them and encourages the transmission of nerve impulses. This process will be largely complete a few weeks before your baby is born. A little later on, her sensory nerves (which control feeling) mature, first appearing on your baby's hands and in her mouth. By 24 weeks, fetal brainwave patterns, monitored electronically on an electroencephalogram (EEG) are similar to those of a newborn infant. The brain cells that have been programmed to control conscious thought are beginning to mature, and research suggests that from this time onward, your baby starts to develop a primitive memory. Certainly, she can now respond to noises in your body, your physical movements, and also to loud outside noises. Her brain is mature at about 22 to 24 weeks, but the rest of her central nervous system will not reach full maturity until 36 weeks.

Memory and consciousness

We now know that babies can see, hear, experience, taste, and, on a very primitive level, learn in the womb. Studies have found that from around 24 weeks, your baby is an aware, reacting human being who is capable of experiencing emotions, too.

Your baby is sensitive to light from the second trimester, and by the fourth month she has developed basic reflexes and facial expressions. At five or six months, she is as sensitive to touch as a newborn, and by the middle of the second trimester she can hear. Through research into premature babies and those in the womb, it is now clear that your baby's nerve circuits are as advanced as those of a newborn, and that her brain is mature enough to support consciousness.

SWEET DREAMS
By 30 weeks, babies have an intense dream life, spending more time in the dream state of sleep than they ever do after they are born. This is significant because dreaming is definitely a cognitive activity, a creative exercise of the mind, and because it is a spontaneous and personal activity.

Even more amazingly, language acquisition begins in the womb as babies listen repeatedly to their mothers' intonations and learn their mother tongue. Studies conducted using an acoustic spectograph, which records and analyzes babies' first cries, show that as early as 25 weeks, a newborn already has rhythms, patterns, and other speech features that can be matched to his mother's voice!

They are capable of responding to voices that they heard while in the womb, and reacting to familiar songs, rhymes, and voice patterns.

25 weeks

Your baby becomes more dextrous, reaching out to hold her feet and tugging on her umbilical cord. She may have a "favorite" hand—an early indication of left- or right-handedness.

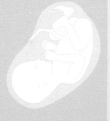

MY BABY

My painful back

During pregnancy, back pain is one of the most commonly reported discomforts. As your baby grows, and your uterus expands to around 1,000 times its usual volume, your balance is affected and the ligaments in your lower back and around your womb are stretched and pulled out of alignment. This leads to changes in posture that encourage your back muscles to work harder, as well as a change in your center of gravity. Pregnancy hormones may also contribute to back pain—relaxin (see p.152) works to loosen the ligaments between your joints to make them more flexible for the birth, but their new and extended mobility can also create discomfort in your lower back.

You may also experience pain in your pelvic area, radiating from your pubic bone in the front. In this case, you may be suffering from symphysis pubis dysfunction (SPD), which occurs when the joint where the bones of your pelvis meet separates too far, becoming inflamed and painful. This will require specialist treatment, so report any pain in this area to your doctor or midwife.

Adopting good posture, with your chin up, shoulders back, and bottom tucked in, can also help to keep things aligned. Lifting carefully—bending at your knees rather than at your back—can help to prevent damage to your back, too.

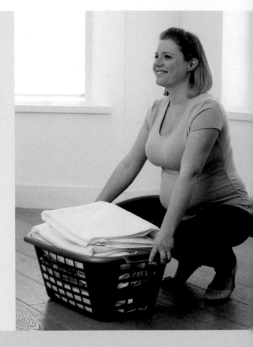

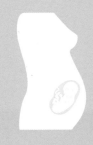

26 weeks

You may experience some back pain and discomfort in the round ligaments surrounding your uterus. You may also experience some rib pain, headaches, and leg cramps.

Relieving back pain

Back pain is not a necessary part of pregnancy, so don't think you have to put up with it. Try these tips:

• If you do experience discomfort, try a "cat/cow" stretch on all fours, rounding and flattening your back. This is great for releasing the muscles of your back and soothing discomfort.

• You can also try standing away from the wall, facing forward, and then leaning forward so that your hands are pressed against the wall at shoulder height, and your back is flat. Push back your hips and bring your weight on to your heels.

• If you haven't already done so, take a careful look at your work station. You may need a new chair to support your lower back, or a change in the level of your desk. Avoid heavy lifting of any description, which can exacerbate the problem. You can be referred for physiotherapy if your back pain is severe, so don't hesitate to mention this symptom to your doctor or midwife.

• Make sure you have a firm mattress, and always sleep on your side, with your knees and hips bent (the fetal position).

• Put a pillow between your knees when you sleep, which will help relieve the pressure on your back. Swimming is a good way to relieve back problems, and acupuncture can also be helpful.

• Stress and poor sleep can cause tension that will make back pain worse; try to nap whenever you can, and experiment with relaxation therapies (see p.286) to ease discomfort.

• Watch your posture when sitting. Try rolling a small towel into a sausage shape and placing it in the hollow of your back to ensure it's well supported.

A regular sleep cycle

At this point in your pregnancy, your baby will begin to have clearly defined periods when he is awake or asleep. In fact, they may become so routine, you'll know exactly when to expect to feel him kicking.

Most babies have a 20-minute sleep-and-wake cycle, which will become obvious as the weeks go by. We don't know what causes this cycle, but it may be that your own rhythms influence it, or he develops his own internal clock. There are clear periods of rest, sleep with rapid eye movements (REM), wakefulness with activity but no eye movements, and then wakefulness with a great deal of activity and eye movements. Less than 10 percent of your baby's time is spent being truly "awake," but that doesn't mean he isn't moving and kicking for more of the time.

NIGHTTIME ACTIVITY

Many babies are naturally more active at night, when you are calm and still; during the day, your movements gently lull him to sleep, making him wake only partially rather than being fully active. If his activities are disrupting your sleep, you can try a warm bath to calm him down, or try changing your position from one side to another. Some research indicates that soft, soothing music will also encourage sleep patterns in him. Whether he is awake or asleep, he will move about 50 or more times each hour, flexing and extending his body, and moving his head, face, and limbs. Some researchers have noted some very odd behavior, too! Your baby may "walk" around the womb by pushing off with his feet. These periods of activity are followed by various levels of sleep and then a sort of dreamlike state between sleep and wakefulness. When you feel him wake and move around, talk to him; there is plenty of research to suggest that not only will he hear you, but he will be comforted by and learn from your voice.

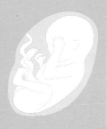

26 weeks

The nerve formation in your baby's ears is complete, and she will be more sensitive to sound. She may startle when she hears loud noises, and become quiet when you play soothing music.

How your baby's teeth are formed

At just six weeks, your baby will have tooth buds, which are clearly arranged in the area where her mouth will be. Your diet and the nutrients it contains play a strong role in your baby's tooth formation, and it is essential that you get plenty of calcium (see p.49) in your diet, as well as the mineral phosphorus, which is found in whole grains, milk, fish, and many vegetables. The fluoride, calcium, and phosphorus in your blood are all passed to your baby and added to her tooth structure as her tooth buds continue to develop. Your baby's teeth begin to mineralize (harden and develop enamel) from around 15 weeks, but her enamel will not be "mature" until between two and nine months after her birth. As calcium builds up around 19 weeks, the first primary (or "milk") teeth to harden are the central incisor teeth and the last are the back molars. Her permanent teeth will start to form at around six or seven months of pregnancy, so that by the time she is born, the development of both her baby and her adult teeth is well underway.

At birth, babies usually have all 20 milk teeth, which will erupt over the next few years with a first bottom tooth usually appearing between four and nine months. About one in 2,000 babies will be born with a visible tooth at birth.

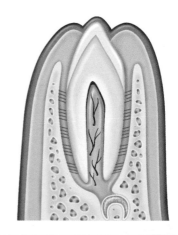

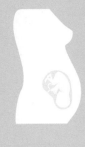

27 weeks

You may begin to suffer from hemorrhoids and varicose veins as the hormone progesterone makes your veins more flexible. In most cases, these will disappear after birth.

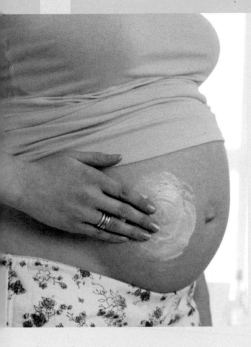

Stretch marks

Stretch marks occur when your expanding skin is stretched to its limit and tiny tears appear in the supporting layers of skin. These appear as red welts, later fading to pink and then silver. Stretch marks are common in pregnancy, with about 75 to 90 percent of women experiencing them on their abdomen, breasts, thighs, and/or buttocks. They can appear early on in pregnancy, as you begin to put on weight, but most commonly arise in the second or early third trimester, when your skin is subject to the most stretching.

Some women are more prone to getting stretch marks; for example, there is a familial link, so if your mom had them, you are likely to as well. Women with darker skin are less likely to suffer. Sudden weight gain can make stretch marks more prominent, so it's a good idea to eat well and exercise to help avoid this and give skin time to adjust.

There are no scientifically proven ways to prevent stretch marks, but there is a huge variety of creams that claim to do so. They ostensibly work by moisturizing the skin to keep it well hydrated and more pliable. In most cases, stretch marks fade naturally by about six months after the birth, but if not, your doctor may be able to prescribe special creams or arrange light abrasion or laser treatment.

What we did about stretch marks

I only had three stretch marks—right in the middle of my belly—but then my mom didn't experience them either, and she had seven children. We can hope to avoid stretch marks by avoiding rapid weight gain and keeping our skin hydrated but, sadly, we can't change genetic predisposition. FF

I didn't get any stretch marks. I massaged ayurvedic and aromatherapy oils onto my body, hips, and breasts daily, which worked wonders! It's important to use oils throughout pregnancy right up until the birth, because stretch marks can occur at any time. TL

I didn't get many stretch marks, apart from a few small ones on my stomach that just went away on their own. LJ

I was given a very expensive, divine-smelling lotion by a colleague. The aim was to apply this daily to prevent stretch marks. I rigorously stuck to a routine of warm bath in the evenings, followed by a very oily five minutes applying it all over. My skin felt soft and moisturized, and the aroma would linger for hours. Unfortunately, I still developed stretch marks! These are now a very faint reminder of my lovely pregnancies. MG

I never had stretch marks in any of my pregnancies. Lucky genes, I think. CH

I was lucky and got no stretch marks at all! Maybe drinking plenty of water helped to keep my skin hydrated. I also massaged my belly daily with moisturizing lotion to keep it supple. My bump was fairly small, so that may have helped. NK

I wasn't quite so particular about applying skin oil in my second pregnancy and, having had no stretch marks with my first, now have a couple of small ones on my tummy. VB

27 weeks

Your baby is now 14.2–14.6in (36–37cm) from her crown to her heel, and will weigh almost 2lb (900g). If she was born now, she would have a very high chance (about 85 percent) of survival.

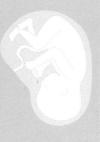

MY BABY

Seeing light

Between 26 and 30 weeks, your baby's sensitive eyes, which have been fused firmly shut to prevent them from damage and to encourage their development, will begin to open. Even with the eyelids open, a fine membrane, which will completely disappear during the final month of pregnancy, protects the delicate structures of the eyeballs. Her eyes are almost completely developed at this stage, and she can now see.

It's too early for your baby to respond to light in a fully coordinated way, but she may turn toward very strong lights or, if startled by a sudden loud noise, she may respond with a blink, just as

children and adults do. Studies have found that babies' heart rates accelerate when they see bright light, even at this stage of pregnancy. You can try shining a bright light on your tummy, and your baby may respond by kicking or suddenly moving. Experts recommend that you avoid performing this exercise too often, particularly in late pregnancy, as it can damage her retina, which is the part of her eye that allows her to focus.

Vision is the last sense to develop, and although your baby will be able to see light and make out shapes, her sight won't be fully developed until she is almost two years old.

By 27 weeks, her eyes may have taken on a little pigment, which will give them

their color, but this process won't be complete for another month or two. All babies have blue eyes in the womb, and they will not achieve their final color until a few months after birth.

She will now open and close her eyes regularly, although this pattern isn't necessarily related to when she is sleeping and awake. By the time you are 32 to 33 weeks pregnant, your baby will begin to close her eyes when she is sleeping and open them while awake, and begin to "track" her own movements and follow lights outside the womb. Her eyes will be open when she is born, although the bright light may cause her to squint. Before long, you'll have your first opportunity to gaze at each other.

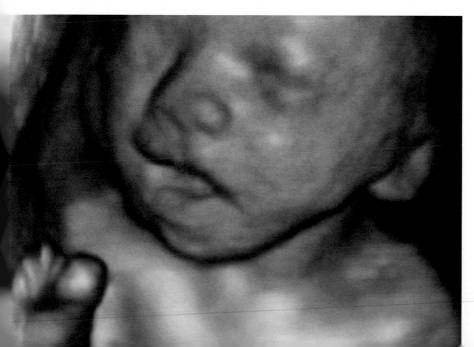

"Your baby's eyes are almost completely developed at this stage, and she can now see"

The third trimester

Your third trimester is a period of dramatic growth for your baby, and a time when you will naturally begin to slow down and prepare yourself for the countdown to birth and new motherhood.

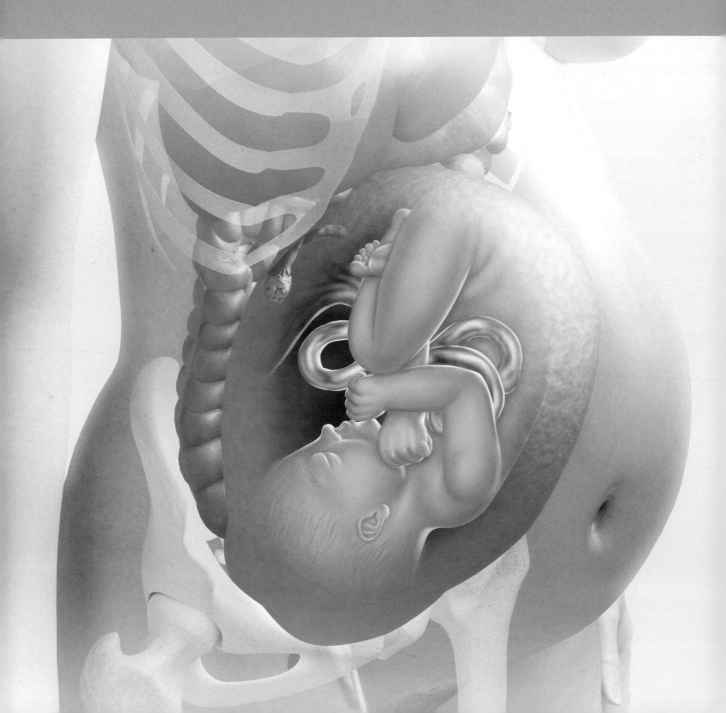

"Take time to savor these last weeks of pregnancy, and enjoy the preparations for your new arrival"

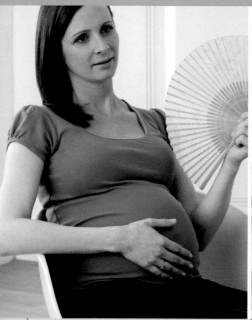

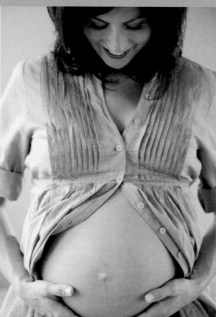

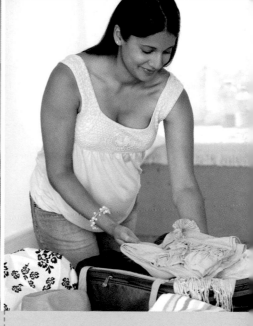

TIME TO RELAX
Part of the preparation for labor involves resting for the big day—and the weeks that follow. Don't hesitate to take things easier.

GETTING LARGER
When it seems impossible to believe that your bump could get any bigger, your baby will experience yet another growth spurt.

GETTING ORGANIZED
As your third trimester progresses, you'll need to get everything in place for your labor and life with your new baby.

GETTING READY FOR LIFE
In the third trimester your baby will usually take on his final position for the birth, and drop into your pelvis. He's running out of space and is eager to make an appearance.

Your third trimester is usually a time of growing excitement and anticipation. You may worry a little about the birth and how you will manage, although you may also be tired of being pregnant and wish that time would pass more quickly. It's not unusual to experience a new set of symptoms as your growing baby puts pressure on every system in your body.

Your baby's development is largely complete, although his organs and senses continue to be fine-tuned. He is busy putting on weight in preparation for life outside the womb, and is practicing his breathing, exercising his muscles, and listening carefully to the sounds he hears from the world outside. This is a wonderful time to bond with your baby, chatting and singing to him, and stroking your bump. You'll notice that he responds to familiar activities and sounds.

Most women feel very tired in the final trimester—try building regular naps into your day. It's normal to continue to gain weight, but it normally slows down a little. You may feel short of breath, as your diaphragm is pushed out of place by your expanding uterus.

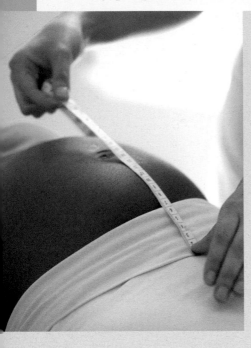

Monitoring my baby's growth

As you enter the third trimester, you may find that your weight gain slows down a little, but your baby will still be growing. Your doctor will regularly measure your abdomen to check his growth (see box, below). Most women put on an average of 10lb (4kg) during this period, but depending upon your pre-pregnancy weight, you may put on a little more. It's normal to feel "huge"—as your uterus continues to expand, your baby grows, and your body lays down fat stores in advance of the birth and in preparation for breastfeeding. Try to remember that the weight you have

gained is comprised of many different elements, and is most certainly not all "fat." At full term, your baby may weigh an average of 7.5lb (3.4kg), with the placenta, fluid, increased blood, amniotic fluid, your expanded uterus, fat deposits, and breast tissue adding about another 19lb (9kg). Most of this will naturally disappear very soon after the birth.

Encourage a healthy weight gain by keeping an eye on your diet. You may find that eating little and often is more comfortable, since your uterus is putting pressure on your digestive system, but try not to fall into the trap of snacking on junk rather than fresh, nutrient-dense, foods for your mini-meals. Try to eat plenty of iron, healthy fats, protein, and complex carbohydrates.

Measuring your fundal height

During prenatal visits, your abdomen will be measured to assess your baby's growth. A measurement will be taken (in centimeters) from the top of your pubic bone to the top of your uterus (the "fundus"). The resulting figure should be roughly the same as the number of weeks you are pregnant. Measurements that fall anywhere between the two blue lines show that your baby's growth is within the normal range. The results will be plotted on a chart (see right), and will be used to work out your baby's weight.

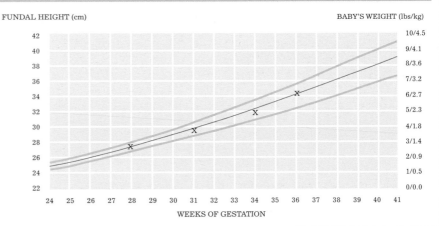

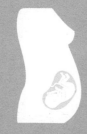

28 weeks

This is a good time to start preparing for your new arrival in earnest, by becoming physically fit and healthy enough to ensure an active, efficient labor.

Muscle power

As you enter the third trimester, your baby's muscles and bones will continue to develop. Between eight and sixteen weeks, he will form very thin muscles under his skin. After this, muscle development speeds up and continues until about 36 weeks of pregnancy. During this period your baby will be very active, which is an important part of encouraging the healthy growth of his muscles. The muscles of his hands and arms develop before those of his legs and feet, until around 32 weeks, when this situation reverses. As he practices using his muscles, they will become larger and better toned, allowing for smoother and more complex movements.

To encourage the optimal growth of your baby's muscles, it's important to include plenty of good-quality protein in your diet (see p.50).

From around nine weeks, your baby's bones have a soft cartilage core that will later be reabsorbed as it converts into hard bone. The process of hardening (known as "ossification"; see p.173) starts in "primary" ossification centers, during the following five weeks or so. Ossification requires plenty of calcium and vitamin D in order to reach optimal density. It is very important that you include calcium-rich foods in your diet, and ensure that you get a daily dose of sunshine, which encourages your body to produce vitamin D. This is particularly essential during the winter months.

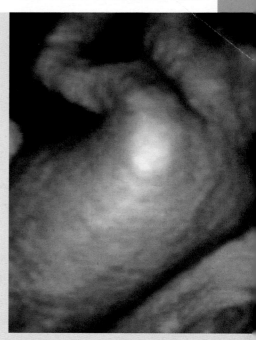

Rhesus negative?

If you have a negative blood type (Rh negative) and your baby is Rh positive, you are considered to have "rhesus incompatibility," which can lead to health problems with your baby. When some of your baby's red blood cells leak into your system, your body can develop antibodies against them, and these antibodies can cross the placenta and destroy the red blood cells in your unborn baby or, more likely, the next Rh-positive baby you have.

In most cases, you won't be exposed to your baby's blood until you give birth, which means that first babies are often

not affected; however, if you have had a miscarriage or a previous Rh-positive baby in the past, suffered from a lot of bleeding early in pregnancy, or had amniocentesis (see p.118) or chorionic villus sampling (see p.119), you may have developed antibodies that could harm your growing baby.

WHAT CAN BE DONE

If you have a negative blood type, your doctor may perform several blood tests to establish whether you have produced antibodies (which means that you have been "sensitized"). If you have not been

sensitized, you will be given an injection of Rh immunoglobulin (RhIg) at 28 weeks, and within 72 hours after your baby is delivered, too. This will also be given after a miscarriage, termination, or any invasive testing, such as amniocentesis. This injection contains antibodies that will destroy any red blood cells from your baby that have entered your blood, which prevents sensitization.

If you have been sensitized during pregnancy or in a previous pregnancy, your baby may require a transfusion after birth, and may need to be delivered early by caesarean section.

28 weeks

Your baby's nostrils are now open, and the development of air sacs in his lungs will continue. He is approximately 15in (38cm) in length and will weigh over 2lb (900g).

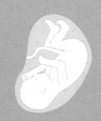

MY BABY

My breasts are changing

One of the first symptoms of pregnancy experienced by many women is a change in breast tissue, and your breasts may feel very sore and tender. As your pregnancy progresses, your nipples may become larger and darker, which some experts believe is designed to make it easier for your baby to find your nipple once he is born. You may also notice small bumps around your areola, which is also normal. These are known as "Montgomery's tubercules."

As you move through the first and second trimesters, your breast tissue will grow in preparation for breastfeeding, and you may find that they begin to leak colostrum. This is the first milk produced by your breasts, which is designed to provide everything your baby needs for his first few months, including antibodies, protection against jaundice, and plenty of nutrients (see below). It may appear as golden-yellow crusting around the end of your nipples, and is a good sign that your breasts are hard at work preparing for your new arrival.

Some women do not experience any significant changes in their breasts during pregnancy; if this is the case for you, don't worry! Your ability to breastfeed will not be affected.

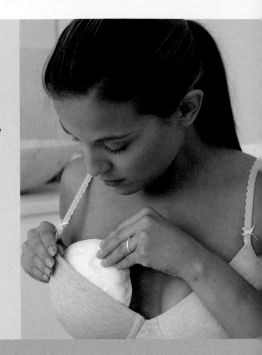

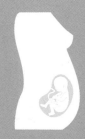

ME AND MY BODY

29 weeks

As your baby experiences a growth spurt, you may be hungrier than usual, but may find it frustrating that you can't eat all you'd like because of the pressure on your stomach.

What is colostrum?

As a result of pregnancy hormones, the internal structure of your breasts begins to change and develop in preparation for lactation and breastfeeding. While the placenta is still in the uterus, high levels of estrogen and progesterone block the action of the key hormones that trigger milk secretion, but you may notice from this stage onward that you are producing some clear liquid that leaks from your nipple.

Before milk is produced, your breasts produce colostrum, a very nutritious, deep-yellow liquid containing high levels of protein, carbohydrates, healthy fat, and antibodies. It is very easy to digest—the perfect first food for your baby. A little goes a long way, too; just a few teaspoons will provide hugely concentrated nutrition, and keep him hydrated before your milk "comes in" a few days later. Colostrum has a laxative effect on your baby, helping him pass his early stools (meconium)—important for the excretion of excess bilirubin (see pp.389–390), which may cause jaundice.

PROTECTING YOUR BABY
One of the antibodies contained in colostrum is secretory immunoglobulin A, known as "sIgA." This literally "paints" a protective coating on the inside of your baby's intestines to prevent potential allergens from invading them. A newborn baby who feeds on colostrum in the first few days of life is better able to resist the bacteria and viruses that cause illness and, because of the sIgA, is much less likely to suffer from allergies. One of the main reasons for trying to establish successful breastfeeding is that you can continue to offer your baby this protection in the first few months of life, before he is capable of producing his own antibodies. Even if you don't plan to breastfeed for longer, it is worth offering your baby this first milk to give him the best possible start.

Capable of breathing

Although he won't actually take his first breaths until he is born and the umbilical cord is cut, your baby's lungs are now capable of breathing, although they are still a little immature. He will be using his lungs to "practice breathe" amniotic fluid (you may notice he frequently hiccups as he does this), and a substance known as surfactant may start to be produced around this time.

Surfactant is a chemical produced by certain lung cells, which acts as a lubricant for the smallest part of the airways, known as the alveoli. It is soapy in consistency—similar to the substance that keeps a soap bubble expanded. Each time we exhale, the alveoli collapse. They open again when we breathe in. The surfactant allows the alveoli to open easily; otherwise, a large amount of friction would be created with each breath.

If your baby was born now, he would stand a good chance of being able to breathe air on his own outside the womb. To be on the safe side, however, an injection of steroids (usually betamethasone or dexamethasone) is offered to women who are in danger of giving birth to a premature baby (see pp.314–315). Steroids help mature the baby's lungs, helping him to breathe more easily.

"If born now, your baby would be able to breathe air on his own outside the womb"

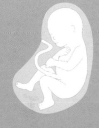

29 weeks

Your baby's muscles and lungs will continue to develop, and his head is getting bigger to accommodate his growing brain— literally billions of neurons are forming daily.

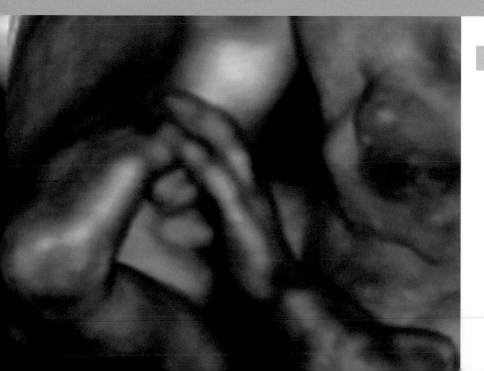

The best nutrients

Your baby is growing, and he needs all the nutrients he can get. He's already almost 15.5in (39cm) in length, from crown to heels, and weighs about 2.5lb (1150g). Good quality proteins—both animal, such as dairy produce and lean meat, and vegetable, such as legumes and whole grains—will encourage your baby's healthy growth and the structure of his brain mass. Essential fatty acids (EFAs), found in oily fish, nuts, seeds and their oils, and flax, are particularly important now; good levels in mothers' diets have been linked with optimal brain development in their babies.

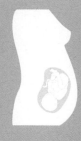

30 weeks

You may find it more difficult to sleep at night, as your bump expands and your trips to the bathroom become more frequent; you may also experience very vivid dreams.

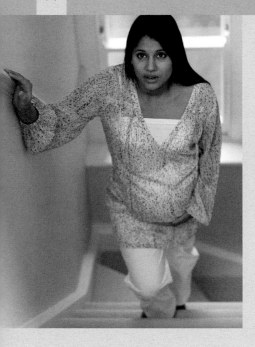

Easily out of breath

As your uterus expands upward, it puts great pressure on the surrounding organs, some of which will need to change their position to accommodate your baby. By now your uterus has grown in length from about 2.6in to 12in (6.5–30cm), and its depth and width have increased dramatically, too. Its weight approaches 2.2lb (1,000g), so it's not surprising that nearby organs feel the pressure.

In particular, your large and small intestines will move upward, and the appendix will move to the right. Your bladder will be displaced upward, and be slightly flattened. Your diaphragm will move up by as much as 1.6in (4cm), reducing the capacity of your lungs, and also pushing your heart upward and a little to the left. This won't impact your heart function, which is working harder because of the increased demands upon it. These changes will also encourage your ribcage upward, and cause it to widen. Your stomach will also move upward, and decrease in size.

Not surprisingly, you may experience some changes in how your body operates, and this is responsible for many symptoms in later pregnancy, including heartburn, breathlessness, constipation, palpitations, and discomfort (such as sharp pains and twinges) in the areas affected.

Did we like our heavily pregnant shapes?

By this stage, I still couldn't believe that I was pregnant and would get a shock every time I glimpsed myself in the mirror. Toward the end of my pregnancy, I felt very heavy and did not like the size of my breasts. I had gone through three different sizes of maternity bras and was really counting the days to going back to my normal shape. MG

I felt my body was a fitting shape for the circumstances, and I truly loved being rounded—I found myself rubbing and holding my bump, not because it was uncomfortable, but to have a closer connection with the baby. It was great when I discovered the relief of a good maternity support belt, so my back didn't suffer. I was not, however, so enamored with being off-balance and developing something of a waddle. CH

I loved my pregnant shape. I was more excited about it during my first pregnancy, when I was very eager to show off my bump; the second time around, it seemed more of an inconvenience, since it got in the way when I was trying to run around after my toddler. TL

I didn't enjoy being pregnant, and I felt it was a total invasion of my body, which stopped me being "me" for a while. However, I wouldn't have missed out on it for the world. I did feel huge, but looking back (and at photos), I'm sure I wasn't as big as I felt. FF

My little one was called the "stealth baby"—she was so well hidden, even my sister did not notice at 24 weeks! I loved my neat bump and it was only after my baby dropped into my pelvis that I started to experience discomfort when I walked. My bump was particularly painful in the groin area. I'm pretty sure that this discomfort was a subversive message for me to slow down a little! NK

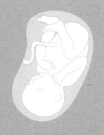

30 weeks

Your baby's digestive tract is nearly mature now, and he will be opening and shutting his eyes regularly. His bone marrow is now fully in charge of producing his red blood cells.

Less room to move

Although your uterus will begin to expand, there is a limit to the amount of space available in your body. Eventually, your baby will be forced to change his position in order to be comfortable in the womb, and to make the most of the space available to him. Because your uterus walls are closing in around him, you may feel his kicks, punches, and other movements much more easily, and some may even be forceful enough to hurt or take your breath away. Soon, however, he will begin to perform more graceful movements, when his space becomes too limited to get the volition he needs to move quickly. You will probably be able to feel his kicks and somersaults by now, particularly when he is most active—which is probably at night!

You can now begin to keep track of your baby's movements; some experts believe that your baby's activity levels are a sign that your pregnancy is progressing normally. That doesn't mean your baby will have to achieve a certain level of activity; you simply need to look for a pattern, and report any decrease in frequency to your doctor or midwife. Spending a little while every day relaxing and just focusing on your baby's movements is a lovely way to encourage your growing bond with him.

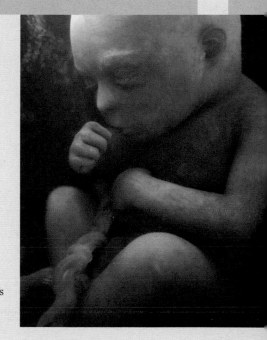

The differences between one baby and twins

Twins and other multiples will be a little smaller than "singletons" and will probably weigh about 1.8lb (800g) each, rather than the whopping 2.9lb (1.3kg) expected of single babies. One twin or triplet is very likely to weigh more than the other(s). Until around now, your babies will have grown at roughly the same rate as singleton babies; however, in the third trimester twin growth slows down a little. The reason for this is that your womb simply cannot expand beyond a certain point, so your babies' growth will be correspondingly limited. However, development will continue at the same rate.

Twins or multiple babies are usually born earlier than singletons. In the case of multiple pregnancies, the placenta becomes less efficient toward the end of your pregnancy. As a result, the ideal length of pregnancy is shorter. If there are plans to deliver your twins by caesarean section, you may begin to discuss the need for steroid injections to mature their lungs sufficiently; this is, however, only necessary if they need to be born before about 34 weeks. Your babies will soon take up a more final position in the womb, since lack of space will mean that they can't shift around as much as single babies.

INCREASED PRESSURE ON YOU
Women expecting multiples may have stronger symptoms and experience more profound changes, as hormone levels are increased and your babies put greater strain on your system. In particular, moms of twins or triplets are more prone to high blood pressure, due to the increased pressure on your cardiovascular system, and also more prone to breathlessness. You may find it almost impossible to find a comfortable sleeping position; in fact, some moms have to sleep virtually upright to get any rest at all. You will probably also be hungrier than a woman carrying just one baby.

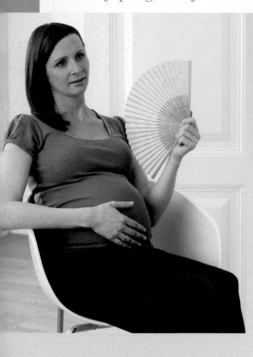

Feeling warm

Throughout pregnancy, your blood volume increases by 40 to 50 percent to accommodate the needs of both you and your baby. This may make you feel rather warm, and possibly give you dizzy spells or make you feel faint.

The increase in blood volume is greater than the increase in your red blood cells, which means that, relatively, your hemoglobin levels can fall. Hemoglobin is the protein in your red blood cells that carries oxygen. Low levels of hemoglobin can result in anemia, which literally means inadequate red blood cells, causing tiredness and other symptoms (see p.384). For this reason, iron supplements may be prescribed to bring your hemoglobin count up to normal. You can encourage this process by eating plenty of iron-rich foods.

The extra blood in your body also means that your system is under greater pressure. Your heartbeat will increase by about 10 to 15 beats per minute, to keep your blood pumping, and your heart will have to work between 30 and 50 percent harder than before you were pregnant. Because your heart is a muscle, gentle exercise will encourage it to perform more efficiently and make you feel more energetic. To produce all this extra blood, your body needs lots of extra fluid, as well as iron, folic acid, and vitamin B12 (which is found in fish and seafood, red meat, tofu, and seaweed).

Measuring your blood pressure

At your initial appointment, your doctor will have measured your blood pressure to give her a figure against which she can compare later measurements, as you proceed through pregnancy. Your blood pressure will be measured at every appointment, to ensure that it remains within a normal range for you. Your blood pressure will normally decrease during your second trimester, but return to normal in the third.

High blood pressure can be a sign of preeclampsia (which occurs when your placenta is not working properly and can eventually damage your liver and kidneys if not treated; see p.386). High blood pressure before 20 weeks is usually "essential" or "chronic" hypertension, which is high blood pressure with no identifiable cause. After 20 weeks, it is probably "gestational hypertension," which simply means pregnancy-induced high blood pressure. Many women have fluctuations in their blood pressure, but if it goes too high, you may be prescribed medication to control it. Consistently high levels can be a precursor to preeclampsia; in fact, one in four women with gestational hypertension will go on to develop preeclampsia during pregnancy or labor. A urine sample to test for protein in your urine will confirm whether you are suffering from this condition.

Try not to worry; although about one in ten women experiences problems with high blood pressure during pregnancy, severe preeclampsia is far less common. Furthermore, most women who experience gestational hypertension have only a mild form of the condition, and do not develop it until near term (37 weeks or later). If you are in this category, you may need to be induced, and are at higher risk of requiring a caesarean section.

31 weeks

You'll gain about 1lb (450g) a week as your baby continues to grow, and probably feel breathless and sometimes a little faint as your blood pressure and/or blood sugar drops.

ME AND MY BODY

A sense of taste

It is believed that your baby's taste buds are largely mature from around 15 weeks of pregnancy and that she is capable of tasting some of the foods you eat—particularly those with a strong taste or smell, such as garlic or spices.

Flavors travel through your bloodstream and the placenta, and into her body via the umbilical cord. When she excretes waste products into her amniotic fluid, it will take on the "aroma" of what you have eaten, giving her an opportunity to taste it when she "inhales" and swallows it later on.

Now that she is regularly practicing her breathing in advance of the birth, she has more opportunity to taste

different flavors. Some experts believe that this early tasting of the food you eat acts as a sort of "flavor bridge" to breastmilk, which also carries food flavors from your diet. Studies show that, in the womb, a baby's swallowing increases when surrounded by sweet tastes and decreases with bitter and sour tastes. The taste of your amniotic fluid varies from day to day, according to what you eat, and eating a varied diet can have added benefits—researchers found that babies who were exposed to certain tastes in the womb via the amniotic fluid were more eager to eat foods with a similar taste when weaning began.

At this stage, your baby is acquiring a good layer of white fat under her skin, and now looks much pinker.

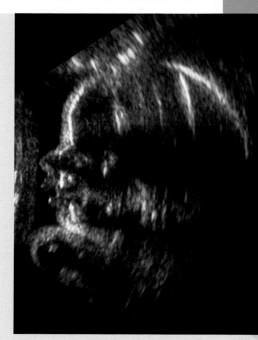

What color will my baby's eyes be?

The color of your baby's eyes depends upon the amount of a pigment known as "melanin," which is present in the iris of her eyes. Blue-eyed babies will have relatively small amounts of melanin, while brown-eyed babies have much more.

In the womb, all babies have blue eyes, which will be lighter or darker according to their ethnic backgrounds. For example, very fair babies may be born with pale or bright blue eyes, while babies with black or dark skin will have eyes that are at the deep gray end of the spectrum. After birth, your baby's eyes will gradually change until they reach

their eventual color between six months and even as late as three years after birth.

Genetics will decide the eventual color of your baby's eyes. Blue eyes are coded for by a recessive gene, while the brown gene is dominant. So, if there are two blue-eyed parents, your baby will have blue eyes. If there is a blue-eyed parent and a brown- or black-eyed parent, your baby could conceivably have eyes that are blue or brown or black, and possibly something in between such as green, gray, or hazel. Two brown-eyed parents could produce virtually anything! This is dependent upon the combination

of genes that the dark-eyed parent carries in relation to eye color. This may seem confusing, but consider it like this. Blue-eyed people always have two blue-eyed genes, because blue is recessive. Brown-eyed people could have a blue gene and a brown gene (because brown is dominant) or two brown genes. Your baby will get one gene from each of you, so your blue-eyed baby could receive a blue gene from her blue-eyed mom and another blue gene from her brown-eyed dad. Two brown-eyed parents could each provide one blue-eyed gene, creating a baby with blue eyes that are quite unlike her parents.

31 weeks

Your baby's ears are now almost completely developed—both inside and out—and she will respond to familiar sounds. She won't be as active, but her movements will be very pronounced.

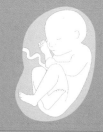

MY BABY

Stopping to feel my baby

Your baby will follow a distinct sleep-wake cycle in your womb, and you may find that your activity during the day encourages her to sleep a little more—or experience a quieter, more dreamlike state—as she is lulled to sleep by your movements. Generally, she will rest for about 45 minutes at a time, but it might feel longer than this to you, because you won't feel every movement. At night, however, it might be a different story! Many babies become active the moment you hope to relax, although it is unlikely that they are doing this to get your attention just yet. We don't know for sure what encourages your baby to move; your quiet periods may just make you more sensitive to her movements, and make you more likely to notice them.

Because it is recommended that you keep an eye on your baby's activities from about 28 or 29 weeks onward—for the simple reason that regular movement is a sign that all is well—you may wish to encourage her to respond when she's been quiet for a little while (see right).

You can do this by stopping and relaxing; it may be that you've been too busy to notice her movements, or that she's rocked to sleep by your activities. There are some more suggestions for how to monitor your baby on the next page.

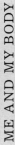

ME AND MY BODY

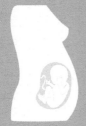

32 weeks

Don't be alarmed if you leak a little urine when you cough or sneeze; the pressure on your bladder and pelvic floor can lead to temporary incontinence. Pelvic floor exercises will help.

How we encouraged our babies to move

Both my babies had their active phases in the evening, when I sat down after a long day's work. When I had any concerns about movement, I would give my tummy a gentle poke—especially where a foot was sticking out. This was guaranteed to cause a stir! MG

Drinking cold water can jolt your baby into moving positions, as will having something to eat. When I worked as a midwife in Saudi Arabia, many pregnant women tried to fast during Ramadan, and often appeared with reduced fetal movements and very "quiet" sonogram recordings (see p.226); however, once they had eaten, their little ones were on the move again, and their sonogram recordings would improve. NK

If my baby was stirring, I would gently press the side of the bump where his feet seemed to be and he would often respond with a movement in return. Near the end of my pregnancy I was concerned my baby wasn't moving enough, so the doctor asked me to eat a big chocolate bar and then come in for an ultrasound. The increased sugar burst worked, and he was more active. I wouldn't recommend this all the time though—all that sugar didn't make me feel too good. CH

Many women say that they feel their babies moving more after yoga classes. TL

Trying to get some sleep was guaranteed to get my baby to move! FF

If I simply pressed on one side of my belly, I could reliably get a heel to poke out the other side! LJ

I was in my third trimester during the summer. Whenever I was out in the bright sunshine, my son became very active. Both my babies responded to their dad's voice. VB

Slowing down

It is not uncommon for your baby's movements to slow down a little, as her space becomes more confined. In fact, this week and the next are when her movements are at a peak. What's normal? As long as you can discern 10 movements across a two-hour period, there should be nothing to worry about. You may have a sleepy baby, who needs nudging from time to time to achieve this.

Studies show that by 24 weeks, your baby's heart rate increases in response to patting or stroking your abdomen. If you want to get her moving, talk to her and stroke the top of your bump, which is where the top of your uterus is.

Loud music should definitely wake your baby, and may even prompt an outraged kick from her in response. Changing your position—moving from lying on the left side to moving to the right, with your bump supported—will stimulate your baby to change hers, in order to remain comfortable within the womb's confines.

Just as you feel more alert after eating something sweet, your baby will also respond when your blood-sugar levels increase. Many women find that their babies are much more active after meals, when they've had a sugar boost.

Your baby's movements will naturally change as her space decreases, so instead of lots of flipping and kicking, you may experience protruding elbows and feet,

and see your abdomen move as she extends a limb or stretches. Her movements may also be felt as squirms, jabs, and tickles, rather than big sensations. Depending upon how your baby is lying, you can usually feel either her head or her bottom, although it will be hard to differentiate between the two at this stage.

It is always a good idea to do a casual check a few times a day, not only to reassure yourself but also to pick up any problems at an early stage, but don't let this become an obsession. If you do have serious concerns about your baby's level of activity, talk to your doctor, who can listen to her heartbeat and arrange for monitoring (see p.226), if necessary.

32 weeks

At 32 weeks, your baby has reached a significant milestone. She is able to suck, which means that if she was born now, she may be able to breastfeed and/or drink from a bottle.

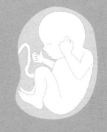

MY BABY

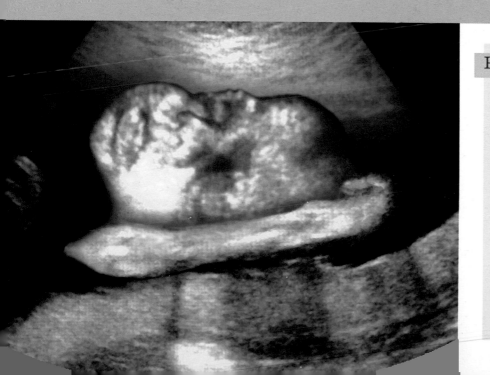

Preparing for feeding

By now, the average baby will weigh about 3.8lb (1.7kg), and measure just over 16.5in (42cm) from her crown to her heel. Not only can she suck, but she will also have acquired the "rooting" instinct or reflex, which will help her to find your breast when she begins breastfeeding after birth. When her cheek or mouth is stroked, she will immediately open it in anticipation of food. Not only will she be able to find your nipple on her own within an hour of being laid on your chest after the birth, but she will automatically "root" when she is hungry, giving you a clear indication that it's time for a feed.

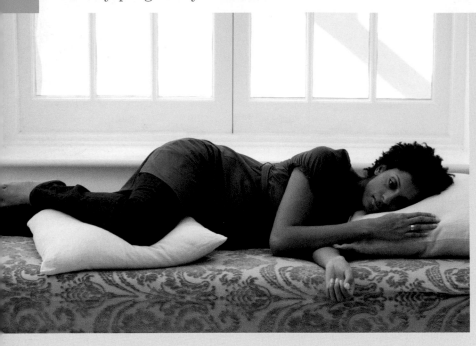

Struggling to sleep

Sleep problems are notorious for disrupting the last trimester of pregnancy, and you may find that you are increasingly tired as you struggle to find a comfortable position, negotiate trips to the bathroom, and possibly deal with the discomfort of restless legs syndrome (see p.86). You may also wake in the night feeling hungry.

It is most important to focus on getting enough "overall" sleep, which means making up for lost sleep at night by taking naps. Try to make sure you are physically tired before you go to bed—swimming, yoga, and gentle walks are good ways to expend energy and relax you. Eating food that contains tryptophan (an amino acid found in turkey, eggs, and cheese) can encourage sleep, and getting plenty of high-energy, slow-release carbohydrates during the day can help keep your blood-sugar levels steady. A snack before bed can help, too. If you are feeling worried, try some relaxation techniques (see p.89), to help you keep calm. Finally, make sure you are comfortable in bed. Layer the covers so that you can add or remove them if you become too hot or cold; use as many pillows as required to support your back, your bump, and any other parts of your body that are uncomfortable.

Sleep in the last trimester

It was feeling too hot that made my nights restless, more than anything else; a damp cloth for my neck and a fan worked best to cool me down. CH

Sleeping on my back was very uncomfortable, which was fortunate—it is recommended that pregnant women not sleep on their backs because it places too much pressure on their major blood vessels. I quickly determined that I was most comfortable sleeping on my side with a body pillow tucked between my knees and under my belly. I have slept that way ever since. LJ

The only way I could sleep was propped up on my side, with a pillow between my knees—but even in this position it took a long time to fall asleep. Despite having a warm bath before bed and a cup of warm milk, I sometimes fidgeted so much that my husband would sleep in the guest room. Actually, though, that helped, since I had the whole bed in which to find a comfortable position. MG

When I woke up around 3am and was unable to get back to sleep, I used breathing techniques, which were very effective. TL

33 weeks

You may notice that you need to get more rest during the day, because the size of your bump can make normal activities more tiring.

Turning head down

This is the optimal time for your baby to change position and turn so that her head moves down into your pelvis, with her bottom facing upward. As your baby will continue to grow, it is advantageous if she achieves the ideal head-down position for a vaginal birth as soon as possible, before she is too big to turn. It is certainly possible that your baby will turn into a head-down position and then flip back upward again, continuing to move until the late stages of the third trimester. But once she has managed to get her head down, it is more likely that she will stay that way.

Your doctor or midwife probably won't take a keen interest in your baby's position for a few more weeks, unless you are expecting twins and a caesarean may be in the cards (see p.312). Many babies don't turn head-down until about 35 or 36 weeks, so there is plenty of time yet. You may actually feel her turning, with a great sliding motion that changes your bump's shape dramatically. Some babies struggle to achieve the right position, and you can experience some painful cramping and discomfort that feels a bit like contractions; this will pass shortly.

If you are very eager to get her to turn sooner rather than later, you can try leaning forward over a birthing ball for about 15 minutes a day. For more tips, see p.273.

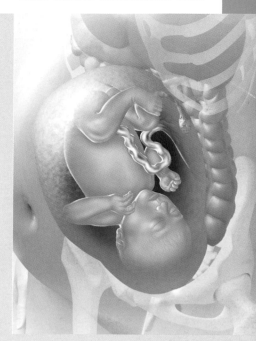

My baby's adrenal glands

In relation to her body size, your baby's adrenal glands are around 20 times larger than yours. These triangular glands are located at the top of each kidney. They have an outer layer (a "cortex") that is responsible for releasing steroid hormones (a hormone that acts as a steroid, such as cortisol). Cortisol is produced in response to stress and low blood sugar. It helps the body to metabolize fat, carbohydrates, and protein and prevents the release of substances in the body that cause inflammation. Part of the adrenal glands also work hard to produce hormones that will work to

coordinate your baby's growth and development, including regulating her salt balance, helping control the availability of sugars, fat, and amino acids in her bloodstream, and producing male sex hormones such as testosterone. There is also some evidence that hormones produced by her adrenal glands will kick-start your labor, sending a message that she is ready to be born.

The outer layer, or "cortex," accounts for the large size of your baby's adrenal glands. In the first couple of weeks after birth, these adrenal glands will rapidly shrink in size.

ADRENALINE
The main function of the adrenal glands is to produce adrenaline. Adrenaline is very important for your baby—it helps her maintain a stable environment in your uterus and cope with any stress accompanying her birth and the world outside the womb.

Adrenaline triggers the "fight or flight" response in your body—it increases the availability of glucose, speeds up the heart rate, and maintains or raises blood pressure. Historically, it would give you the means to fight your enemy or to flee a potentially threatening situation.

33 weeks

Most of your baby's bones are becoming harder, but her skull will remain quite pliable, with plates of bones that can move so she can be delivered through your birth canal.

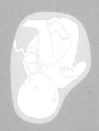

MY BABY

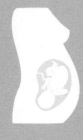

34 weeks

By now, you may be feeling distinctly uncomfortable and more than ready for your baby's birth. This is a prime time for water retention, which will make your ankles, feet, and face swell.

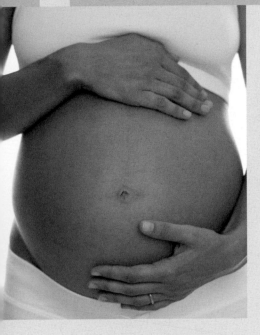

My skin feels tight

As you approach the end of your pregnancy, you may feel that your skin simply can't stretch any further, as your bump continues to grow. This is a very normal experience, even if it can be incredibly uncomfortable and even distressing. Your stretched skin can also feel itchy and sensitive, chafing easily with even loose clothing. The best advice is to use a gentle, hypoallergenic emollient (such as one designed for eczema) and apply it to your bump and any other uncomfortable places a few times a day. There is nothing you can do to ease the sensation of your skin being stretched beyond its capacity to cope, but as your baby drops down into your pelvic cavity, the shape of your bump will change—hopefully not protruding quite so far forward, and pulling out your skin.

By now your belly button may have popped out, or become flat and taut against your skin, as your stomach expands with your baby. You may even experience some pain and irritation around your belly button, as the skin is pulled tight and your clothing rubs against it. A little petroleum jelly on the area should prevent chafing and soothe itching. Rest assured that all will return to normal once your baby is born.

Group B streptococcus

Group B streptococcus (GBS), is a type of bacteria that causes life-threatening infections in newborns, and may also make you very ill. This bacterium can cause "sepsis" (infection of the bloodstream), meningitis (infection of the lining and fluid surrounding the brain), and pneumonia in the first weeks of life. Around 20 percent of women carry GBS in their vagina, which is completely normal, and does not cause any symptoms. This type of bacterium can be carried in your body (usually in the gastrointestinal tract, genitals, or urinary tract) without infecting you. It can, however, be passed on to your baby, particularly during birth, which can cause serious problems with her health. The risk factors that increase the chances of your baby being born with a GBS infection include having previously had a baby infected with GBS, and experiencing symptoms of infection, such as a fever, during pregnancy. You will likely be tested for group B streptococcus with a swab around your vaginal or rectal area at 35 to 37 weeks.

WHAT IF I HAVE GBS?
If GBS is detected on the swab or in a urine culture in your pregnancy (or any previous pregnancy), talk to your doctor to agree on a birth plan that will protect you and your baby. You will be offered intravenous antibiotics as soon as you go into labor or when your water breaks (whichever comes first). If you do not take antibiotics, or they are not administered at least four hours before you give birth, your baby will need to remain in the hospital for a minimum of 48 hours, for observation.

If it is suspected that your baby has GBS, the diagnosis may be confirmed with blood and urine tests. There is no evidence that treating GBS in pregnancy is helpful, since the GBS tends to return once treatment is finished.

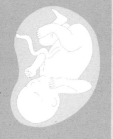

34 weeks

Your baby has a 99 percent chance of survival if she is born now, and is capable of breathing at birth. She may have adopted a head-down position now, as she drops into your pelvis.

Developing immunity

While you are pregnant, your antibodies are passed from your bloodstream, through the placenta, to your baby. These are an essential part of her immune system, and they will identify and bind to harmful invaders such as bacteria and viruses. This, in turn, triggers different immune cells to destroy the foreign substances. The type of antibodies that pass the placenta are known as Immunoglobin G (IgG) antibodies, which are the smallest and most abundant, making up 75 to 80 percent of all of the antibodies in our bodies. They are also the most important for fighting viruses and bacteria, and will help prevent your baby from becoming ill in the womb. Toward the end of pregnancy, your baby will begin to develop a rudimentary immune system, which, with help from your antibodies, enables her to fight off many bacteria and viruses once she is born.

Immediately after birth, she will still have high levels of your IgG antibodies in her bloodstream. Babies who are breastfed will receive more antibodies via breastmilk, which contains all five types of antibodies. Your baby's own immune system will kick into action in the first few weeks of life, but it will not be mature until much later in childhood.

> "Your baby can hear you clearly now, and will recognize your familiar voice; she loves to hear you talk"

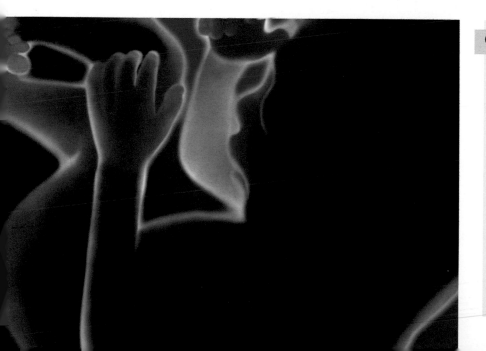

Getting heavier

At about 17.7in (45cm) from crown to heel and almost 4.9lb (2.2kg), your baby is fast approaching her birth weight and height, and will continue to grow, putting on about 1lb (500g) each week until she is born. This is not only reassuring from the point of view that she is sturdy enough—and has adequate fat stores—for survival, but also explains the feelings of heaviness that you will undoubtedly be experiencing. Although you may not put on much more weight this trimester, your baby will continue to grow and move upward into the space beneath your ribs, making you feel more breathless.

My large bump

With your growing baby protruding in front of you, your bump may seem to get in the way of everything you try to do. Even simple, everyday activities might seem really difficult at this time, and may leave you frustrated. It's important to be cautious at this stage; although your baby is well cushioned by amniotic fluid, you could hurt her and/or yourself if you suffer a fall.

Your center of gravity will have adjusted to compensate for the extra weight, but it's still easy to lose your balance, particularly if you can't see your feet or the ground beneath them. For the last few weeks of pregnancy, it's a good idea to be particularly careful as you go about your everyday activities, taking time to move slowly and methodically, and stopping whenever you feel twinges in your joints or abdomen, or if you feel off-balance. At this stage of pregnancy, your mind may be on other things, so you may have to actively remind yourself to take care.

Hold on to railings as you climb and descend stairs; make sure the edges of your rugs are taped to the floor and household items are not left in hallways or on the stairs; bend from your knees when lifting or sitting down; try rolling over to sit on the edge of the bed before getting up, to prevent from feeling lightheaded and losing your balance; and try to remember to keep the lap part of your seatbelt under your bump when traveling, to prevent injury in the event of an accident. Sit down when you get dressed, or when you put on tights and underwear, but avoid low chairs or sofas, which may be impossible to escape! Finally, don't be embarrassed to ask for help if you need it. Most people are only too glad to lend a hand to a heavily pregnant woman. It is important for you to be patient. Try to relax and take some quiet time for yourself, and don't hesitate to communicate your worries to your partner or a close friend. Focus on getting through the next few weeks, and look forward to when your body is back to normal.

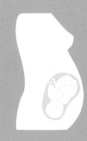

ME AND MY BODY

35 weeks

Your weight gain will stop or slow down around now, and some women even experience a little weight loss toward the end of the final trimester.

Feeling moody

Mood swings become increasingly common around this time, due to changing hormones, lack of sleep, and a natural anxiety about the birth. Try to relax and don't hesitate to communicate your worries to your partner or a close friend. With your labor fast approaching, it's also a good idea to make time for a regular rest, and to practice your breathing techniques. Not only will this help you feel calmer now, but you will be well prepared for the big day. Irritability can also be exacerbated by dehydration, so make sure you are drinking plenty of water.

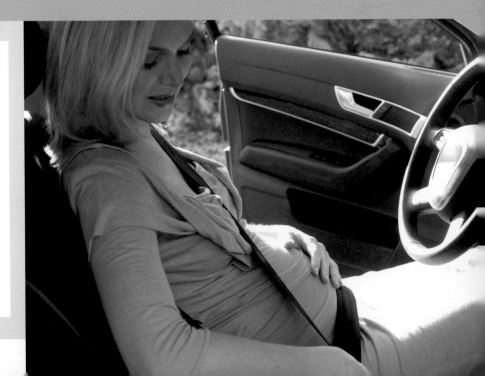

Making faces

From about 16 weeks, your baby has been capable of making a variety of different facial expressions in response to cues in her environment and whatever is going on in her little brain. By now, she's developed a whole repertoire and will grimace, yawn, purse her lips, raise her eyebrows, squint, frown, and even produce something like a beatific smile when she dreams.

Studies performed via ultrasound scanning also show that your baby's facial expressions change in response to external stimuli, and according to the emotions that she is feeling. We know that babies of mothers who are angry or under a great deal of stress can look solemn or anxious, and that babies who hear a loud noise will startle, raising their eyebrows and opening their eyes wide.

A recent study found that twins are incredibly sociable in the womb, and, from 18 weeks of pregnancy, reach out to touch one another's faces and bodies. There is also evidence that by five months of pregnancy, they respond to their sibling's touches with a variety of facial expressions, including smiling at a gentle touch.

What's more, despite the fact that it is probably too dark for twins to see each other in the womb, they appear to mimic one another's expressions.

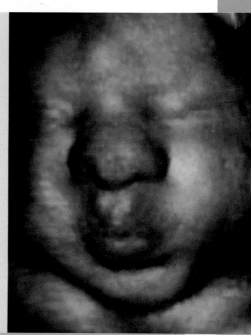

35 weeks

Babies tend to grow at different rates, and your baby may be a little smaller or larger than average. Your doctor can give you a rough idea of your baby's birth size by palpating your womb.

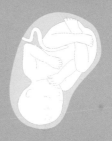

MY BABY

Meconium: your baby's first stool

Your baby's intestines are lined with a thick, greenish-black, tar-like substance known as "meconium," which is created from cells that your baby has shed, lanugo (see p.185), and other substances including bile and mucus. Meconium is not normally released until after his birth, but it is common to see meconium staining of the amniotic fluid in overdue babies. If meconium is seen when the membranes rupture in very premature babies, it can be a sign of listeria infection (see p.54). If your water breaks at home, make sure that you mention any greenish staining of the fluid to your doctor. If you do see this, you will be asked to go to the hospital for assessment. Meconium staining can be a sign that your baby is stressed. A Doppler scan (see p.293) can help to determine if there is anything to be concerned about.

In labor, your doctor will regularly check for the presence of meconium. If she finds any, she will recommend continuous fetal monitoring (see p.293). Pediatricians may be called if meconium has been seen in labor, particularly if is suspected that your baby is in distress. Sometimes distressed babies can gasp as a response to low levels of oxygen, both before and after delivery, causing them to inhale meconium. This "meconium aspiration" can cause pneumonia in newborn babies. If your baby has passed meconium before the delivery, he may have green-stained skin and nails.

In most cases, you won't see meconium until after the birth, when your baby will pass it in his diaper in his first days. It is very messy and sticky, and you'll be glad when her normal bowel movements (see p.350) appear. However, seeing it in her diaper is a good sign because it indicates that her bowels are working normally.

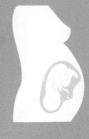

36 weeks

Your breasts may be more tender as hormones produced by the placenta stimulate them to produce milk. Your first milk (colostrum) may begin to leak a little.

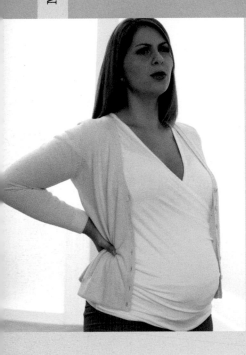

I'm having contractions

Early contractions, which indicate that your uterus is warming up for labor, are known as "Braxton Hicks" contractions (see below). They can occur throughout your pregnancy, only becoming more noticeable—and uncomfortable—in the later stages. In most cases, they are experienced as a "tightening" sensation, which quickly passes.

Many women are tricked into thinking that they are in labor once their womb starts to contract, but the difference is that with these type of contractions, there is no regular pattern, they don't tend to be very painful, and they start and stop without growing closer together or building in intensity. If you are in any doubt about whether you are in labor, see pp.276–277; however, rest assured that only a minority of moms-to-be go into labor before their due date, and far many more are late!

The best advice is to practice your breathing techniques, and take a walk or a nap until the contractions pass; in many cases, they are a message from your body to slow down. You may find that a warm bath helps. However, if a pattern is established and they become closer together and increasingly painful, call your doctor, who will advise you what to do.

Braxton Hicks contractions

Braxton Hicks contractions are a tightening of the muscles of the uterus, lasting for a minute or two, to prepare your body for the birth. However, they don't appear to have any effect on the cervix. If you place your hands on your abdomen during one of these contractions, you'll notice that it becomes very hard and then, after a few moments, relaxes. Braxton Hicks contractions are not part of labor, and not all moms-to-be seem to notice them. They do, however, occur in most women from about seven weeks of pregnancy, but will remain irregular and largely painless until much later on. These contractions get their name from the English doctor John Braxton Hicks, who first described them in 1872. There are a few situations that can bring them on, including dehydration, which can cause muscles to spasm and encourage contractions. Overwork, stress, and exhaustion can also encourage their appearance, while rest, rhythmic breathing, exercise, and gentle stretching can cause them to disappear. Having a full bladder can also cause these contractions, perhaps because it puts pressure on the uterus, which stimulates it to contract.

FALSE LABOR

It is possible to experience a series of Braxton Hicks contractions, which appear more rhythmically, in late pregnancy, and this is known as "false labor" (see p.276–277). You may believe that you are in labor because they can also become more painful and closer together. However, false labor does not cause your cervix to dilate significantly or progressively, and the contractions don't get consistently stronger. It can be hard to tell the difference, but your doctor can confirm that labor has not begun by performing an internal examination.

36 weeks

Your baby may now have a full head of hair—or none at all—and it may be a color that is completely unrelated to the color it will eventually become.

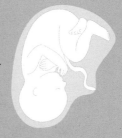

MY BABY

Reaching clinical maturity

By the end of this week, your baby is officially full term; only those babies born before 37 weeks are considered premature or "preterm." Although her lungs are now well developed, she still runs a risk (about 5 to 10 percent) of suffering from respiratory distress syndrome (RDS), so it is best to hold off induced labor or a caesarean for as long as possible. She is now a good size, with an excellent chance of surviving outside the womb with little or no support. However, she will benefit from gaining more weight to insulate and support her after the birth. If this is your first pregnancy, there is a chance that your baby has not yet "engaged," or, indeed, even turned into the head-down position that is ideal for a vaginal delivery. A little more time in the womb will allow her to position herself properly. As her head begins to settle into your pelvic cavity, her legs can stretch a little more, which will encourage their continued growth.

Your baby will mostly lie in a curled-up position, with her limbs folded close against her body, since there is not much space in your uterus at this time. You may notice a change in her movement patterns, because there is less space for your baby to move around.

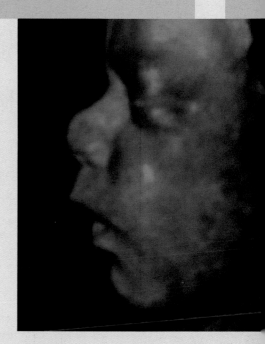

Practice breathing

Although we don't know exactly when this begins, there is evidence to suggest that your baby began practicing her breathing skills from 15 weeks of pregnancy, first by simply moving her chest and drawing in a little amniotic fluid, and then beginning to learn to inhale it at around 20 weeks. By 33 weeks, she will have mastered this skill and will now be regularly practicing it in advance of her birth.

Practice breathing encourages your baby to inflate and deflate her lungs by "breathing" in amniotic fluid, and then "exhaling" it. Some amniotic fluid is absorbed into her body, and then expelled with her waste products into the amniotic fluid; the remainder goes in and out of her lungs as she prepares for breathing air. There is no exchange of air in practice breathing—your baby will continue to get the oxygen she needs from you, via the placenta and her umbilical cord, and return carbon dioxide in a reverse procedure. When your baby is born, she must breathe air for the first time; this can be a tricky process and a fairly stressful moment, since her lungs are often filled with fluid, and she must immediately begin to process oxygen through her lungs and into her blood circulation, which is altered at the moment of birth.

Labor and birth will prepare your baby to take that first breath. Not only does the process of being squeezed down the birth canal empty her lungs of fluid, but the sensory changes she experiences in response to her new environment—and the heightened arousal that occurs after birth—both encourage the release of adrenaline, which kick-starts breathing.

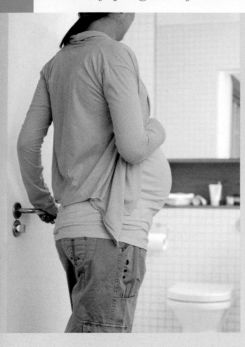

To the bathroom

One of the most annoying symptoms of late pregnancy is the frequent urge to urinate, as your uterus and possibly your baby's head presses down on your bladder, changing its position and shape, reducing its capacity in the short term, and also irritating it. What's more, the weight of your baby and your uterus can make you think you need to urinate, when your bladder isn't even full.

During pregnancy, your pelvic floor muscles are also stretched and made more elastic (by progesterone), making it more difficult to control the urge to urinate, and to stop the flow once it starts. For this reason, many women experience "stress incontinence," a temporary condition that involves urine leaking when the bladder is put under pressure (by jumping or running) or the muscles around it tighten—when you laugh, cough, or sneeze, for example. Practicing your pelvic floor exercises can help to keep the muscles toned and minimize the problem. It's also a good idea to lean forward when you urinate, to ensure that your bladder is entirely emptied and to avoid allowing your bladder to get too full. If you do leak regularly, just be aware that when your water breaks, the fluid can trickle or drip out as urine does—so you might confuse the two. It helps to remember that amniotic fluid is clear and odorless and will flow fairly continuously, whereas urine is straw colored with a distinctive smell.

How the placenta ages during pregnancy

At various stages of pregnancy, the "placental grade" may be assessed, which refers to the age of the placenta. This is determined by the number of white spots on its surface. These spots are calcifications, which are signs that the placenta is becoming harder and less effective. The calcified parts eventually die, which puts your baby's health at risk when nutrients and oxygen are restricted, and his waste products are no longer adequately collected.

In a healthy pregnancy, in which your placenta is constantly nourished with nutrients and oxygen from your bloodstream, it will continue to do an effective job until your baby is born.

PREMATURE AGING
The placenta can be affected by "premature" aging, which is a serious condition that could result in your baby not getting the nutrients he needs. This may be evident because he isn't growing adequately or his movements slow down significantly. Your baby may need to be delivered early to ensure his health and safety. This condition occurs most commonly in women who smoke, suffer from diabetes or high blood pressure, or develop an infection by small bacteria known as "Nanobacteria." It may help to ensure that you are getting enough antioxidants via prenatal vitamins, and through your diet (in fresh fruits and vegetables). Some experts believe that antioxidants help prevent premature aging of the placenta.

If you fall into a high-risk category, your doctor or midwife will keep tabs on you, checking your placenta regularly via ultrasound.

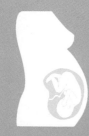

ME AND MY BODY

37 weeks

Your uterus now reaches just over 6in (16cm) from your belly button. If your baby's head is facing down, you may regularly feel sharp (and sometimes painful) kicks to your ribs.

Amazing reflexes

Your baby is busy practicing her skills for life outside the womb: sucking, sleeping, looking around, and urinating. This includes reflexes—instinctive, involuntary, and almost instantaneous reactions—which are designed to protect her and ensure her survival. Your baby will have more than 70 different reflexes at birth. Her doctor will check only a few of these after her birth, since some are more important than others.

Some key reflexes include the Moro reflex (or startle reflex): your baby will thrust her arms outward and then seem to embrace herself while curling her fingers when you fail to support or hold her head or neck. There is also the

Palmar grasp: your baby's fingers curl and cling when you touch the palm of her hand. The Plantar grasp (also known as the Babinski reflex) is when your baby's toes spread open and her foot turns inward when you stroke the sole of her foot.

Your baby will suck when something is placed in her mouth because of the sucking reflex; this ensures that she will suck to feed. She will display the rooting reflex when you stroke her cheek—she will turn toward you, looking for food. The stepping reflex can be seen by placing your baby's feet on a flat surface, which will encourage her to "walk" by placing one foot in front of the other.

Most of her reflexes will naturally disappear before she is six months old.

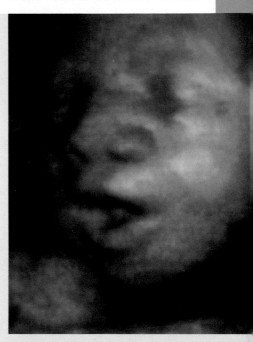

My twins are ready to be born

Twin pregnancies are considered full term at 37 weeks, when your babies' lungs are almost fully mature. Many women (about half) naturally go into labor around or before this time. If your pregnancy extends past this point, your doctor may decide to induce you at 38 weeks, depending upon how your twins are progressing. This is because it was believed that leaving them any longer in the womb could lead to complications. However, although a recent Canadian study found that waiting past 40 weeks increased the risk of the babies dying by 2.5 times, there was little difference

between delivering at 37, 38, or 39 weeks for long-term survival. Thus many doctors now wait until 39 weeks to induce, unless they think that your babies should be delivered earlier.

In most cases, however, moms of twins go into labor much earlier than 37 weeks, rather than later. When this happens, the priority is to keep the twins in the womb as long as possible, and ensure their lungs develop through the use of steroids (see p.315).

Twins tend to be lighter than singleton babies, and you can expect your babies to weigh around 5lb 14oz (2.7kg) at birth.

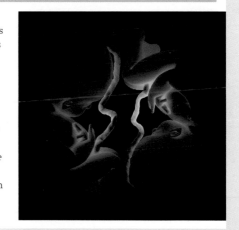

37 weeks

Your baby's growth will begin to slow a little, but she will continue to put on weight until she is born. Her face is filling out and she has recognizable eyelashes and a thicker neck.

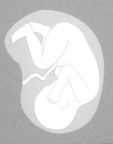

MY BABY

Measuring my baby bump

Toward the end of your pregnancy, your doctor or midwife will assess your baby's growth to assess her well-being in the womb. Her growth will have been measured regularly since about 28 weeks (see p.200), which simply involves measuring the distance between the top of your pubic bone and the top of your uterus (fundus), and plotting it on a chart to make sure that it falls within a normal range. Any aberrations in this figure, which may lead your doctor to suggest that your baby is not growing at the expected level, will probably lead to a referral for an ultrasound, in which your baby can be accurately measured and her well-being assessed.

If there are doubts about her growth or well-being, your doctor may suggest a "non-stress" test and/or biophysical profile (BPP) testing, which observes how your baby responds to stimuli and looks out for signs of fetal distress. In the non-stress test, an external transducer is placed on your abdomen to listen to your baby's heart rate, looking for "accelerations" that last about 15 seconds. The result is considered to be "reassuring" if your baby's heart rate accelerates (speeds up) twice over a 20 to 30 minute period, and there are no large decelerations (slow-downs).

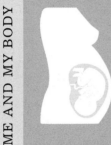

ME AND MY BODY

38 weeks

Your uterus may be as high as 7in (18cm) above your belly button. You may find some relief from discomfort when your baby "drops" into your pelvic cavity and becomes engaged.

Getting through these last few weeks

Managing those last weeks when you're really big and uncomfortable can be a challenge. Try these suggestions:

• Make sure a hospital bag for you and your baby is packed and ready by the front door. Place a waterproof sheet on your bed, just in case your water breaks at night. Keep busy by getting your shopping done, some food stored in the freezer, your route to the hospital planned, your car's tank full of gas, and your birth plan and important phone numbers on hand (in case you go into labor while you are out). And then rest!

• Focus on all the pleasant things you can do alone with your partner before two becomes three—or more.

• Enjoy a little pampering, and get plenty of relaxation. If you are calm and in a positive frame of mind, your labor will be that much more straightforward.

• Although it may be tempting to catch up on household chores and get things organized, you are much better off resting while you can, to prepare yourself for the hard work of labor. Don't be afraid to take nice long naps during the day.

• Take time to refresh your birth plan, and practice breathing techniques and positions for labor to reassure yourself that you are as prepared as possible.

• If you have other children, make sure you have contingency plans for childcare, should you go into labor unexpectedly.

• At this stage, even if you are very frustrated with still being pregnant, the best option is to wait for nature to take its course. Intervention at this stage may lead to a caesarean delivery, which is probably not what you have anticipated.

Slower heart rate

Your baby's heart rate has changed throughout pregnancy, and has been monitored carefully by your doctor or midwife at your routine prenatal appointments. Have you ever wondered what's "normal"?

When your baby's heart begins to beat at about seven weeks, her heart rate will be about the same as yours—80 to 85 beats per minute (BPM). For the remainder of that month, your baby's heart rate will increase by about 3 BPM per day, until about 10 or 11 weeks, when her heart rate will reach approximately 175 BPM. From here, it declines significantly until halfway through your second trimester, settling between 120 and 180 BPM.

In the last 10 weeks of pregnancy, her heart rate will gradually slow again, to somewhere between 120 and 160 BPM, although this can fluctuate at certain times of the day, including when she is sleeping or very active. A drop in her heart rate is often a sign that labor is about to begin, and is usually nothing to worry about. If it accelerates dramatically at any stage, it may be an indication that your baby is in distress (see p.279), and the decision may be made to deliver your baby quickly, by emergency caesarean section.

> "A drop in your baby's heart rate is often a sign that labor is about to begin— usually nothing to worry about"

38 weeks

With a bit of luck, your baby will now be head down in your uterus, with her head descending well into your pelvic cavity on its way to being engaged. She will weigh about 6.6lb (3kg).

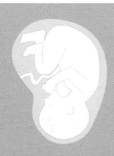

MY BABY

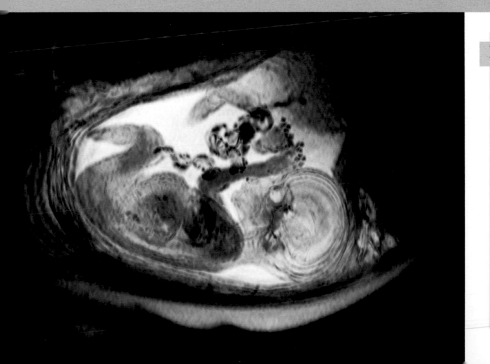

No tears

Although she's now beautifully formed and ready for the challenges of the outside world, one thing she is not prepared to do is cry tears. Most babies cry when they are born—and are, actually, encouraged to do so, to kick-start the process of breathing with big, deep breaths; however, she will not develop tear ducts until a couple of weeks after the birth, so her cries will not be accompanied by a welling up of tears.

Interestingly, she may have been crying for some time now. One researcher was astonished to find babies making "crying faces" at just 18 weeks' gestation.

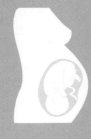

39 weeks

Try not to count the days; only about 5 percent of babies are born on their due dates, with about 75 percent being born later. If this is your first baby, chances are she will be late.

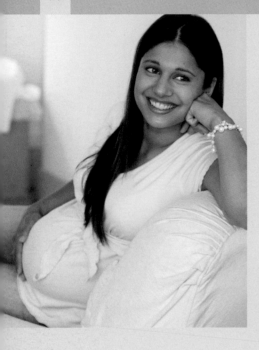

I'm excited . . . and scared!

It is completely normal to feel apprehension at this point in your pregnancy. You may not only feel ill-prepared for your baby's arrival and at the prospect of becoming a parent, but also nervous about the impending labor. Part of you may be desperate to get your pregnancy over with, while another part may be reluctant to let go of this big bump—a familiar companion over the past nine months. Mixed feelings are a common feature of late pregnancy, and partly governed by hormonal activity and natural anxiety.

The most important thing you can do is to put yourself in nature's hands and let her do the work. Your baby will come when she is ready, and you will adapt to motherhood just like you have to every other challenge in your life. You have created the ultimate miracle—a new life—and your instincts will not only take over and help you to nurture, love, and care for your new arrival, but you will find that your life is enhanced on every level.

Relaxation and positive visualization (see pp.286–287) can encourage a positive labor and birth experience. Give yourself a pep talk—you were capable of making a baby, so you are most certainly capable of delivering and caring for her!

How we expected our labors to go

My first baby was breech and delivered by caesarean section, which wasn't nearly as bad as I had anticipated. My second birth was vaginal, and wasn't any better or worse than I had imagined, but I did have complications as a result of my previous caesarean. In all, I am a lot more open-minded now about birth, and am able to encourage my students to be open to every eventuality. TL

One of the worst things about labor is not knowing what it's going to be like. That's not to say that preparation doesn't help, but my first labor was more

unsettling than the subsequent two, simply because I didn't know how long it was going to last, how intense the labor pains were going to be, and how well I could cope. As it happens, it moved along swiftly and before I knew it, I was close to delivering. LJ

As an obstetrician, I was always apprehensive and anxious about labor, since I had seen and been involved in cases where things had not gone according to plan and complications arose. I tried hard to be positive, but it is very difficult when you know what can go wrong. On

the whole, I felt that my labor was much better than I anticipated, and I was discharged two days later, after a vacuum-assisted delivery, with my baby boy. MG

Labor was much quicker than I anticipated! There was no buildup to my contractions, so it was quite a shock for my husband, me, and my new baby, who ended up in the NICU for a while. There were a few dramas in an emergency situation, and at one point we thought we had lost her, but she is now a thriving four-and-a-half-year-old with no problems whatsoever. NK

39 weeks

The average baby is about 20in (51cm) in length, from crown to heels, and weighs around 7.5lb (3.4kg). There are huge variations, but 5.5–8.5lb (2.5–4kg) is considered average and healthy.

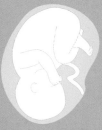

MY BABY

Swollen genitals

Don't be surprised to find that your baby's genitals look enormous when he is born; many new parents are shocked to find that they are so out of proportion with the rest of their new baby's body. This is, however, entirely normal, and things will settle down within a few days or weeks after his birth.

Your baby's genitals are enlarged for a few different reasons. First of all, babies are born with extra fluid in their bodies—probably the result of having inhaled so much amniotic fluid in the womb and being waterlogged—and this is excreted during the first few days of life. Your baby will lose about 10 percent of his birthweight in the days after birth, and this loss is mainly water. Water is retained in specific areas of his body, in particular his face and genitals.

Just before your baby is born, you will pass a large dose of hormones across the placenta and into his or her bloodstream via the placenta. These hormones help with the birth process. They will encourage the genitals to swell temporarily, until the hormones are excreted from the system. Finally, a male baby may have excess fluid in a sac around one or both of his testicles, which is know as "hydrocele." This condition can last a little longer, but should disperse within a few months or, at most, a year after birth.

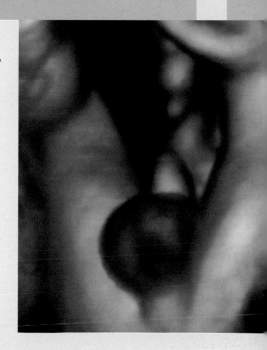

The "molding" of your baby's skull

Your baby's head has taken on an unusual shape. The bones that comprise your baby's skull are designed to move so that her head can pass through the tight birth canal when she is born. The bones of her skull fit together, but they are not firmly attached or "fused." Your baby also has two soft spots, known as "fontanelles," which allow her head to decrease in size as she travels downward.

When your baby takes up her position in the final stages—usually upside down with her head in your pelvis—the bones of her skull change shape to fit your pelvis, in a process known as "molding."

This means that her head can look lopsided—flatter on one side than the other—or pointed. Her cheekbones and her ears may also look out of alignment. If your baby is born via an assisted delivery, her head may take on even more unusual shapes. The good news is that molding is reversed within a week, when your baby's head will take on its standard "round" shape. Her fontanelles will not close for a while yet (see p.173), to allow for the growth of her brain in the first year or so of life. It's worth noting that even after birth, the bones of your baby's head will remain thin and flexible, and

her skull can change shape if pressure is placed upon part of it for long periods of time. Because babies tend to spend a long time on their backs (sleeping, feeding, and playing), they can develop a flattened spot on the back (and sometimes the side) of their heads, known as "plagiocephaly." This does not affect the growth of the brain, but it can cause uneven growth of the face and head.

It is important to avoid leaving your baby in the same position for more than a couple of hours—in her car seat, for example. Try putting her on her tummy or side for brief periods—always supervised.

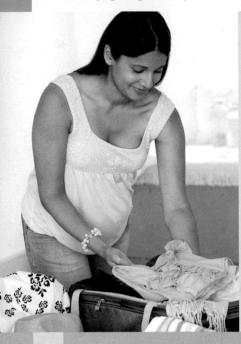

Any time now…

Many new moms (and dads) are surprised to find that their baby isn't delivered on the date that has been established—and written on the calendar—for 40 long weeks. We know now that most babies don't make an appearance until after their due date, but that doesn't mean that you shouldn't be prepared for any eventuality.

Have your hospital bag packed, and your birth plan at the ready. Although most women have a fair bit of warning before active labor (see pp.294–297) begins, there are women whose labors are extremely quick, giving them little or no time to get things organized. Make

sure you've got last-minute, flexible care planned for any other children, and that your birth partner is on call. Rushing around making last-minute arrangements is stressful and will create anxiety that may discourage the progress of your labor, and result in more discomfort.

Equally, however, don't sit by the door with your hospital bag on your knee. Eat well, get plenty of rest, and enjoy being as active as you can, which will stimulate contractions and help to move your baby into the right position for labor. Distract yourself by meeting up with friends, doing a little light shopping, or even booking a massage to relax you before your life changes forever. It can, and will, be any time now. . .

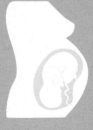

40 weeks

As your labor and delivery approaches, your uterus may have reduced in size a little, as your baby shifts her position and moves down into your pelvis.

Our babies' due dates

My third baby arrived right on his due date, which surprised me more than the other two—who overran by almost a week each. His arrival was so rapid that we barely got to the hospital in time. I vividly remember between contractions urging my husband to call the babysitter to look after our toddlers, and we made it to the hospital with only 26 minutes to spare before he was born. CH

I was induced by having a sweep at 9pm the night before my baby was due, had my water broken before midnight, and she arrived on her due date. NK.

I went into labor the night before my planned caesarean section. Since my son was breech, I still had the caesarean, but a little earlier than planned. In my second pregnancy, my daughter was delivered at 34 weeks by caesarean. VB

I was so eager for the arrival of my first-born that I started getting impatient around 36 weeks; thank goodness she was born five days early. Of course, that set me up for the (false) expectation that my second would also be born ahead of his due date. After two false starts in three days, he was born three days late, and my third was born exactly on time. LJ

My first baby was four days early, because of a planned Caesarean section. My second baby, delivered vaginally, was 10 days late! TL

With my first pregnancy, I went into labor two days before my due date. With my second pregnancy, my daughter was in no rush to be born! I started having a leak of fluid three days after my due date, but still no sign of labor after 24 hours. I had to be admitted for induction, and this took another 24 hours. Finally, I had my water broken and she was born 12 hours later, but well worth the wait! MG

Full-term baby

Every sense, organ, and body system in your baby is now mature. Your baby's average crown-to-heel length will be 20.2in (51.2cm) and the average weight will be 7.6lb (3.5kg). She will have a plump, rounded appearance and chubby cheeks. She has all of her little bits in place, including eyelashes, eyebrows, fingernails, and perhaps even some hair. She is able to breathe, and although her sight will take some time to develop after her birth, she will be able to see you when she is born. She'll be able to move, feed, respond to the world around her, and, most importantly, begin the process of bonding with her mom and dad.

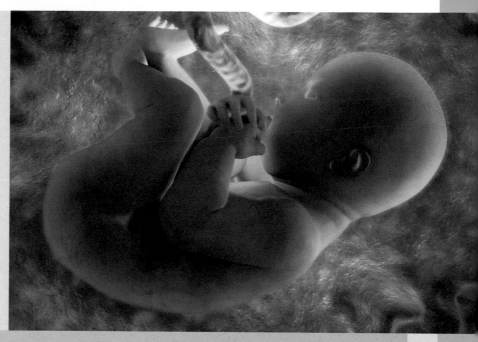

40 weeks

At full term, your baby is ready to go. She may have gained a little weight and length, but her growth has largely slowed as she prepares for her birth.

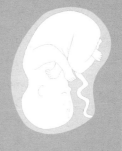

MY BABY

How your baby takes her very first breaths

In just a minute or two, your baby will have to adapt from her entirely liquid home in the womb to an air-filled environment where she will have to take her first breaths. Although she has been practicing breathing in the womb, there has been absolutely no transfer of air. Her lungs have learned to inflate and deflate, but her circulation has been wired to bypass her lungs, and her oxygen has been supplied by you.

This sudden transformation is nothing short of miraculous. In an incredibly short time, her circulatory system—including her heart—will be redirected, fluid will be expelled from her lungs, and she will draw in air, which her body will have to learn instantly how to use.

HOW THIS PROCESS OCCURS
Your baby is stimulated to breathe by the rapidly flowing oxygen levels in her blood. Her chest will have been compressed in the birth canal, and its sudden release may contribute to her need to breathe. Babies born by caesarean do not have the fluid "massaged" out of their lungs by traveling down the birth canal, and may take a moment or two longer to expel it, but from there, the process is the same. When your baby first breathes, her lungs expand to almost full capacity, and it is at this point that the relationships between all of her chest organs change dramatically. At the same time, the blood vessels in her umbilical cord are made redundant, and if they have not already constricted, they will do so when your baby takes her first breath. Her first cry is evidence that she has made the transition from your uterus to the outside world safely. You may feel a huge sense of relief when you hear it, and chances are your new baby is triumphant!

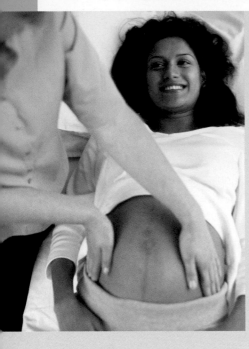

Being assessed

When you pass your due date, you may have more frequent prenatal appointments, during which your doctor or midwife will carefully monitor the health and well-being of both you and your baby, ensure that your placenta is still in good working order and able to supply your baby with the nutrients and oxygen she needs, and monitor your baby's heart rate and movements to ensure that all is well.

Your baby's heartbeat may be monitored using a Doppler scan or an ultrasound, which will be used to assess various factors, including your baby's continued growth, her position and your placenta's position, your baby's activity levels, and the volume of amniotic fluid. If there are any concerns, induction may be suggested, but in most cases your doctor or midwife will be happy to wait until up to 42 weeks before going down that path. Although this is a point of some controversy, there is some evidence to suggest that your placenta may stop working efficiently after 42 weeks (known as "placental insufficiency"), and your doctor or midwife may be eager to get your baby out into the world. You may be very happy to consider this prospect, particularly if you are becoming anxious and tired. The good news is that you are unlikely to have to wait more than a week to meet your new baby at last.

Coping with induction

You may feel concerned if you have to be induced. Consider these points to reassure yourself:

• Having all the facts about induction can help you prepare for and get through the process. Make sure your birth plan includes your wishes about induction and brief your birth partner about the process. Ask questions about what's being planned and done, so you can feel in control.

• Some women believe that anything short of a completely natural birth is a failure and a poor reflection upon themselves. However, it's very important to remember that your ultimate goal is to have a happy, healthy baby—as safely as possible. Pregnancies that go far past their due dates are at a much greater risk of complications, and induction is a reasonable, noninvasive way to get your labor jump-started and going.

• If your baby is in the right position, try some deep squats to help her descend and encourage her head to press down on your cervix. This will act as a signal for your labor to start.

• The secret here is patience. Induction of labor can take a long time if your body is not prepared for it—even days. Buy a few good books, and then tell all of your friends and relatives to await news from you instead of seeking it. Get your bags ready, have your birthing props on hand, and try to stay positive!

• Try to remember that induction does not always mean a whole lot of medical intervention. Sometimes something as simple as a membrane sweep (see p.281) is enough of a trigger to start labor.

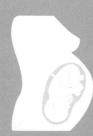

41 weeks

Some evidence suggests that your placenta become less efficient after 42 weeks, and your doctors may be eager to encourage your baby's birth before complications arise.

Late arrival

Babies who are born after full term (37 to 40 weeks) are considered overdue; when they go beyond 42 weeks, they become "post-mature" (see below). While you may be anxious about your baby's health and very eager to get on with the business of delivering her, it is important to remember that babies are all unique, and have their own individual timetables. Throughout this pregnancy calendar we have described the physical and cognitive developmental changes that have occurred throughout your pregnancy, week by week; however, the truth is that your baby may be far ahead of this agenda, or may fall a little behind. In the vast majority of cases, your baby will arrive when her body is sufficiently mature for her to do so. Although you may be anxious to hold your new baby in your arms, she will come when the time is right for her.

Having a "late" baby is not a bad thing. Most late babies who are still in a healthy environment—with a placenta that is still working well—weigh more, which can make them sturdier and more resilient to the challenges of the outside world. They may also appear to be more alert than babies who are born earlier, with stronger Apgar scores (which relates to a test done as soon as your baby is born; see p.325). Their lungs will be fully mature, and they will have benefited from being nurtured longer. They are likely to have more hair than a baby born on or just after the due date, and also be a little plumper.

If your baby has not arrived by 42 weeks, your pregnancy is considered to be "prolonged," and action will normally be taken to get things going by inducing you. This usually starts with a membrane sweep (see p.281), which involves inserting a finger into your vagina and clearing the tissue between your cervix and the amniotic sac. You can refuse induction, but it is worth remembering that complications are much more likely to occur after 42 weeks (see below), and it may be a risk that is not worth taking. You can, however, attempt to get things going yourself, and there are plenty of ways that this can be undertaken (see p.275).

Post-maturity and what it means for your baby

Fewer than six percent of babies are born post-mature, and it is not known why some pregnancies last longer than others. You are more likely to have a post-mature baby if you have experienced one or more in the past, or if the condition runs in your family. It is also believed that post-mature babies occur more commonly in well-nourished women, and there is evidence that pregnancies last longer in the summer than in the winter.

Post-maturity can be a concern because your amniotic fluid may decrease, and your baby may stop gaining weight and you may not be able to provide her with enough oxygen to get through the labor—this is because of placental aging (see p.218). She may suffer from low blood sugar (hypoglycemia) because she has too few stores to keep her going, and she is at greater risk of breathing in meconium (see p.215). The risk of stillbirth increases after 42 weeks.

AFTER THE BIRTH
Signs of post-maturity in your baby include dry, peeling skin, overgrown nails, abundant hair on her head, creases on her palms and the soles of her feet, minimal fat deposits, and yellowish/greenish skin coloring from meconium staining.

It's worth remembering that although your baby is later than expected, she may not have any problems at all. An assessment will be made, examining her physical appearance and comparing it to the length of your pregnancy. In most cases, no treatment will be required, although low blood-sugar levels may need to be addressed, and your baby may require aspiration to remove any meconium that has entered her lungs. Post-mature babies are very likely to be healthy, alert, and, most of all, well worth the wait.

41 weeks

At 41 weeks, the average baby weighs more than 7.7lbs (3.5kg), but could weigh considerably more (or, sometimes, a bit less). She will be about 20.5in (52cm) or more in length.

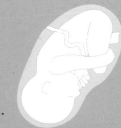

MY BABY

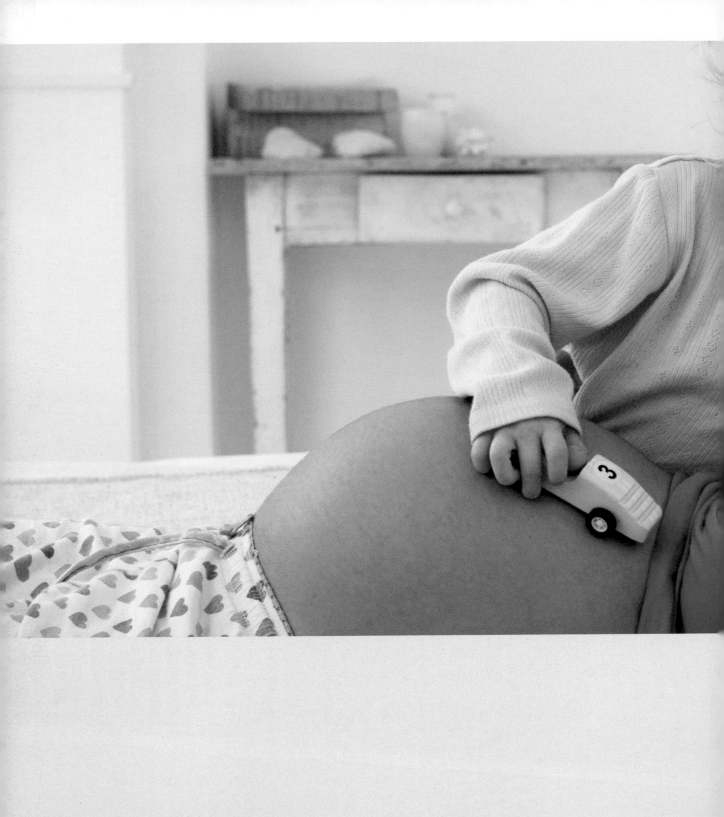

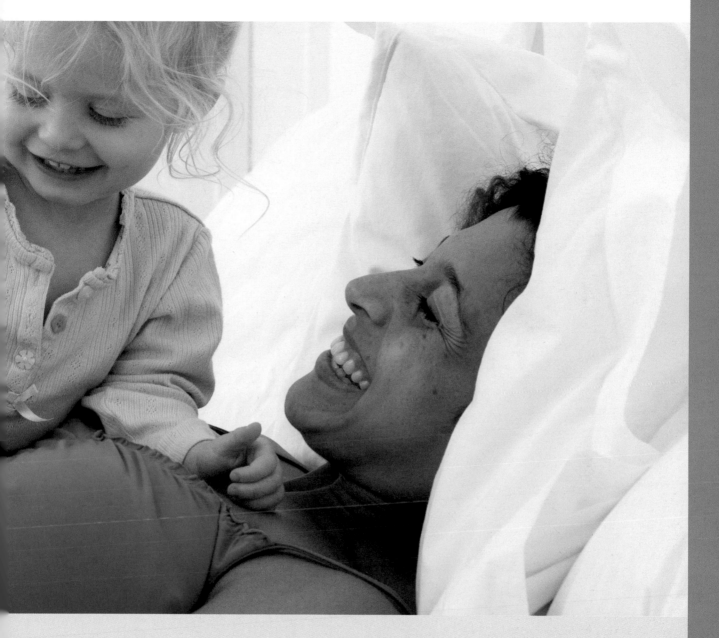

Preparing for motherhood

Planning and getting organized for your baby's birth in advance is not only great fun, it's absolutely essential for busy moms-to-be.

Working mom-to-be

Juggling pregnancy and work can be a daunting prospect at first. Keeping your employer informed means you can work together to plan your leave and ensure your environment is safe and comfortable during pregnancy.

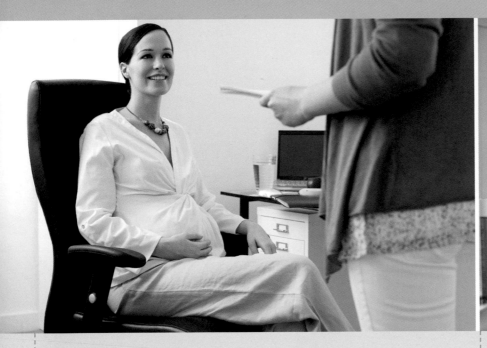

MEETING YOUR NEEDS
A work-station assessment looks at ways to ensure your comfort, health, and safety as pregnancy progresses, by rearranging your computer equipment for example, and making sure that you have space under the desk to move your legs freely.

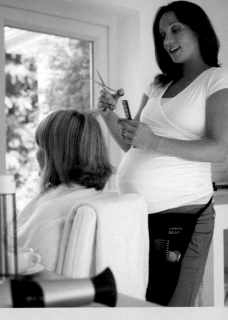

EASING THE STRAIN
If your job involves a lot of standing, talk to your employer about switching to less tiring tasks, or find ways to sit down when you can.

When you become pregnant, one of the first things you are likely to consider is how having a baby will impact your working life. Finding out what you're entitled to can ease anxiety about how you'll cope and help you to plan ahead.

Maternity rights

When you have a baby, you are entitled to take a certain amount of time off work to recover from the birth and to care for your newborn. You may or may not be paid during this time off. You also retain the right to return to the same, or an equivalent, position at your company, with equivalent pay and benefits. It's against the law for your employer to dismiss you or lay you off for any reason connected to pregnancy, childbirth, or maternity leave. Each province and territory has its own legislation regarding job protection during pregnancy as well as maternity and parental leave, so you should check with your company's human resources department for the specifics in your area.

Maternity and parental leave

There are two types of leave available to new parents that will give you job-protected, unpaid time off work. Both are regulated by your provincial or territorial government, so the amount of time that you are eligible for will depend on where you live. Maternity leave, sometimes called pregnancy leave, is available for birth mothers only, and ranges from 15–18 weeks. Parental leave can be taken by either parent and ranges from 12–52 weeks. In some jurisdictions, parental leave can be shared between the parents. In most provinces and territories, you must have completed a specific period of continuous employment with a company to qualify for leave. Your employer does not have to pay you during your time off, although some of them do. You need to inform your employer at least 15 weeks before you plan to begin your leave. Speak to your human resources department about your specific situation.

Maternity and parental benefits

You may also be entitled to receive benefits that will pay you while you are on leave. Benefits are provided by the federal Employment Insurance Act (EI)—you are eligible if you have worked a minimum of 600 hours in the last 52 weeks and have been contributing to the EI program. The basic benefit is 55 percent of your average insured earnings, up to a certain yearly maximum. Some employers have a benefit plan that will "top up" this amount.

Eligible birth mothers are entitled to a maximum of 15 weeks of paid maternity benefits. If you decide to stop working before your due date, you can start receiving your benefits up to 8 weeks before your due date.

Parental benefits of up to 35 weeks are also available for either eligible parent, and can be shared between them. If the birth mother decides to take both the maternity and the complete parental benefits, she can receive a total of 50 weeks' benefits. Parental benefits can be claimed starting the day of your baby's birth.

EI benefits are considered taxable income, which means that both federal and provincial or territorial taxes will be deducted from your payment. You will need to apply for EI benefits as soon as you stop working, either in person at a Service Canada Center or online at www.servicecanada.gc.ca.

Benefits for the self-employed

Thanks to recent regulations, self-employed parents can now apply for EI coverage for maternity and parental benefits. You need to register for the EI program, pay an insurance premium, and have earned a specified minimum amount of self-employed earnings during the calendar year before the year you submit a claim. Visit www.servicecanada.gc.ca for more details.

Benefits for Quebec residents

Instead of EI, self-employed and salaried residents of Quebec are covered by the Quebec Parental Insurance Plan (QPIP). Birth mothers can receive up to 18 weeks of benefits. Fathers can receive up to 5 weeks of paternity benefits. In addition, there are parental benefits of up to 32 weeks which can be used entirely by the mother or shared between both parents. There are two benefit plans available: the basic plan pays lower benefits for a longer period, and the special plan pays higher benefits for a shorter period. Go to www.rqap.gouv.qc.ca for more details.

Returning to work

Inform your employer at least 4 weeks before you plan to return to work. It's wise to look into child care options while you are still pregnant to see what options are available. Check to see if you are eligible for the Canada Child Tax Benefit, which can help with child care costs.

Combining pregnancy and work

I was in my final year of pediatric training during my first pregnancy; I worked the same number of hours, was expected to take the same number of overnight calls, and ended up working up until the day I delivered! In fact, I vomited all the way through 19 weeks of pregnancy—largely, I believe, because I took overnight calls that required me to get up quickly and run down hospital hallways in the night. With no time allotted for rest, getting up slowly, or eating something when you first get up (all standard advice), it was common for me to return from attending a middle-of-the-night delivery and vomit in the hallway trashcan before returning to lie down and wait for my next summons! LJ

I was a resident doctor during both of my pregnancies. In my first pregnancy I worked full time and found early mornings the worst part of the day—it was hard to get out of bed and I felt very nauseated as soon as I did. I hadn't told colleagues that I was pregnant because I had suffered a miscarriage before. Fortunately, my pregnancy progressed well and I stopped working at around 36 weeks. MG

I was more conscious of safety at work when I was pregnant and more protective of myself, trying to stick to my 9-to-5 hours, rather than overwork. CH

I felt well through both pregnancies, but coping with long hours was hard. When I noticed contractions while working, I realized I needed to slow down! I stopped working around 36 weeks. VB

Preparing siblings

Finding out that a little brother or sister is on the way can be both exciting and concerning for an older child. With some thoughtful planning, you can help him feel secure of his position in the family and happily embrace the new addition.

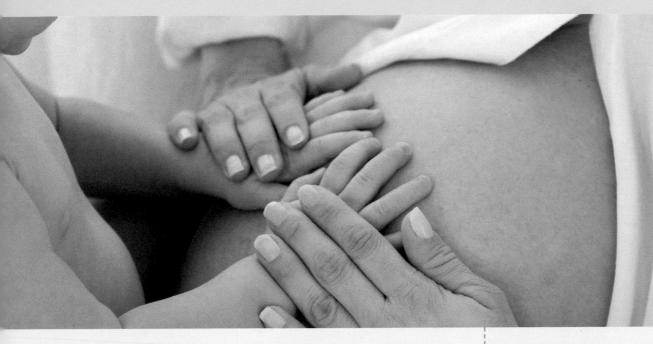

Before telling an older child that you are pregnant, take some time to think about how best to prepare her for the arrival of her sibling. Bear in mind that she may feel concerned about how the baby will affect the family—after all, up until now she has been the center of attention.

Telling your child

You may decide to wait until after your first ultrasound, when you may feel more certain that the pregnancy is going well, before breaking the news to your older child. When you tell your child may also depend on her age—very young children have an elastic sense of time, and can find it hard to understand that their new

brother or sister won't be making an appearance for eight or nine months. On the other hand, telling your child early on in pregnancy gives her time to come to terms with the idea of a new baby. If you do tell your toddler early on, link the date of the birth to a significant event around the same time, such as a birthday or a religious festival, to help her understand that there's a while to wait.

When you break the news, keep things simple. Explain to your child that a baby is growing in your tummy and will be arriving around a certain date. Tell her that your tummy will become very big and you may become more tired than usual. Reassure her that you have plenty of love and time for more than one child. You may want to point out that although

HELPING YOUR CHILD CONNECT
Let your child stroke your growing tummy, talk to the baby, and feel her kick to help make the event more real for her.

her new sibling will be lots of fun in years to come, he may be hard work at first, and that she can help to care for the baby if she wants. Giving her a defined role and making it clear what is ahead will encourage her to feel involved and help ease the transition.

INVOLVING YOUR CHILD
Encourage your older child to share the experience with you. Show her your ultrasound pictures as well as your growing tummy and read her story books about a new baby arriving in a family to

"Older children need to be given ample warning of the new baby so they have time to prepare and some idea of what to expect"

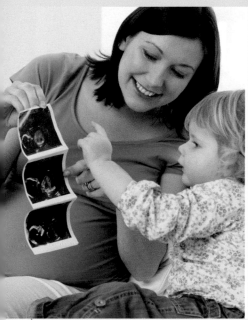

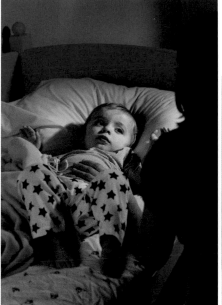

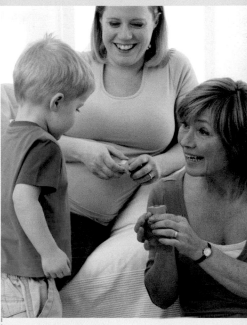

SHARING YOUR NEWS
Excite your child's interest with your scan pictures, and let her come to a prenatal appointment to hear the baby's heartbeat.

SETTLING YOUR TODDLER
If your toddler needs to move out of his crib into a bed, give him plenty of time to adjust to his new surroundings before the baby is born.

A HELPING HAND
Spending time with a grandparent before the birth will ensure your child is relaxed if she looks after him when you go to the hospital.

encourage her understanding and prompt questions about how life will change once the baby has arrived.

Help your child to feel involved by asking her to help you choose equipment, clothing, room colors, and furnishings for the new baby—but give her a limited range of options to choose from, all of which you are happy with!

Nearer the time of the birth, talk to her about who will take care of her when you are in the hospital; and let her know that she has a couple of treats lined up to give her something to look forward to.

Meeting the baby

Buy a small gift for your toddler to give her new sibling, and one for the baby to give her. This makes it a celebration, and helps your child feel favorably toward the new baby. You could also put aside a couple of small gifts for your toddler so she doesn't feel left out when friends arrive with gifts for the baby.

Show her how to stroke your baby gently, and hold your child while she holds the baby, helping her support the baby's head. Set some rules too, such

as not pulling the baby's hair, putting anything on her face, giving her anything to eat or drink, or picking her up. Having said that, always supervise them together.

Your child has been the center of your attention so is bound to feel some jealousy. Help her to feel involved by assisting with small jobs, such as passing a diaper. Make sure, too, that you spend time with her, occasionally asking someone else to watch your baby while you play a game together. When you have to focus on your baby, for example when feeding her, set up your toddler with a snack or toy.

What will my baby need?

The weeks after your baby's birth will be taken up with feeding, changing, bathing, settling, and getting to know your newborn. Get organized in advance by buying the essentials so you can concentrate on your baby when she arrives.

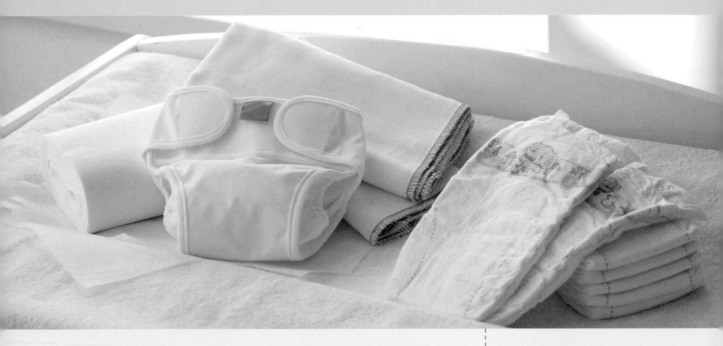

Aim to buy everything you need for your baby while you still have the energy to shop. Consider what you can borrow or buy second-hand.

Buying diapers

One thing that is essential as soon as your baby is born is a supply of diapers, which she'll need until she is two or three years old. You can buy reusable or disposable ones (or a combination)—there are advantages to each. Your baby will go through 10 to 14 diapers a day, or more, in the early weeks, but don't buy too many of the same size—she will outgrow the smallest sizes quickly and, if you have a big baby, they may never fit. It's

impossible to know exactly what size your baby will be, but you could ask your doctor to give you a rough idea so hopefully you buy the right size at first.

REUSABLE DIAPERS

There's a wide range of cloth diapers, which nowadays use Velcro tabs instead of pins. You will need 20 to 24 diapers, since they take time to launder and dry. You'll also need a diaper bucket with a lid to put soiled and wet diapers in; plastic or rubber outerpants (about six, since they can be rinsed between wearings); and diaper liners, which form a barrier between the diaper and your baby's bottom, and can be lifted out to dispose of stools. You can choose sensitive detergents to protect your baby's skin.

WHICH DIAPER?

Once you've decided which type of diaper you want to use, buy enough for a couple of weeks to keep you going after the birth.

DISPOSABLE DIAPERS

Buy these according to your baby's age. There's little variation between brands although some use fewer manmade chemicals. You can buy "bikini"-style diapers for newborns, which fold down or are cut to sit below the umbilical cord to allow it to heal without irritation.

WIPES AND MORE

When changing diapers you will also need the following:
• Thin washable cloths or cotton balls to clean your baby's bottom, and a

"If you don't manage to buy everything you need before the birth, don't panic—you'll still be able to shop after your baby is born"

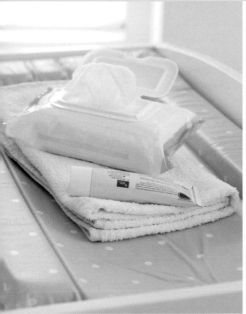

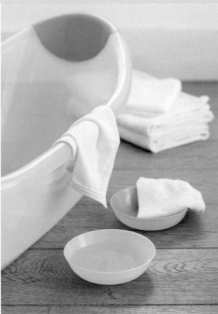

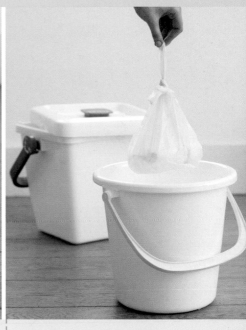

YOUR CHANGING STATION
Choose a designated spot where you can keep together all the equipment you need to change your baby's diaper.

BATHTIME ESSENTIALS
A baby bath is ideal for stress-free bathing. Stock up on soft towels and washcloths to make bathtimes comfortable.

DISPOSING OF DIAPERS
A bucket or diaper bin is convenient for disposing of throwaway diapers, or to store reusables before washing.

Caring for the environment

I tried to be green, but didn't have any success with the washable diapers. However, I ended up doing the next best thing, which was using more environmentally-friendly diapers. I also made sure that I used as many natural products on my babies as possible, avoiding chemicals in washing products, soaps, oils, wipes, and everything else, whenever possible. When they were weaned onto solids, I chose organic food when it was possible. TL

I have to admit that I was greener with my first baby, using cloth diapers throughout. But, as the work load piled up with second and third babies, I did resort to disposables, biodegradable though they were. CH

When I had my children 10–15 years ago, the environment wasn't such a big area of concern. I certainly believe that consideration for the environment is important, but even when it comes to things like disposable versus reusable diapers, the sense I get from researching the subject is that one is not clearly better than the other in terms of its impact on the environment. LJ

I probably didn't try hard enough to be kind to the environment, and I must admit that I feel a little bit guilty about not giving the "green" diapers a try. NK

travel-size pack of baby wipes.
• A barrier cream to prevent or treat diaper rash; choose one with zinc oxide.
• Diaper sacks for disposing of dirty diapers when you're out.
• A changing bag.
• Plastic changing mats: one for at home and a foldaway one for your diaper bag.

Keeping your baby clean

Invest in a few essential basics for bathing your baby:
• A sturdy baby bath is a good purchase if you have the space (although you can also use the bathroom or kitchen sink, or even the full-sized tub).
• A bath thermometer.
• A mild baby bath/shampoo combination product.
• Thin washcloths that allow you to clean in your baby's skin creases.

• Three or four baby towels with hoods to keep your baby warm while drying her or before you put her in the bath.
• A non-slip mat (if you plan to bathe her in a full-sized tub).

Baby clothes

Babies outgrow their clothing very quickly, so try to avoid buying too many items in the smallest size. Baby clothes are also a popular gift for new moms, and you may find that your baby ends up with a wardrobe full of items that she quickly grows out of. Tell family and friends that you'd appreciate gifts in slightly larger sizes for your baby to grow into, and then purchase a few basics in the smaller sizes. Avoid anything that is complicated to fasten—for the first few weeks you will find onesies and one-piece pajamas most convenient; they allow easy access for diaper changes and keep your baby snug. Go for soft,

comfortable, machine-washable fabrics without fussy or itchy seams or tags.

Bear in mind that baby shops stock clothing seasonally, so a bathing suit in the next size up may not be useful when your baby grows into it during the winter.

Baby clothes also tend to come in similar color combinations, and for good reason. Clothing that can be mixed and matched without requiring a whole change when one item becomes dirty is ideal. Choosing a selection of socks in the same color also means that you can avoid wasting time looking for a matching pair. Even the tiniest babies have an uncanny knack of losing socks and hats.

A good first wardrobe will include:
• 5–8 short-sleeved onesies. In the winter, they act as an extra layer to insulate your baby; they can be worn alone in warmer months. Choose cotton all-in-ones with snaps at the crotch.
• 5–8 sleepsuits. Choose loose-fitting all-in-ones, with snaps.
• 2 drawstring nightgowns.

ESSENTIAL ONESIES
This staple item is a versatile part of your baby's wardrobe, providing extra warmth as an undergarment in the colder months, or worn on its own on hot days. As your baby grows, long-sleeved onesies can be added to wear with pull-up pants.

ONE-PIECE PAJAMAS
These are perfect for young babies, providing warmth, comfort, and easy access for diaper changing. As a matter of fact, your baby is likely to wear little else—both night and day—for the first few months. Look for front-opening suits with convenient snaps.

JACKETS AND COATS
The key to dressing your baby is to go for layers. A sweater can be easily added indoors in the winter and for trips outside on fresh spring days. Choose lightweight coats with cozy hoods and soft fabrics for added warmth and comfort.

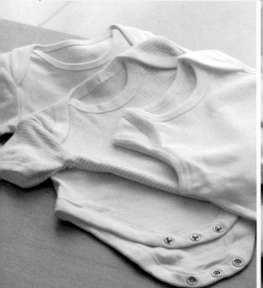

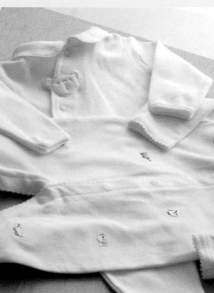

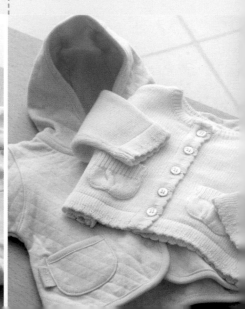

What we couldn't do without

If you have enough room, a changing table with storage space is essential in my opinion; it helps you to look after your back after having a baby. I had a mobile changing table with a small basin under the mattress for bathing my baby. Every evening I would wheel the table into the bathroom, and give my son his bath before bedtime. I also strongly recommend a comfortable nursing chair for the nursery or your bedroom. Whether you breast- or bottle-feed, there are times (especially in the middle of the night) when you need to be comfortable and rested in order to feed your baby. MG

Onesies and pajamas dominated my baby's wardrobe. I seemed to be constantly taking layers on and off to keep him warm—but not overheated—as we went about our daily routine. CH

I would recommend scratch mittens to prevent your baby from inadvertently scratching herself while she gains control of her limbs. An all-in-one outdoor suit is perfect, particularly if it has mittens and a hood attached. Baby shoes are definitely not necessary for months to come, and dresses for girls are unlikely to see the light of day for the first few weeks—and even months. NK

Both of my babies were born in heat waves, so I didn't need anything apart from diapers, onesies, and short-sleeved pajamas. TL

Hats are important for newborns when outside to stop them from losing heat from their heads. Overall, the best clothing is soft and comfortable, without buttons and frills. Easy-to-fasten (and unfasten) snaps and baby-friendly zippers are much more practical, particularly for late-night changes and when your baby is not in the mood for a change of clothing. LJ

- 1–2 sweaters or jackets. Go for light options, and avoid anything that has to be pulled over your baby's head.
- 1 warm coat or snowsuit. Choose a brand with a detachable hood, if possible, and an easy fastening.

WRAPPED UP WARM
A fleecy snowsuit is a must-have item for babies born in winter months. Some come complete with attached booties, or add socks and mittens as required. Remove snowsuits once indoors to prevent your baby from becoming hot and uncomfortable.

- 5–8 pairs of socks or booties. If your baby is wearing footed pajamas, you may not need these, but you may want to keep her toes warm if she's in her onesie. Socks also double up as scratch mittens.
- 1–2 hats (or bonnets). Choose one with

ALL-WEATHER ACCESSORIES
Hats, mittens, and socks are the essential extras for your baby's wardrobe. Soft, warm hats and mittens keep your baby cozy outside on cold days; in the summer, wide-brimmed hats protect her from the sun. Socks and booties will ensure her feet don't get cold.

a wide brim for summer, or something soft that covers the ears in the winter.

What else does your baby need?

Whether you breast- or bottle-feed your baby, you will need some equipment and/or clothing to get started (see pp.242–243). You also need to buy a bed, bedding, and other sleeping items (see pp.244–47), and you may want to have a changing table.

Toys aren't essential at first, but you may want a couple of items to stimulate her. Toys for newborns take into account that she can see only a short distance and won't see everything in full color for a few weeks. The following are ideal:
- A brightly colored mobile for your baby's crib or bassinet.
- A light rattle: try wrist or sock rattles.
- Soft toys that crinkle, ring, or rattle when touched, with a variety of textures.
- A soft, washable cuddly toy: babies can form attachments in the early weeks.
- Musical toys.
- Comfort toys, blankets, and pacifiers.

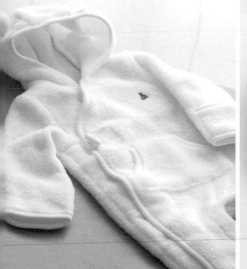

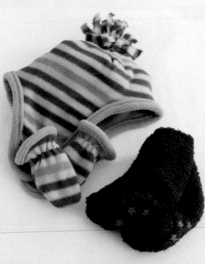

How will I feed my baby?

There is no doubt that breast milk is the ideal first food for your baby, and with a little guidance most women manage breastfeeding successfully. If this is not for you, formula has all the nutrients your baby needs to grow and thrive.

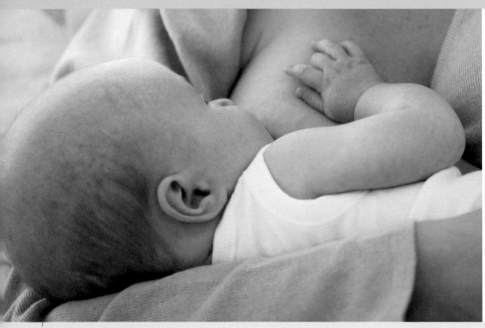

READY TO BREASTFEED
Once you've established breastfeeding, you will find it a wonderfully convenient way to feed your baby—you will have the right amount of food at exactly the right temperature without any preparation, whenever and wherever she is hungry.

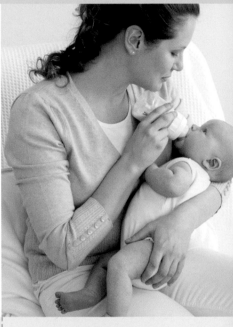

GIVING YOUR BABY A BOTTLE
If you choose to bottle-feed, formula contains all the nutrients your baby needs. You'll need to learn how to clean the equipment and make up a bottle.

It's definitely worth putting some thought into how you will feed your baby. If you want to give breastfeeding a try, there are several ways to prepare before the birth. Read up on breastfeeding and look into prenatal classes on the subject—some courses hold extra sessions on it. These sessions are a great opportunity to discuss techniques and, often, to meet breastfeeding moms and watch them in action. Of course, if you wish to bottle-feed, you will need to prepare by buying bottles, formula, and equipment.

Breastfeeding

Not only is breastfeeding free, extremely convenient, and the most natural way to feed your baby, but it also protects as well as nourishes your baby, and has benefits for you, too.

BREAST IS BEST
The composition of breast milk changes constantly to allow for your baby's individual growth and changing nutritional needs. Apart from nutrition,

breast milk has a lot of added bonuses. Research has found that breastfed babies have fewer incidences of vomiting and diarrhea, and that breast milk protects against gastroenteritis, as well as ear infections, respiratory illnesses, pneumonia, bronchitis, kidney infections, and septicemia (blood poisoning). Breastfed babies also have a reduced risk of chronic constipation, colic, and other stomach disorders, and the fat contained in human milk, compared with cow's milk, is more digestible for babies and allows for greater absorption of fat-soluble vitamins into the bloodstream. This is important because healthy fats, including essential fatty acids (EFAs; see p.51) are necessary for healthy growth and optimal development, particularly in the brain. What's more, calcium and other important nutrients are better utilized when they come from human milk. Human milk also promotes healthy growth, largely due to the presence of certain hormones in breast milk; and while antigens in cow's milk can cause allergic reactions in a newborn, such reactions to human milk are rare.

The long-term benefits are clear, too. Breastfed babies have a reduced risk of developing childhood diabetes and obesity, and breast milk is also thought to offer protection against allergies such as asthma and eczema.

Most important, breastfeeding your baby reduces her risk of sudden infant death syndrome, or SIDS (see p.357): research has found that breastfed babies accounted for just three out of every 87 deaths from SIDS.

There is plenty of other interesting evidence about the unique benefits of breastfeeding. The way babies suck on the breast is quite different from using a bottle, for example. This is thought to help the development of your baby's facial structure and encourage straighter teeth. Moreover, studies indicate that brain and nervous-system development is improved in breastfed babies, who may develop higher IQs. For this reason, breastfeeding is sometimes referred to as the "fourth trimester" because of the way in which it assists brain growth and development in newborns.

The emotional benefits of breastfeeding are also well documented. Breastfed babies enjoy a warm, emotional relationship with their mothers, and skin-to-skin contact is believed to promote bonding. With so many obvious benefits, it is definitely worth making breastfeeding your first choice.

WHAT YOU'LL NEED

Although one of the benefits of breastfeeding is the fact that it is readily available and does not require special equipment, there are a few items that help it run smoothly. A comfortable chair with sturdy arms and a supportive back is essential, and a U-shaped feeding pillow can make the experience more comfortable. You will need two or three well-fitted nursing bras that you can fasten and unfasten with one hand, and breast pads to deal with leaking breasts. Some women find breast shields useful for periods when their nipples become sore. An emollient nipple cream can also prevent chapping and relieve any discomfort. If you are planning to express your milk (see p.347), you will need the following:
• A pump (electric or manual); electric pumps can often be rented from a hospital or medical-supply store.
• 2–4 feeding bottles to store your expressed milk (see p.240).

Our breastfeeding experiences

As a pediatrician, I was not only well informed about the benefits of breastfeeding, but had the added advantage of additional training by breastfeeding professionals at the hospital as part of my job. So I knew exactly how to ensure that each of my children learned how to latch on correctly. This helped me to avoid cracked, sore, bleeding, or blistered nipples. My firstborn had a very weak suck and required frequent feeds for much longer than most, but I knew the importance of keeping her nursing long enough to gain weight. LJ

I planned to breastfeed exclusively for the first few months, but found my baby was still hungry after feeds and wasn't putting on enough weight. I ended up topping up with formula after feeds from about six weeks, so that she could have extra if she needed it. It's important not to pressure yourself or feel like a failure if breastfeeding doesn't go according to plan. If you've given it your best shot and you have to bottle-feed or combine feed, don't beat yourself up about it. Your baby will be fine! TL

I had planned to breastfeed both my children, because I am well aware of the benefits of breast milk for babies. Although I had a slippery start, with sleepless nights, sore nipples, and a constantly hungry baby, I breastfed both of my babies on demand and I would say that the secret to success is definitely perseverance. MG

I did manage to breastfeed all my children, but it took a great effort of will, plenty of reminders to myself that I didn't want to miss out on this experience, and good support from experts to get over the first few days when it was so painful. CH

I always planned to breastfeed, and although my little one lost over 10 percent of her birth weight in the first few weeks, I still managed to breastfeed for a year without ever trying formula. I also returned to work after four months, so spent a lot of time expressing milk for my husband to feed our daughter by bottle! I found that if I stayed well hydrated and drank fennel tea (which acts to increase milk supply), I always had plenty for my baby. NK

I was determined to breastfeed, but it required dedication to manage the discomfort of the first few weeks, and the endless feeds during growth spurts. VB

"Reaching an informed decision about how you will feed your baby will ensure that you are doing what is best for both you and your baby"

• Suitable nipples (see below).
• Cleaning equipment (see below) and a brush to clean the pump, bottles, and nipples.
• Plastic bags or bottles for storing and freezing your milk.

Bottle-feeding

Some women struggle with the concept of breastfeeding, or find it difficult in practice. The good news is that formula offers your baby all of the essential nutrients she needs, in exactly the right quantities. All of the leading brands are fairly similar in terms of their ingredients. Most formula is based on cow's milk that has been modified to resemble breast milk as closely as possible, with the same quantities of protein, fats, and carbohydrates, as well as vitamins and minerals. As long as you buy formula that is appropriate for your baby's age; make up bottles exactly as instructed on the packaging; take care when heating your baby's bottle; and are scrupulous about hygiene, bottle-feeding is a healthy, practical way to feed your baby.

Newborn bottle-fed babies normally have six to eight feeds a day, with a total intake of 32 fl oz (945 ml) over this period. As well as powdered formula, it's handy to keep some cartons of ready-made formula in the cupboard (the same brand if possible) for emergencies.

Buy everything you need for bottle-feeding before the birth, including a dedicated brush for cleaning and nipples for different stages, and make sure you know how to make up your baby's feeds.

BUYING BOTTLES
For newborns you will need six to eight smaller bottles, since younger babies do not consume much milk at one sitting. There are a variety of bottles available, including ventilated and disposable ones, and some that self-sterilize. Investigate the options and choose one that you think will be best for your baby and your lifestyle. You may decide, though, to change the type of bottle you use if your baby has a problem such as colic (see p.359).

CHOOSING A BOTTLE
Apart from the standard plastic bottles, you can also choose from vented bottles, which are designed to reduce the amount of air your baby takes in while feeding; glass bottles that are chemical-free; and BPA-free plastic bottles.

STOCKING UP ON FORMULA
Always follow the instructions when making up formula, using the scoop provided. Make sure, too, that you buy the right formula for your baby's age.

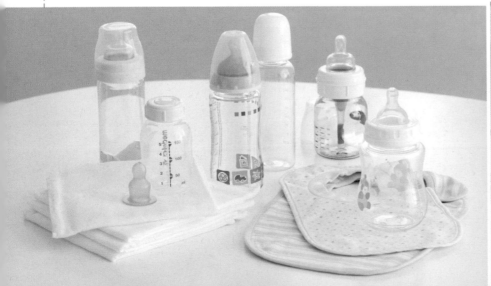

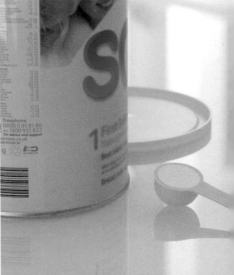

What's in formula

The production of all infant formula milk is closely regulated to ensure that it contains exactly the right ingredients for your baby to grow and thrive. As a result, most formulas have the same ingredients, which include fat, protein, carbohydrate, vitamins, and minerals. Some formulas have added extras, such as omega oils to encourage the health of the brain and nervous system; or pre- and probiotics, which are said to ensure healthy levels of good bacteria in the gut.

Choose an iron-fortified formula that is appropriate for your baby's age to be sure it contains the right amount and type of protein for your baby. There are two types of protein in milk: casein and whey. Formulas intended for newborns have a greater ratio of whey, about 60 percent whey to 40 percent casein, which replicates the balance in breast milk; whey protein seems to provide more protection against infections, so is ideal for newborns. Some formulas aimed at "hungrier" babies have more casein, but these tend to be harder to digest, and unless your pediatrician specifically recommends these products, normal formula is sufficient for your baby.

Avoid formula that is low in iron, as this isn't suitable for most babies who need good quantities of iron in their milk to grow and develop properly.

Some babies have problems digesting the lactose (sugar) or proteins in milk. In this case, a lactose-reduced formula may be suggested, or one that is hydrolyzed, which means that it has been prepared to remove most, or all, of the cow's milk proteins. Goat's milk, sheep's milk, rice milk, and nut milk formulas are not recommended, and soy milk formula should not be introduced before the age of six months.

You will need an equal number of caps and nipples for your bottles. Nipples come with different sized holes to control the speed the milk comes out. Choose slow-flowing nipples for your newborn, and then gradually change to faster ones as your baby gets older. You can buy nipples made of silicone, which is durable, or latex, which is thought to be closer to the feeling of a human nipple. You can also choose from a traditional bell-shaped nipple or a special orthodontic one, which manufacturers claim closely resembles a human nipple—although you may find that your baby is the one who decides which shape is best.

CLEANING BOTTLES

Keeping your baby's bottles clean is essential, and you will need to wash all her bottle-feeding equipment when she has finished a feed. First, you will need to wash thoroughly the bottle, nipple, lid, and any other parts in hot, soapy water. For this, it's worth buying a good nylon bottle brush that is specially designed to remove trapped milk from both nipples and bottles, with a smaller brush at one end that can work its way into the narrow nipple.

Washing bottles in hot soapy water is sufficient for safe feeding, but some people choose to take cleaning a step further by sterilizing bottles, as well. Baby-gear stores sell electric steam sterilizers or equipment to use in the microwave, or you can simply boil your bottle-feeding equipment on the stovetop without any special equipment. You can also sterilize bottles in a dishwasher that reaches a high temperature of 180°F/82°C.

WHAT ELSE DO I NEED?

You will need a designated measuring scoop (which comes with powdered formula) and a knife to level off the powder. It is important that the liquid measurements on your bottles are easy to read (particularly when you are making up feeds in the night), since it's essential to make up formula accurately to get the right nutrient balance.

Finally, whether you are breastfeeding or bottle-feeding, you may want to invest in several bibs. Babies can be very messy, spitting up and regurgitating milk, as well as drooling and dribbling, and your baby may be more comfortable if there is a barrier to protect her from getting wet. Investing in some cotton burp cloths is also a good idea. These can be placed over your shoulder (or on your lap) when you're burping your baby to soak up any milk that comes up; and they can also be used to wipe away any dribbles from your baby's face and neck after feeds.

YOUR STERILIZING SYSTEM
If you choose to sterilize in addition to washing, purpose-made sterilizers are an efficient way to sterilize pumping and feeding equipment.

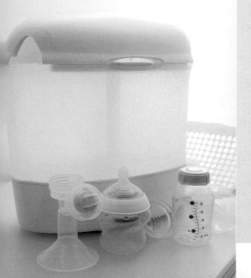

What will I need?

If up until now you have concentrated on what you need to buy for your baby, spare some time to think about the few items you will need for yourself to simplify the job of feeding and caring for her.

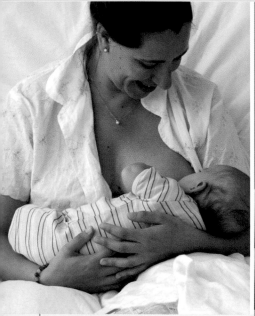

QUICK ACCESS
Comfortable, loose night and day wear that can be easily opened or lifted to feed your baby is a must while breastfeeding.

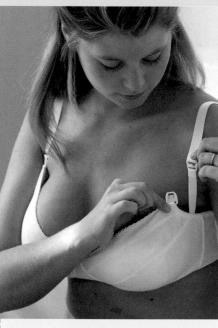

A SUPPORTIVE NURSING BRA
Your breasts may be a size or so larger while feeding; wearing a properly fitted nursing bra will support your breasts and help milk flow.

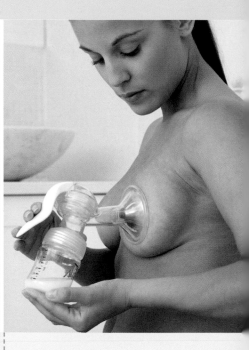

GET PUMPING
Expressing, whether with a hand pump (above), electric pump, or your hands, provides a useful supplementary milk supply.

You won't need much for yourself to help you do the job of caring for your newborn, but there are a few key items that you may find helpful.

Breastfeeding moms

You may wonder what you need for breastfeeding apart from yourself and your baby, but there are a few items that you should have ready. Most important is a comfortable chair with support for your arms and back, and ideally a footstool so you can put your feet up if you want to. Some well-placed pillows can support you and your baby, or you can buy a horseshoe-shaped nursing pillow that fits around your body to lay your baby on (which can be especially useful for feeding twins). Position your chair where you can listen to the radio, watch television, and reach a cold drink to stay hydrated.

Of course, you will need to be able to access your breasts easily, so make sure you have some loose-fitting, comfortable clothing and zips or buttons that undo easily, as well as nightwear that doesn't have any fiddly fastenings. One of the essential items for breastfeeding is a properly fitted nursing bra that can be opened with one hand (see p.83). Comfort is key here; you may want to wear it at night if your breasts need some support. Disposable or washable breast pads can be useful too if your milk leaks.

You will also need to buy any equipment you need for expressing your milk (see p.347).

"Where you sit to feed your baby, set up a little nest with supportive pillows, a foot rest, and a side table for drinks, snacks, and a book"

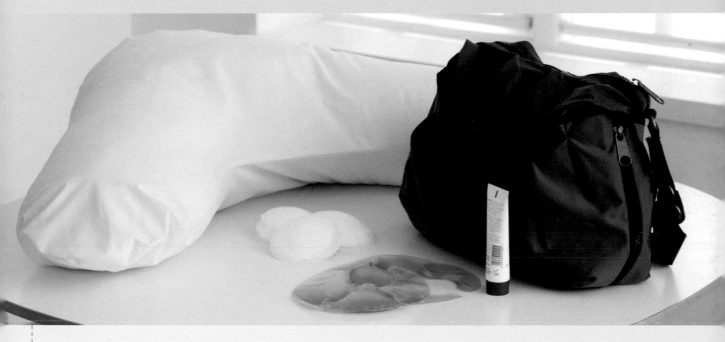

FOR YOUR COMFORT
If your body feels a bit battered after the birth, or your milk supply is taking time to settle down, invest in a few aids, such as a soothing gel pad to sit on, a nursing pillow to help support your baby, and breast pads and nipple cream to make feeding easier.

Bottle-feeding moms

You won't need any equipment other than formula, bottles, and cleaning supplies (see pp.240–241), and containers for holding formula to make up bottles when you're out. It is just as important, however, to be comfortable while you're bottle-feeding to avoid straining your back. Choose a comfortable chair with a firm back to feed your baby and have pillows for support if you need them.

Diaper bag

As soon as you take your first forays out with your new baby, you'll realize the importance of this item! Your diaper bag should contain everything you will need to keep your baby content and you organized. Choose a sturdy, washable bag with easy-to-access compartments and pockets, so you can keep your personal items separate. A wide, comfy strap is helpful since your bag is likely to be fairly heavy. Keep it stocked at all times so you can make spur-of-the-moment trips out of the house. As well as the items you need for your baby, including diaper-changing supplies, spare clothes, and formula to make up feeds if you're bottle-feeding, you might want the following for you:

- A clean shirt (in case of breast leaks).
- A small bottle of water and a snack (to keep you going).
- Some tissues.
- A shawl or blanket (for warmth and/or discreet feeding).
- Your camera—to catch those unmissable firsts.
- Breast pads and nipple cream.
- Spare sanitary napkins (particularly in the days immediately after the birth).
- Your cell phone and enough money to get you home in an emergency.

Where will my baby sleep?

You do need to put a bit of time and thought into where your baby will sleep—even if at first it's just creating a space in your bedroom—and how to ensure that her sleeping environment is comfortable, safe, and cozy.

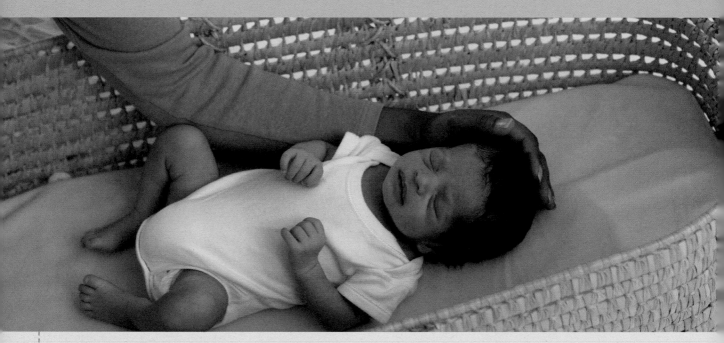

A SNUG ENVIRONMENT
A Moses basket will keep your newborn cozy and secure in her first weeks. It's also easily transportable so you can keep her close by you as you move around the house and by your side during the night.

Sleep is a big issue for new parents, and you will want to ensure that wherever your baby sleeps is an inviting and calm environment so that she grows to associate sleep time with a comforting and welcome part of her day.

As well as making the area where your baby sleeps comfortable and thinking about what type of bed and bedding she will have, you also need to be sure that she is safe while sleeping (see p.357). Experts now recommend that your baby sleep in the same room as you and your partner for the first six months, as this is one of the factors shown to reduce the risk of SIDS. Keeping your baby close by means that you will be quickly aware if your baby is in any discomfort and can attend to her right away.

Baskets, cradles, and bassinets

Many babies sleep more soundly in a smaller, cozier environment in the first two to three months, and will enjoy the snugness of a Moses basket, crib, bassinet, or cradle. However, these are quickly outgrown, so you will need to have a bigger crib at the ready.

Most Moses baskets and bassinets are portable, so you can keep your baby close by while she sleeps—reassuring when she's a newborn and you want to keep her in sight. Choose a basket with sturdy handles so you can carry it easily, and a strong base to support the weight of the basket when you're holding it.

"Your newborn may wake every two to three hours during the night at first, so it makes sense to keep her close by you"

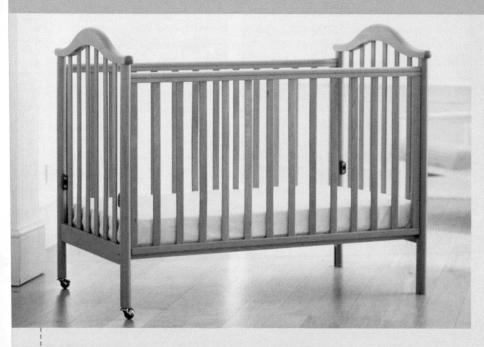

USING A CRIB
There's no reason why you can't start your baby out in a crib. A crib with an adjustable mattress enables you to raise the base so you can put your baby down or lift her out with ease.

entertain herself when she gets a little older. If your baby seems a bit lost when you first move her to a crib, you could try to ease the transition by placing her Moses basket or bassinet inside it at first until she gets used to her new environment. Some cribs are on wheels so its location can be changed easily. If you choose a mobile crib, make sure the wheels are lockable so the crib can be secured when your baby starts to bounce and move more. Cribs with a base that can be raised up allow you to lift her without putting undue strain on your back. Choose a frame with a non-toxic finish, such as beeswax.

Many cribs with drop-sides have been recalled recently, so you may want to purchase a new crib, rather than using a hand-me-down crib. All cribs that were made before September 1986 do not comply with current safety standards and should not be used.

Bassinets are another good option for newborns. They sometimes come as part of a travel system so they can be part of a baby carriage, which can be particularly useful when you want to transport your baby without waking her. If you use this system, you may need to change the mattress for nighttime sleeping.

Many bassinets and cradles rock or glide to help your baby get to sleep. They can also be used for a bit longer than a Moses basket, usually lasting until your baby is about six months old. However, cradles aren't as mobile, which can be inconvenient, and there's the danger that your baby will become accustomed to being rocked to sleep and find it hard to move to a crib without this facility.

Cribs

A good, sturdy crib is a worthwhile investment; your baby will be able to use it until she moves to a bed at around two or three years old. Not only will its familiarity help her to sleep, but she will have ample room to move, and even

YOUR BABY'S MATTRESS
Even if you do have a second-hand crib frame, it is important to buy a new mattress for your baby since old ones can harbor dust and damp, which increases your baby's risk of SIDS (see p.357). A variety of crib mattresses are available on the market today in all price ranges. Some have springs, while some are spring-free. Some are made of memory foam, and there are organic cotton mattresses, as well. Just be sure that the mattress you choose is the proper dimensions for the crib you select. (The

Transporting my baby

Daily outings are a common feature of life with a new baby, so it's worth investing a little time and energy to find travel equipment that is safe, comfortable, and, of course, appropriate for your lifestyle.

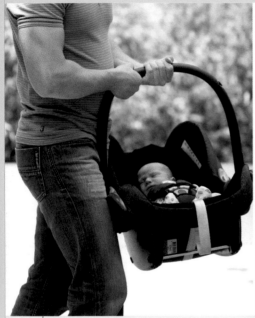

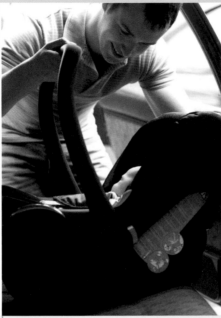

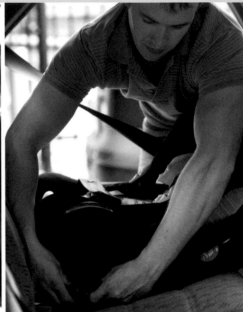

CARRYING YOUR BABY
A car seat with a sturdy handle allows you to carry your baby safely. Make sure her harness is fastened at all times.

FACING THE REAR
All babies under 22lbs (10kg) must be placed in rear-facing car seats in the back seat of the car; it's the safest place for a newborn.

STRAPPED IN
Anchor your car seat base to your car with a seatbelt or your car's UAS system, and go to a car seat inspection clinic.

Buying equipment to transport your baby around will be a major purchase, and with so much choice, it can be very confusing to try to work out what is most practical for you, your lifestyle, and your budget.

Give yourselves time to look around at what's available: You'll probably be using the items you buy every day for the foreseeable future, so it's important that you're happy with them. Look online at the models you're interested in and read safety reports and reviews. Talk to other parents, too, about which systems they use and how they rate them.

Car seats

Even if you don't spend a great deal of time in the car, your baby will need a car seat to be transported home from the hospital; in fact, most hospitals will not allow you to leave until you've confirmed that you have one. When you're looking at car seats, your top priority should be that it is safe for your baby and is compatible with your car. The safety advice is that you should not use a second-hand baby car seat, especially one whose history you don't know,

because it might have been involved in an accident. If you still have an older child's car seat, check its expiration date; plastic degrades over time, making it unsafe to use after a few years.

CAR SEAT FEATURES
• Your baby's car seat can act as a chair when you are on the move, and for short periods at home when you move her from the car into the house, so it needs to be sturdy and well padded for comfort. Make sure it has an easy-to-manage handle for carrying, and that the seat provides

proper support for your baby's back. Babies will need a rear-facing car seat until they are at least 22 pounds (10kg), regardless of age.

• A five-point harness, with straps that come over the shoulders, across the middle, and under the legs, is essential for optimal safety. Always fasten your baby's car-seat straps, even when you're in the home. It can be easy to forget to do this, especially if your baby is covered with a blanket; but establishing good safety habits now can protect her from accidents later on when she's more mobile.

• Try out the seat fixtures before you buy it—some are trickier than others, so you need to be confident that you will be able to get your baby in or out quickly if needed—or with minimal disruption. All car seats should have washable covers.

• An added bonus is attachable toys and other entertainment that can distract your baby on longer journeys.

• A child-restraint system called UAS (Universal Anchorage System) has been introduced in newer cars. It consists of fixed anchorage points in a car into which a child seat can be fitted. Check the seat and your car's manufacturer's manual to be sure that your seat and car are compatible.

• If you have bucket seats, you may need to insert a wedge of Styrofoam or something similar to give the seat a firm base.

WHICH TYPE OF SEAT?

There are two styles of infant car seats: infant-only rear-facing seats and convertible seats. The infant-only seats snap into car-seat bases that you install in your back seat. You remove the car seat with the baby each time you leave the car, then attach it to a stroller frame or travel system, which allows sleeping babies to continue napping. Convertible seats can be installed rear-facing now and forward-facing when your child is tall enough and heavy enough. Babies must be unstrapped from convertible car-seat seatbelts and carried out of the car, since the seats remain in the car at all times. Although it's possible to put a newborn in this type of seat (weight requirements for individual models vary), it's in your best interest to use a infant-only seat at first. These seats are specially designed to hold the tiniest babies, so they offer better protection, and they'll prevent you from having to wake a sleeping baby who nodded off on the drive home.

Baby carriers

A baby carrier or sling is a practical and easy way to carry your newborn, and has the added bonus of leaving your hands free for shopping or housework.

Slings are great for soothing babies, who love the feeling of closeness to you and being able to hear your heartbeat. Look for one that provides plenty of back support for your baby, and with wide straps so it's comfortable for you. Think about whether your partner will use the sling as well, and experiment with a few different styles to find one that fits you both comfortably, and that is easy to get your baby in and out of. Ask the store for a demonstration to see how easy it is to get the sling on and your baby in and out.

• A popular carrier for newborns is one that supports your baby in an upright position. During the first few weeks, you can keep your baby facing inward; then when she gains more head control—and curiosity about her surroundings—you can turn her around to face outward.

• If you are breastfeeding, a sarong-style sling enables you to carry your baby in a

---

Getting around together

There aren't that many must-haves for babies, so it is a good idea to focus on those items that will make your life with your baby easier, safer and more enjoyable.

• When fitting your car seat, it should be held tightly by the seat belt, with very little sideways give. If the seat— or its base—moves around, it is not safe. When purchasing strollers, consider whether you'll need to negotiate stairs or public transport. There are lighter, foldable models designed for newborns, and this may make getting around a little easier.

• Using a sling for long periods can cause backache, particularly as your baby begins to fill out and gain weight. Exercising and practicing yoga can strengthen back and abdominal muscles, which can help to prevent discomfort. Sarong-style slings are supposed to distribute your baby's weight more evenly and put less stress on your lower back.

• There are so many combinations of strollers for sale that choosing one can be very confusing. Take your time to research all the different options. Good stores will have specialists who can give you advice and guidance as to what to buy to ensure that you get the equipment you really need.

• Having a stroller with an infant car-seat attachment is a good option for juggling everything when you're out.

• Consider a backward-facing stroller. This allows you to see your baby, to make eye contact, and to respond to each other while you're on the move. Recent research directly links backward-facing buggies with improved communication skills in babies.

natural breastfeeding position, and you will also be able to take her out more easily for diaper changes.

SLING SAFETY

Safety is an important consideration with a sling. You need to ensure that your baby's face is uncovered and visible at all times, and it's very important to check her frequently. If you're breastfeeding your baby in a sarong-style sling, change her position after a feed so that her head faces up and is clear of both the sling and your body. Health Canada recommends that you be especially vigilant if your baby is premature, younger than four months, or has a pre-existing medical condition.

Strollers

An easy-to-manage, comfortable stroller is a must for all parents; however, the huge range of strollers and baby carriages on the market can make figuring out which one is best for you and your baby fairly challenging. Essentially, you want to choose a model with sturdy wheels, an easy-to-use brake, a manageable five-point harness, and comfortable, washable fabrics.

Ask a sales assistant to show you how to open up the stroller and use the brake, and how to fold it away, and then ask to try it yourself. In particular, you want to be sure that the brake is secure and easy to use. This is the feature you will use often, and even the gentlest of inclines can lead to a runaway stroller!

Think about your lifestyle when looking at models. For example, if you think you'll be doing plenty of walking, choose one with adequate, built-in storage for your diaper bag, toys, and, of course, your shopping. If you need to use public transportation a lot, a less bulky model will be most convenient. Or you may want a model that you can jog with or take on long walks on uneven terrain to help you regain your fitness levels; in which case, choose one that is robust and with good suspension to keep your baby comfortable over bumps. Generally, strollers with high handles lessen the strain on your back.

There is a wide variety of models available, including those with seats that can be altered to face outward or toward you, and some that are on a narrow, high frame that allow you to maneuver them easily, and give your baby a better view of you. Strollers as part of a travel system, where the base takes either the stroller seat or a car seat, are also practical, but the frames can

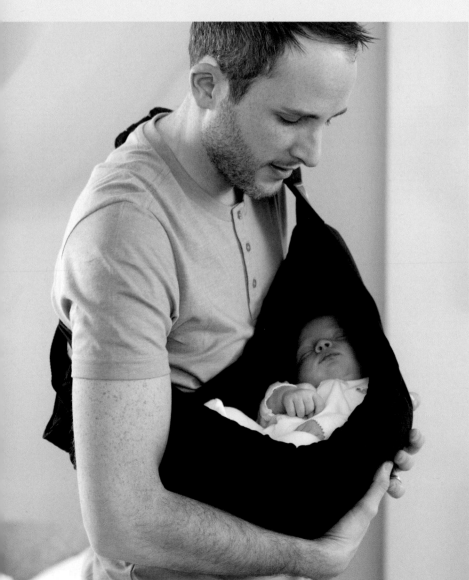

SOFT SLINGS
Hammock-type slings are a comfortable way to carry a soundly sleeping newborn. Make sure your baby's face isn't covered by any material, and that you can see her at all times to make sure that she is breathing well.

often be heavy and difficult to erect. If you're considering a travel system, try out all the different parts before you buy it. Lastly, don't forget to check that whichever model you choose fits easily into the trunk of your car. Also consider a car-seat frame, which holds an infant car seat and folds up compactly, making it easy to put in your trunk.

DOUBLE STROLLERS

If you are expecting twins, or need to transport a toddler and your baby, you'll need a double stroller. There are two types: a twin stroller with seats side by side, and a tandem stroller with one seat behind, or below, the other. Both have pros and cons. In twin strollers, your children can see each other and, as they grow, entertain each other; while tandems can be easier to fit through smaller spaces, such as store aisles, or to push along narrow sidewalks, but are tricky to get up and down steps.

Consider, too, whether you need a model where one or both seats recline completely for a newborn, and that you can erect and fold the stroller easily—

bearing in mind that you will have your hands full with two young children.

BABY CARRIAGES

Many parents prefer traditional style baby carriages, which enclose their baby in a snug space and so provide both a comfortable and comforting environment. Some parents like to use these in the house for impromptu naps, too. Look for styles that have a bassinet that detaches from the base, which can be removed while your baby is sleeping without disturbing her. These can also double as an ideal travel bed for the first few months.

UMBRELLA STROLLERS

Light, foldable strollers are not really appropriate until your baby is at least six months old, because she needs to lie flat during the first few months until she can sit up unaided. However, some foldable strollers have a fully reclining, well padded seat with a sturdy back, which can be used for a newborn and then be adjusted later on when your baby can sit up.

> "Your baby's stroller will be one of your major baby purchases; take your time to look at what's available and find one you're completely happy with"

BASSINET STROLLER
A traditional bassinet top that attaches to a sturdy base is ideal for your new baby, providing a secure and comfortable ride.

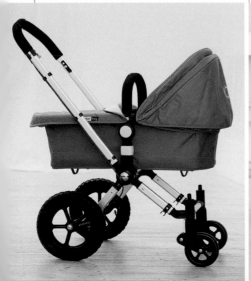

ADJUSTABLE SEAT
Some strollers recline fully for newborns and can be adapted as your baby grows. Seats that face inward are reassuring for your baby.

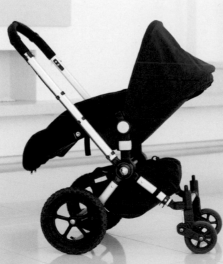

TRANSPORTING TWO
A side-by-side double stroller is one option for twins. Make sure the model you choose is able to fit through your front door!

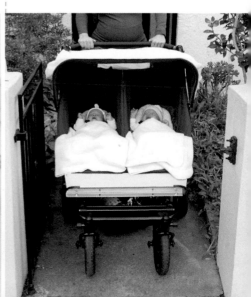

Common concerns

It's natural to have a whole host of concerns—about your baby's health, whether you will be a good parent, and how you'll manage breastfeeding. Caring for a baby is a big responsibility, so it's not surprising you need some reassurance.

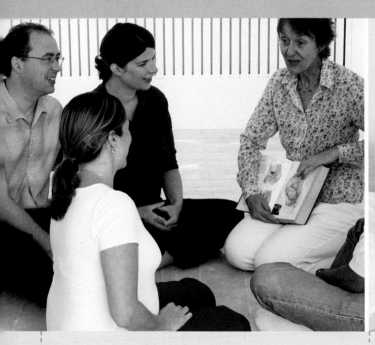

BEING INFORMED
Attending prenatal classes is a great opportunity to find out all you can about labor and birth. The more informed you are, the less anxious you are likely to be.

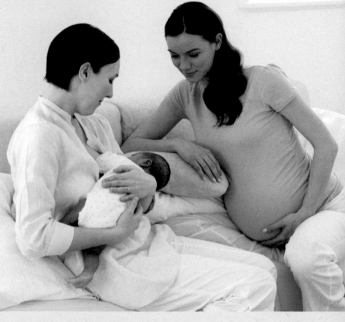

THINKING AHEAD
Watching new moms feed their babies and asking them about their experiences with breastfeeding will help you feel as prepared as possible when it comes to feeding your own baby.

It can be helpful to know that many pregnant women have similar anxieties. However, don't let a worry eat away at you: Call your doctor or midwife for a reassuring chat.

Will I be able to breastfeed?

Many women become concerned before the birth about how they will do with breastfeeding. You may have heard stories from friends who didn't manage to master the technique, and found it particularly stressful. Or you may worry that you won't be able to sustain your baby on breast milk.

In the past, women were given little information or advice about the best way to feed their babies, and formula was actually considered to be healthier, with more nutritional value than breast milk. With significant improvements in formula, breastfeeding was discouraged and considered old-fashioned. Not surprisingly, as women were presented with a viable option, many gave up breastfeeding early on, or didn't attempt it in the first place.

We now know that breast milk gives your baby the best possible nutritional start in life (see pp.238–239), and your breasts are designed to produce exactly the right amount of milk for your baby.

The good news is that today, with help and support from your pediatrician and/or a lactation consultant, you can learn to breastfeed successfully (see pp.343–345) and provide your baby with all the food she needs for her first six months.

"Feeling protective of your baby motivates you to make healthy lifestyle choices to help your baby grow and develop well"

Will my baby be healthy?

The vast majority of women—in fact, more than 95 percent—give birth to perfectly healthy babies. Of course, there are occasions when a baby's health or development in the uterus raises concerns. However, with modern ultrasound techniques and screening tests, most problems are raised early in pregnancy, and most of these are treatable—some even while your baby is in the uterus. If you have any particular concern, talk to your doctor or midwife; they may arrange further monitoring if it is necessary.

COULD I HAVE HARMED MY BABY?
This is probably the most common concern for moms-to-be, who are often unaware that they are pregnant during those first few weeks, and merrily continue to drink, smoke, or take prescription drugs.

While it's of course true that the early stages of pregnancy are important for your baby's development—particularly before your placenta, which helps to protect your baby (see p.158), is properly formed—rest assured that the majority of babies are unaffected by early maternal transgressions.

Bear in mind that during previous generations there was little research into the impact of drugs, alcohol, nicotine, and hazardous foods on pregnancy. Our parents and grandparents were likely to have eaten and drunk things that today we know are best avoided. The vast majority of babies were perfectly healthy, despite this.

As soon as you do know you are pregnant, you should of course take precautions to ensure your baby's health (see Chapter 2, pp.48–103), but try to avoid worrying too much about what you did previously, and instead give your baby the best possible advantage by making lifestyle changes and concentrating on enjoying a healthy pregnancy from now on.

HAS MY BABY STOPPED GROWING?
Your doctor will assess your baby's growth (see p.200) and listen to her heartbeat throughout your pregnancy. You will also be given at least two routine ultrasounds to check that your baby is growing as expected, so any problems will be highlighted early on.

There is a condition known as intra-uterine growth restriction (IUGR; see p.388), which is identified when your baby's ultrasound measurements show that she is in the smallest 10 percent for her gestational age. This is a rare condition, occurring in only 3 percent of pregnancies. IUGR can be caused by smoking, poor nutrition, carrying twins and other multiples, or problems with the placenta. If this is identified, your pregnancy will be monitored carefully, and, if it's thought necessary, your baby may be delivered early so that she can receive extra care and attention.

CAN HAVING SEX AFFECT MY BABY?
You cannot hurt your baby by having sex, although some positions may cause you more discomfort. As long as you have not experienced unusual bleeding during pregnancy and you haven't been identified as having a "weak" cervix (see pp.384–385), which carries a heightened risk of miscarriage, there is absolutely no reason why you can't continue to make love regularly. In fact, climaxing during pregnancy increases the blood supply to your pelvis (and therefore your baby), as well as encouraging the release of your body's natural feel-good hormones, which in turn is beneficial for your baby's health and well-being.

I'm worried about the birth

You may find it impossible to believe that your vagina can stretch enough to deliver a bouncing baby, and most women experience at least some anxiety about this prospect. The idea of going through hours of pain, even for a much-wanted baby, can be very daunting. In reality, labor is a natural process, and women have been giving birth successfully since the beginning of humankind. Of course, labor and birth are uncomfortable and painful, but finding out about all the methods of pain relief (see pp.284–291) available to you can help you face it with less anxiety. Also, if you have your heart set on a natural birth, there is no shame in changing your mind and using medication when the time comes. Ultimately, your goal is to deliver a healthy baby, and the means by which you achieve this are irrelevant.

There is no doubt that horror stories abound, however, it's best not to listen to negative experiences; in reality, while some women do have a difficult time, this is not the case for the majority. One interesting study found that of 137 factors that affect a woman's satisfaction with her birth experience, 4 stood out in particular. These were a woman's personal expectations; the amount of support she received from caregivers; the quality of the caregiver-patient relationship; and the woman's involvement in decision-making.

In other words, your labor actually is very much within your control, and approaching it with confidence and belief in your ability to cope will not only make it a more positive experience but, as research suggests, a more comfortable one, too.

WILL I GET TO THE HOSPITAL ON TIME?

As your due date draws nearer, it's time to think about what will happen when your labor begins and exactly how and when you will go to the hospital. If you find that you're starting to worry about whether you will be able to make it to the hospital for the birth, rest assured that in reality, sudden deliveries make up only a tiny percentage of all births—less than 1 percent—so you will almost certainly make it to the hospital on time, especially if this is your first baby.

The average labor is between eight and twelve hours, and sometimes much longer for a first baby, so you should find that you have plenty of time to relax at home during the early stages before heading to the hospital; in fact, this is recommended, because you're far more likely to feel comfortable in your own home. Your doctor will offer clear guidelines for when you should head to the hospital (see pp.295–296). If you follow these guidelines—and, as long as your baby's head isn't making an appearance already—you should have plenty of time to get there. It goes without saying that being prepared for any eventuality will reassure you (see page 318 for what to do if your baby does decide to make an unscheduled, speedy exit). On the other hand, being well informed about how your labor is most likely to progress should dispel any fears or anxieties you have about getting to the hospital on time.

Instead, try to focus on the techniques you might use to help you relax during early labor.

WILL THE HOSPITAL BE HYGIENIC?

There is always a small risk that your baby (or you) could pick up an infection in a hospital, and there are a few things you can do to avoid this. The first is to call your hospital's labor and delivery department to discuss your concerns with a nurse, who can describe their

LOVING RELATIONS
Rest assured that having sex is highly unlikely to harm your baby. On the contrary, the feelings of relaxation and loving support that intimacy brings can reduce stress, contributing to an optimal environment for your baby.

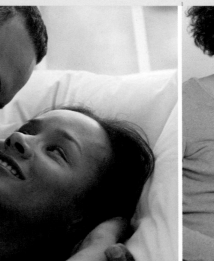

WATCHING YOUR PROGRESS
When labor starts, work with you partner to gauge your progress and help you relax during the early stages.

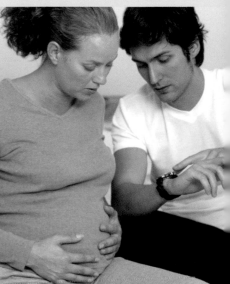

protocol for maintaining hygienic conditions. You can also make a note on your birth plan regarding handwashing and use of antibacterial hand gels. Be warned, this may not go down well with hospital staff who are trained to do just that, but it does highlight your concerns.

You and your partner also can be scrupulous about personal hygiene in the hospital. You can use your own bedding for your baby, if you wish, and bring along sanitizing wipes and hand sprays to use in the bathroom. Ultimately, however, the risks are low, and this is one area not really worth worrying about. If, in the worst scenario, you or your baby do acquire an infection, it will be treated and your prognosis will be very good.

Will I be a good enough parent?

It can be hard to imagine yourself caring for a helpless newborn and managing successfully to meet all her needs as she grows and develops. In fact, you will discover that parenting is very much a "learning on the job" experience: You will find that much of the time you naturally respond to and fulfill your baby's needs, although there will, of course, be occasions when you don't get something right at first. This is normal and allows you to grow and learn as a parent.

While there can be no doubt that the early days of parenthood are challenging and that you will face many more challenges as you guide your daughter or son through childhood and into adulthood, it can be reassuring to consider that there is no "right" way to parent. As long as you nurture, care for, protect, and love your child unconditionally, you will be doing what's best for her.

Along the way you will find you pick up tips from more experienced friends and family, and will also find that often you can be guided by your instinct. When you feel overwhelmed or uncertain, you'll find that there are many health professionals who can encourage you to make the right decisions: If you want to be a good parent, you will be.

WILL I LOVE ANOTHER BABY?

If you already have a child you may wonder how you will extend that love to a new baby—it can be hard to imagine how you could possibly love anyone as much as you love your first child. You may also be concerned about how the family dynamic will be altered, perhaps disrupting your happy little unit and beautifully settled routine.

These feelings are natural, but be reassured that love doesn't have limits; you will find that your love extends naturally to all of your children—and your partner—and continues to grow and change with each new arrival. When your newborn arrives, you'll probably wonder how you could ever have doubted that you wouldn't feel the same way about her as you do for your other children. Even if you find that the bonding process is different—which can be due to factors such as the type of labor and birth you had—over time your love for your baby will grow. For many parents, this happens in a rush, while for others it can be a slow process as they get to know their baby over weeks and months.

How pregnancy made us feel

During my first pregnancy I longed to have a girl and I was worried that I would not bond if I had a boy. All my fears were groundless—I adored my baby boy on sight. CH

I have to confess to worrying about everything. I worried something would be wrong at every ultrasound, and was anxious that there would be something wrong with my baby when she was born. Of course, everything was fine. TL

We worried whether our baby would be OK because she was suffering from IUGR (see p.388), and not growing sufficiently. I was worried about how I was going to breastfeed for a year when I would have to return to work after only three months. But, where there is a will, there is a way! NK

I was pretty relaxed, maybe because I had "seen it all before," and knew that the likelihood of something untoward happening was small. I did, however, worry about stillbirth, but I suppose this is one thing that everyone dreads. However, if you have a low-risk pregnancy, the chance of stillbirth is low, at around one in 500. So if I was thinking logically, I shouldn't have worried. The chance of this happening is significantly less than 1 percent. MG

As a pediatrician, I hear many concerns from first-time moms—mostly about labor: whether they will be able to deliver naturally, and even worries about modesty and lack of control. As my job is to reassure parents, I knew that there was little risk of anything going seriously wrong. Of course, I did have some nervousness and anticipation, but only until my babies were in my arms. LJ

With my first baby, I was anxious that there would be complications because I saw other women suffering at work. It spoiled things for me, so with my second daughter I made a conscious effort to be more relaxed. VB

Getting organized

Preparing yourself and your home well in advance of your baby's due date can make things much easier when your baby comes along—when you will be wholly preoccupied with caring for your tiny new arrival.

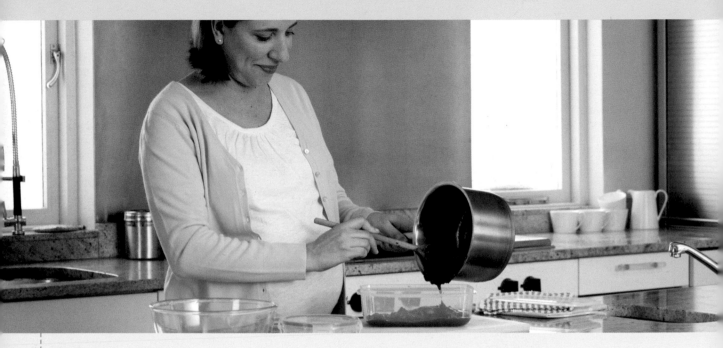

STOCKING UP
Delving into the freezer for a ready-made home-cooked meal can be a godsend once your baby has arrived. A new baby in tow can leave you without a moment to cook, or you may simply be too exhausted to even think about preparing food—either way, you will congratulate yourself on this particular foresight.

Pace yourself in the run-up to the birth. Make a list of what you want to get done, and cross off tasks one at a time—but don't push yourself. Ultimately, whatever you don't manage to do now is unlikely to have a huge impact. The weeks before the birth are the ideal time to rest and get yourself in the right frame of mind, so by all means, get organized, but do it sensibly, taking time to put your feet up.

Cooking in advance

Making some favorite meals to store in your freezer is probably the best thing you can do right now. Although it may be

hard to believe that a tiny baby can render you incapable of preparing a meal, this may well be the reality! Having a pre-prepared, healthy meal on hand when your arms are full, or when you simply lack the energy to make something from scratch, can be invaluable. Date and label the meals and, to save extra time, store them in foil containers so that you don't have to clean them afterward. If you have the energy now, you could even bake a few treats, too, to reward yourself—and provide for visitors—after the birth.

This is also a good time to go through your refrigerator and cupboards and throw away anything that is past its use-by date, as well as stock up on any basics that are running low. Chances are,

"Nesting may be an alien experience to you, but go with it; the most important thing is to channel your energy productively"

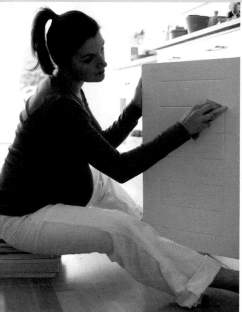

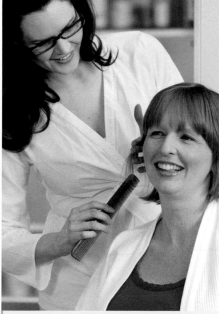

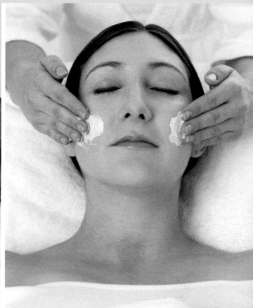

SQUEAKY CLEAN
If the urge to clean the house from top to bottom grabs you, don't resist—but be careful not to exhaust or strain yourself.

TIME FOR A TRIM
Now is the time to get a haircut or trim. An easily managed style is best for after the birth when time to groom will be in short supply.

A PAMPERING TREAT
Indulge yourself now with a relaxing facial or massage to help you wind down and get in the right frame of mind for the birth.

you won't be making major shopping expeditions in the weeks after your baby is born, so getting organized now can make a massive difference later on.

Better still, if you haven't done so already, now is the time to set up an internet grocery shopping list at the supermarket of your choice, so that you can order your shopping for the week with just a few tweaks and a push of a button. As well as household basics, consider everything you are likely to need for your baby, including diapers and wipes, and add them to your list.

A little nesting

Nesting is a peculiar phenomenon that some women experience, which usually occurs during the third trimester of pregnancy. This supposedly primal instinct throws you into a flurry of activity to prepare your environment for your baby's arrival.

The cleaning, tidying, organizing, and preparing that nesting entails is thought to be a natural symptom of pregnancy, and although you do need to be careful not to overdo things and exhaust

yourself, satisfying this urge can be a part of the emotional preparation for becoming a new parent.

SPRING CLEANING
If you are feeling energized, take advantage of this and invest in some natural cleaning products to give your house a toxin-free spring clean. Cleaning is going to be at the bottom of your list of priorities once your baby arrives, and you will enjoy your first weeks with your baby more if you aren't distracted by lots of clutter and dust. Ask a friend or

family member to come for the day to help you out and to make it a more sociable occasion. Don't overdo things and, of course, make sure you leave the heavy lifting, ladders, and big stretching to someone else.

Change the beds, launder the linen and towels, and open all the windows to air out the house; get the rugs out on the line, and let the light in!

Jobs worth doing

If your energy levels are flagging and you'd rather not spend your last precious days cooking and cleaning, there are still plenty of things that can be done to prepare you for life with a baby.

• Get your hospital bag packed (see pp.260–261) so that you don't have the task hanging over your head. Having it ready and waiting will mean that you won't have a stressful scramble at the last minute. Put it by the front door and leave it there.

• Make a list of everyone you would like to contact after the birth to announce

your baby's arrival. Make sure that numbers are programmed into your or your partner's phone; or set up an email group so that everyone can be notified together—complete with a picture of your new arrival.

• If you want to be more formal, prepare a written birth announcement—address and stamp envelopes, or design something that can be sent via the internet, slotting in your new baby's photo and details at the last moment.

• Sort your baby's clothes into sizes, so when she is born, you won't have to search through piles of onesies to find one that fits. Wash new baby clothes, to ensure that they are fresh and that any chemical finishes that could irritate your baby's sensitive skin are removed. Use a dye- and fragrance-free detergent to protect your baby's skin.

• If you plan to use cloth diapers, spend time now finding out about local companies that provide a laundering service and sign up. Using a service saves hours of laundering time, which makes it easier to commit to reusables. If you are using disposables, look for

supermarket offers and stock up. Invest in the first two sizes, rather than simply newborn ones—your baby may be bigger or grow more quickly than you think.

• Get your finances in order by paying bills, setting up direct debits, ensuring that payments are made directly to your bank account, rather than in check form, and consider signing up for online banking. Anything that makes your life easier after the birth is worth a shot. You may also want to draw up a new budget, particularly if you're starting maternity leave and will be on a reduced salary. Having to cut costs and accustomed luxuries may make you gulp, but this allows you to plan ahead, and saves stress later on.

• If you are planning to go back to work at some point and haven't already made arrangements for your baby's childcare, this is a good time to investigate the options and organize some visits to daycare centers, or even interview a nanny. Even if you have a lengthy maternity leave, it's a good idea to plan childcare as early as possible, since many centers have long wait lists.

GETTING TOGETHER
A baby shower hosted by friends is a great opportunity to celebrate in advance of the birth—and you may find that you get some useful items that you can cross off your own list.

PREPARING YOUR CHILD
If your older child will be staying at his grandparents for the birth, make sure he knows the plan, and consider a trial run.

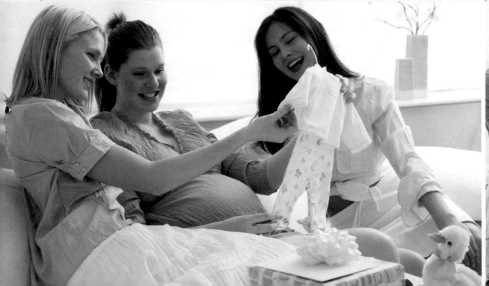

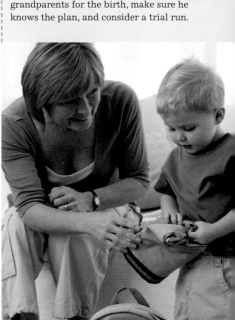

• Take some time for you. This is the ideal time to meet up with friends, get a manicure, pedicure, or massage, and fit in a little last-minute shopping. Take naps, go out for a meal with your partner, and have lots of early nights. You might want to go for a gentle swim and read a good book, as well as look ahead and sign up for a mom-and-baby yoga or exercise class. This is your time, and probably the last solo time you'll have for a while. A little pampering goes a long way toward raising spirits and putting you in a good frame of mind.

Enlisting help

The first weeks (and even months) of new parenthood can be exhausting, and you will benefit from some support. You might want to arrange for a family member—perhaps your mom or sister—to stay and help out for a few days after the birth. Or, if you would prefer to have time alone with your baby and partner at first to help you all to bond, short visits from friends and family can give you welcome respite from rocking and soothing your baby, or help with getting meals ready, laundry done, or time off to sleep.

Organize help well in advance, and consider setting up a schedule so you know who is available when. Don't turn down any offers of help; even having someone empty the dishwasher or hold your baby while you shower can be invaluable. If you are expecting twins, it is important that you arrange for another pair of hands, even if you have to pay for them.

If you have other children, make some arrangements for them to have some treats out of the house; not only will this give them something to look forward to, but you'll have a break from caring for more than one.

Keep in touch with your prenatal class members. Sharing stories, swapping advice, and socializing with other moms with babies of a similar age can be relaxing and provide you with useful skills. Get the number, too, of some local lactation consultants and the local La Leche League chapter, who can help you to deal with any breastfeeding problems.

Finally, talk to your partner now about how you will both manage the division of labor in the household once you have a baby to care for, too. If possible, arrange for a cleaner to help out with housework for an hour or so a week so you have more time to enjoy your new family life. Providing support for one another will make your relationship with your partner that much stronger.

Counting down to labor

As you approach labor, you may begin to feel overwhelmed by everything you need to get done: A practical approach can help things seem more manageable. Some simple advance planning and time spent talking to your partner and family about anything you need them to help out with will help you relax and feel that things are under control, and enable you to spend some much-needed time winding down before the birth.

• Avoid any arrangements that involve long-distance traveling, and try to stay in the vicinity of the hospital or birthing center where you plan to deliver. If you have younger children, make sure you have contingency plans for their care, in case you don't go into labor on schedule!

• This is a wonderful time for some gentle yoga to relax you and help you prepare for the birth, both physically and emotionally. Breathing exercises and listening to positive visualizations or meditation CDs can put you in a calm and tranquil frame of mind.

• Try to arrange for your partner to have as much time at home with you after the birth as possible. This period of being together as a family builds bonds and also helps you to keep on top of the day-to-day running of your home.

• Speak openly with friends and family about what would help you after the birth. You may want company and babycare advice, or simply someone to do the shopping or bring over a meal occasionally so that you don't need to cook. If you don't tell people what's needed, they won't know how to help.

• Try to clear the decks of all the day-to-day chores, tasks, appointments, and work, so you have less to deal with later. Stock up on the things you know you'll need, so you don't get caught out by an early arrival, and most of all, sleep while you still can! Entering new parenthood in a state of sleep deprivation is not a good idea.

• Review your birth plan and talk it through one last time with your birth partner. By reassuring yourself that it is all in order, you can relax more fully as you wait for events to unfold.

• Be on red alert from 36 weeks, with bags packed and people on standby to care for older children. Get your partner to do a test drive to the hospital to check out parking and alternate routes, and check for road construction or sports arenas that may play havoc with your plans! Fill your gas tank, install your car seat in the back seat, and arrange an alternative birth partner—just in case your partner doesn't manage to get there in time. Most of all, get as much rest as you can.

Packing my hospital bag

Aim to have your hospital bag packed and ready by the front door at around 36 weeks. Babies do not always arrive when scheduled, and you'll feel much more confident and relaxed knowing that everything is prepared.

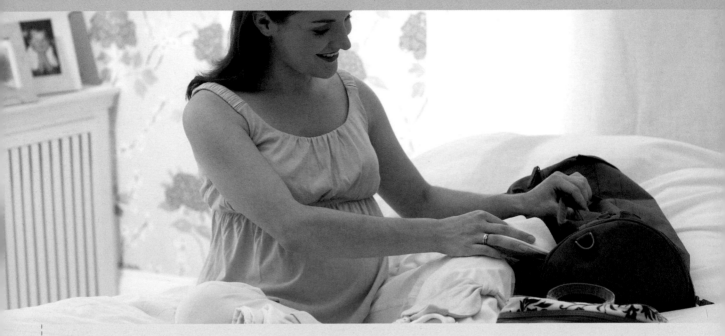

TIME TO PREPARE
Getting together everything you and your baby will need for the birth and afterward is an exciting task because it brings the reality of your baby's imminent arrival a significant step closer.

Your hospital bag should contain everything you and your baby will need for your stay in the hospital. In addition to the basics, include anything you think might be relaxing during labor, such as music or reading matter. It's also worth packing some home comforts: You may be living out of your bag for at least two days, so it's nice to include things that will give you a link to more familiar surroundings.

Pack a little more than you think you need, in case your stay is longer than you anticipated. Although your partner will undoubtedly be able to pick up items that you may have forgotten, you are likely to feel much more relaxed if you know that you have all your essentials ready to go.

Packing for you

Think about practical and personal items when packing. You will want to include at least some of the following:
• Your birth plan, and a copy in case there is a change of staff and your original goes missing. Your birth partner may like a copy to refer to as well.
• A robe, slippers, and socks. Choose something that makes you feel attractive! You may wear your robe on forays around the labor and delivery ward as you try to stay active during labor, and to cover up for the flurry of guests who may come to meet your new arrival.
• Lip balm—lips have a tendency to dry out during labor.
• An old T-shirt or nightie for labor:

Most hospitals provide a gown, but you may be allowed to wear your own clothing if you prefer.

• Snacks and drinks (if allowed) and bottled water. Staying hydrated is essential for labor and breastfeeding; although water will be available at the hospital, you may want to bring a bottle.

• Relaxation aids, such as relaxing or inspiring music and pillows.

• Any natural pain-relief therapies, such as massage oil, a reflexology chart or map, a HypnoBirthing CD or book, or a TENS machine.

• Soap, washcloth, and towel; makeup; a hairbrush; toothbrush, and toothpaste.

• Any regular medication (check with your doctor first if you are planning to breastfeed).

• A book or magazine, or a diary to record your thoughts during labor and when your baby is born.

• A digital camera or video recorder, if allowed—your partner may have this covered, but you may want your own.

• Something to wear home: Your figure won't snap back into shape, so choose loose and comfortable clothing.

• 1–2 front-opening, clean nightgowns or pajamas for after the birth. You'll need easy access for breastfeeding and skin-to-skin contact.

• A couple of nursing bras, some breast pads, and nipple cream.

• Maternity pads.

• Old or disposable underpants.

• Earplugs (for a noisy ward!)

• Your cell phone (if allowed), or your address book and change for phones.

Packing for your baby

Your baby will need the following:

• A soft hat. (All young babies should wear hats outdoors for the first few weeks to ensure that they maintain their body temperature.) Hospitals generally provide any clothes your baby needs while she's in their care.

• Check with your hospital before packing diapers, wipes, or other toiletries for your baby, because some maternity wards supply these necessities for you.

• Your baby's car seat. The hospital will not discharge you unless they see that you have strapped your baby into the car seat safely for the drive home.

• A baby book, so you can record details like the time and date of birth, her length and weight, and slip the piece of paper with her footprints on it into place right away.

• Comfortable clothing for her journey home. Some babies don't love car trips, so you need to make sure that there isn't anything that will irritate her skin or make her too hot.

• A "comfort" toy.

What you will and won't need in the hospital

Work on the premise that your labor may take some time, and bring along anything you may need for the journey.

• If allowed, snacks are important to keep your blood-sugar levels stable and energy levels high; choose whole grains and plenty of fresh fruit and vegetables, as well as some nutrient-dense sandwiches. A little chocolate, some cookies, or even a hard candy can be useful for a quick boost when you need it most. Store your snacks with an ice pack to keep them fresh. Don't forget to bring along some bottled water; staying hydrated in labor can make the process easier. Freeze it in advance so that it will be nice and cold when you need it.

• You can purchase "layette sets," which provide everything your baby will need for one wearing. A couple of these will see your baby through the first few days if you don't want to keep your baby dressed in the clothing supplied by the maternity ward.

• Go "disposable" whenever you can during your hospital stay: disposable diapers and bibs can be a bonus, letting you clear away mess completely with a minimum of fuss. It will also save you from creating a mountain of laundry!

• Choose organic or, at the very least, completely fragrance-free toiletries for your baby, and use sparingly. Your baby's skin will be very sensitive after the birth.

• Don't forget your camera. This must be the most important item you'll need once your baby is born!

• A yoga mat or blanket can protect your knees when you take on different labor positions. A birthing ball may be available at the hospital; if not, bring one along. You can sit on it, bounce, and rotate your hips during contractions to ease pain and open your pelvis. Don't forget warm socks; your feet can become very cold in labor; water spray for your face to keep you cool; very loose underpants (that won't rub the wound in the event of an unexpected caesarean); and a straw for drinking, so you don't have to get upright when you don't want to.

• Pack two bags: one for labor, and one for after the birth. Bring along a facial sponge or washcloth, which is good for cooling down; moisturizing lotion for massage during labor; cards, board games, and a book, in case your labor is longer than anticipated; and heavy-duty sanitary pads (if you prefer your brand to hospital pads). Pack a fully charged iPod or CD player; you may not be able to plug in electrical equipment in the labor ward.

Getting ready for labor

You may well feel a mixture of excitement and anxiety as you wait for labor to start. Preparing yourself both emotionally and physically will help you to enter labor with a positive and confident frame of mind.

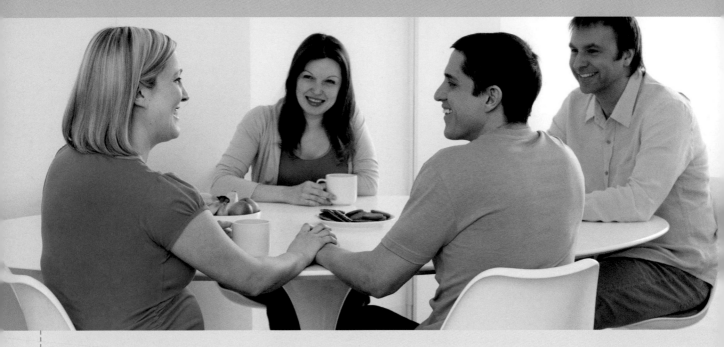

SHARING EXPERIENCES
Sharing your excitement and anticipation with couples you've met at prenatal classes, or friends who have children of their own, can be helpful; your common experiences allow you to identify with each other and offer mutual support.

Giving birth is a natural process that occurs hundreds of times each day—and over 350,000 times a year in Canada—and in the vast majority of cases is entirely straightforward. But no matter how reassuring the statistics, if you're about to go through labor for the first time, you are bound to feel a little apprehensive; after all, it's unknown territory for you. The best way to alleviate any anxiety is to take a few simple steps to prepare yourself mentally and physically for what lies ahead.

Knowing what to expect in a variety of scenarios will help you feel more confident and empowered. For example, being aware of what a forceps delivery or a caesarean entails will mean that the reality will be less of a shock.

As well as being informed, there are other ways to prepare yourself for labor and birth. Staying healthy and active throughout pregnancy will give you the stamina needed to cope with labor. As labor draws nearer you can start to focus more on the event itself and take other steps to prepare yourself physically, mentally, and emotionally.

Preparing yourself mentally

Being mentally prepared for labor helps to ease anxiety and also gives you a greater ability to cope if your labor doesn't go as you had hoped.

Take some time to reflect on the end of your pregnancy and look forward to what lies ahead. Some women feel almost a sense of loss at the thought of no longer having a baby on board after becoming so used to having a bump. Pregnancy sets you apart and makes you feel special, so it can take a while to get used to no longer being pregnant. Making this mental adjustment can help you feel more prepared for labor.

Let your birth partner know that you need him or her to be supportive in the lead-up to labor as well as for the actual event. Let them know how helpful it is to talk to them about your concerns, and to have their practical support, for example by helping you relax by giving you a soothing back massage.

Go through your birth plan one last time and make sure you're happy with it, and talk it through with your doctor or midwife, as well as with your birth partner. If everyone knows what to expect and is supportive of your choices, you'll feel more confident. Think, too, about all the possible scenarios that could happen during labor, and how you would deal with them. Feeling mentally prepared will help to ease your mind as labor approaches, and you'll be more confident that you can deal with whatever arises.

Talk to your friends about their experiences and ask them to offer constructive advice. Seek out those who are upbeat and optimistic to talk to about labor and birth.

THE RIGHT FRAME OF MIND
There are many strategies you can adopt to help you deal with the pain of labor, and it's definitely advisable to think in advance about how you might cope. In many cases, women who have difficult experiences are often shocked because they simply didn't know what to expect, or how to accommodate unexpected events during labor.

Whether or not you're planning a natural childbirth, it's useful to learn some techniques to help you overcome fear or discomfort during labor. It is often the actual fear of pain that causes tension and anxiety, which in turn can make pain worse and harder to deal with. Research the various options for pain relief (see pp.284–291), and think about which ones might be best for you.

ALTERNATIVE TECHNIQUES
Alternative techniques such as HypnoBirthing (see p.137 and p.287) and positive visualization, both aimed at putting women mentally in control, have been shown to result in shorter, more comfortable labors. Likewise, using positive affirmations prior to and during labor are believed by some to help you feel open to the experience of labor, which in turn helps you to let go of tension. Repeating statements such as "My baby will find the best position for birth" and "My body knows how to give birth" can help you to face labor with greater confidence in your abilities.

Other techniques, such as acupressure and reflexology (see pp.286–287) can be learned prior to labor and used both in the lead up to and during labor, making you feel more in control.

FEELING RESTED
It's important to stay strong and emotionally focused both before and during labor, and a key way to ensure this is to get plenty of rest and relaxation before the event, especially during the weeks immediately prior to labor. Although sleep is required for physical reasons—preparing your body to cope well with the event—it is also necessary to ensure that you are not emotionally vulnerable.

If you are finding it difficult to relax, there are plenty of proven relaxation techniques you can try to help you, such as yoga, gentle exercise, aromatherapy massage, and HypnoBirthing techniques (see pp.284–287). All of these will have an impact on your frame of mind, helping you to relax and increasing your positivity, which in turn will mean you are better equipped to manage your fears and anxiety.

Many women work until the last moment, often making the decision to save their maternity leave until after the baby is born. However, a few weeks before they're due, some women decide to stop working and focus on getting regular rest, eating healthily, going for gentle walks, and preparing for labor. If you begin labor under-rested, stressed,

Believe in yourself

What would be the best possible way for your labor to go? Think of the best possible scenario and capture it in your mind. See a happy, calm labor and imagine meeting your beautiful baby at the end of it. Whenever you feel anxious, replay these scenes in your mind.

● Keeping active (walking, swimming, and yoga, for example) can help to encourage the release of hormones that keep you feeling more positive. However, as pregnancy progresses, it's important to achieve a balance between rest and activity so that you don't enter labor tired. Breathing and relaxation techniques, as well as massage, will also encourage a positive approach.

● Do seek out birth stories from new moms who have had a good experience. However, if someone begins to tell you about a difficult birth, politely stop them. This is unhelpful to you and may simply make you feel anxious without any need to be.

"Although every labor is unique, being physically and mentally prepared can have a direct, positive bearing on your labor experience"

and possibly still buzzing with work issues, you are less likely to stay focused and adapt to the challenges of labor. Look after yourself as much as possible in the weeks before your baby is born to put you in the best frame of mind to experience a positive labor and birth.

Getting physical

Labor is physically grueling. Your body is built for it, but it's fair to say that the fitter you are and the more energy you have, the easier it's likely to be. There are also ways to prime certain body parts so that they are more resistant to the rigors of childbirth. Read on. . .

SOUND SLEEP

Getting plenty of sleep is one of the best ways to prepare yourself physically for labor. Many women are unaware of the physical toll that labor can take on the body—particularly a long labor—so making sure that you rest as much as possible in advance, going to bed at a decent time and napping in the day, too,

particularly in the last trimester, can help your body prepare.

Bear in mind that your sleep is likely to be disrupted during the last trimester, since you will probably need to get up in the night to go to the bathroom, and may find it hard to get comfortable and settle. Also, many women go into labor in the early hours of the morning. So not only are you likely to lose a night's sleep before the big event, you will also probably be exhausted after labor just when you need to adjust to life with a new, frequently waking baby.

If you find it hard to settle during the night, use pillows to support your bump, or keep your feet raised on a pillow; if you lie on your side, arrange pillows behind your back for extra support. Also, consider wearing a sleeping bra if your breasts feel heavy and uncomfortable. Whenever possible, nap for an hour or two in the day, and arrange to have a relaxing massage, or ask your partner to give you one, to reduce tension that may keep you awake. A little activity during the day will also ensure that you are physically tired enough to sleep at night.

CONSERVING ENERGY
Don't underestimate the importance of feeling rested prior to labor. Going to bed on time, and stealing a nap in the day if you feel like it, will mean that you will enter labor and life with your new baby with optimal energy reserves.

KEEPING SUPPLE
Gentle stretching and exercise even late in pregnancy will ensure that your body is well prepared for labor.

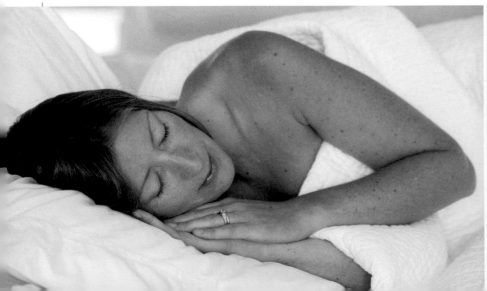

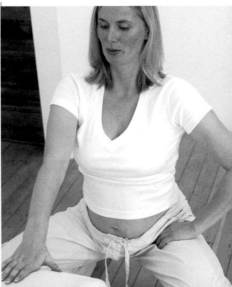

KEEPING ACTIVE

While it is important to rest in the weeks leading up to the birth to ensure you have the energy reserves to get through labor, it's equally important to get some gentle daily exercise. Staying active helps to relax you, thereby reducing tension, which in turn eases any physical discomfort. Furthermore, the release of the "feel-good" hormones known as endorphins that occurs during exercise helps to lift your mood and put you in a more positive frame of mind.

Regular movement helps to open up your pelvis in advance of the birth, and also encourages your baby to adopt a head-down position, which is more likely to result in a speedier and more effective labor.

Swimming, yoga, and aquarobics classes designed for late pregnancy, and gentle walks are all ideal forms of exercise as you prepare for labor. Be aware that your ligaments will start to soften before the birth, which means that you become more prone to injury, so make sure that you take time to stretch and warm up before exercise and cool down properly afterward. Listen to your body, take things at a slow pace, and stop if you experience any discomfort.

A HEALTHY DIET

Eating well in the last few weeks of pregnancy will keep up your energy reserves. It can be harder to eat large meals now, because your uterus may be pressing on your stomach, causing you to become full quicker. In this case, frequent nutritious snacks can give you the sustenance you need.

Healthy, whole-grain carbohydrates release energy slowly, which can help to keep you going during labor, so try to make these the backbone of your diet in the final weeks. If you aren't feeling particularly hungry, go for nutrient-rich foods, such as fruit; lean proteins; nuts and seeds; vegetables; and whole grains such as brown rice, quinoa, whole-wheat breads, hearty muesli, and even popcorn. Avoid rich, fatty foods, which can exacerbate heartburn, indigestion, and nausea. Avoid refined carbohydrates, such as white bread, white rice, and pasta, which provide short-term energy, but leave you feeling tired soon afterward.

MASSAGING YOUR PERINEUM

The area between your vagina and anus, known as the perineum, will be stretched during labor and birth. You can help to make this area more supple by massaging it with a little olive oil about four to six weeks before your due date, which helps to increase its elasticity by encouraging the blood flow to the area. Also, the hormones progesterone and relaxin are carried in your blood, and these will help to soften the surrounding muscles and ligaments and encourage controlled stretching.

Several studies have found that perineal massage reduces tearing, and fewer women require an episiotomy (see p.311). Perineal massage is also believed to reduce discomfort after the birth. However, you will need to avoid this type of massage if you have a yeast infection or herpes, because it may exacerbate symptoms.

PELVIC FLOOR EXERCISES

Ideally, these will have been a regular feature of your prenatal regime. Now though, pelvic floor exercises, or "Kegels" (see p.67), should be done in earnest to prepare the muscles supporting your uterus for labor and birth. Not only do these exercises condition the muscles that you use to push down during contractions, but research suggests that you will also be less likely to experience tearing of the perineum if you practice them regularly in the weeks leading up to labor. What's more, pelvic floor exercises encourage a supply of oxygenated blood to the pelvis, which can help to reduce the discomfort caused by contractions.

RASPBERRY LEAF TEA

Studies show that drinking raspberry leaf tea (or taking it in tablet form) from 35 weeks helps to prepare your uterus for labor. Raspberry leaves contain an alkaloid known as fragine, which is believed to work directly on the uterus, strengthening and toning it in readiness for labor. Research also suggests that taking this in the weeks prior to delivery helps to shorten the first stage of labor by making contractions more effective; and there is evidence that it may reduce the need for an assisted delivery (see pp.310–311).

However, very little medical research has been done on the effects of raspberry leaf on pregnant women and their babies, so it's best to avoid this remedy unless you're already full-term and your ob/gyn gives you the go-ahead. After the birth, the tea is believed to help the uterus contract back to size.

EAT LITTLE AND OFTEN
If you can't face big meals in the later stages of pregnancy, try grazing on small snacks, such as a fruit salad, throughout the day.

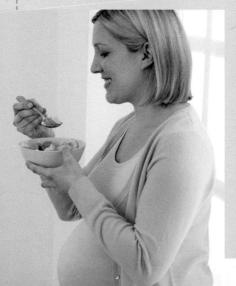

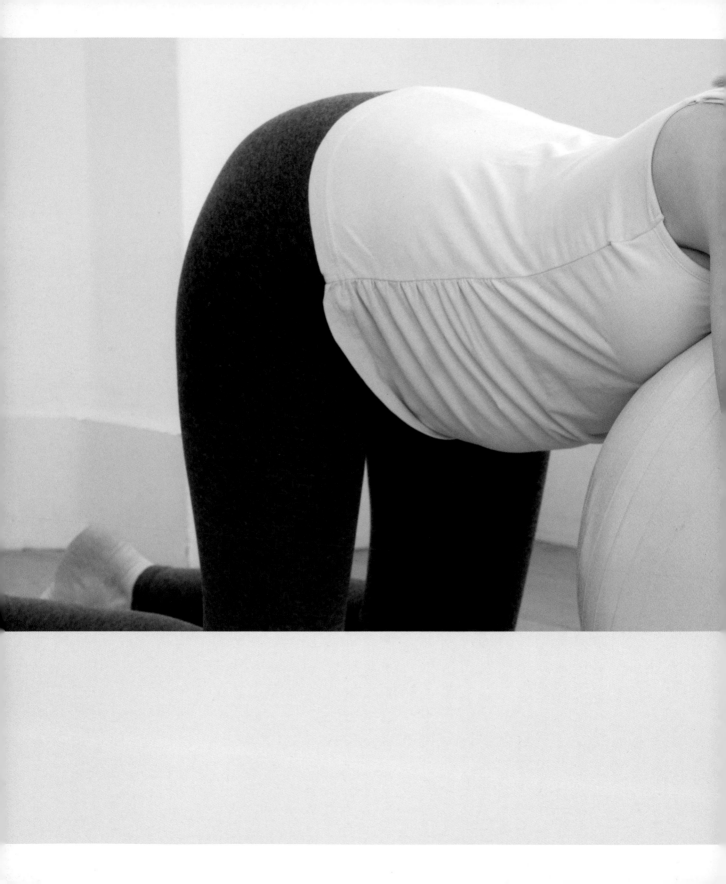

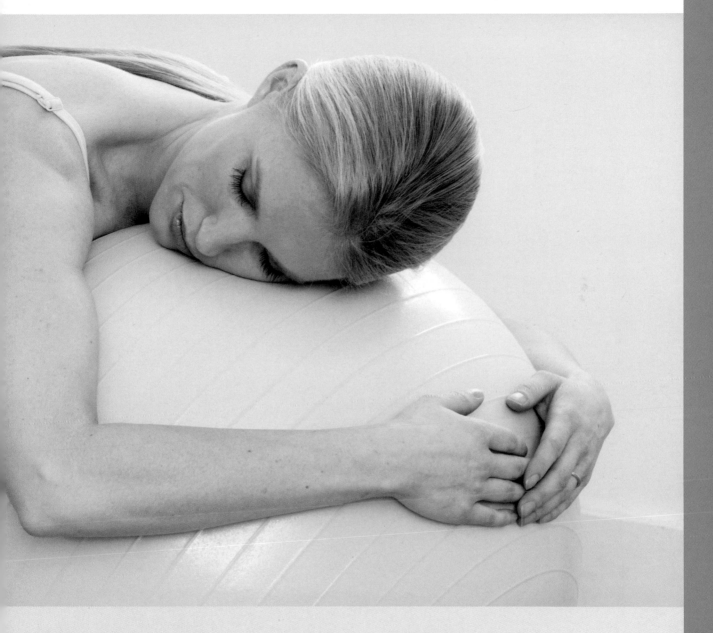

My labor and birth

The wait is almost over . . . knowing what to expect in labor and about pain-relief options can help you face the experience positively.

The process of birth

After nine months of being confined in a relatively tight space, it's time for your baby and body to work together to move your baby through your cervix and down the birth canal for the tumultuous moment of birth.

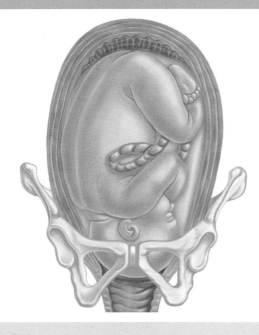

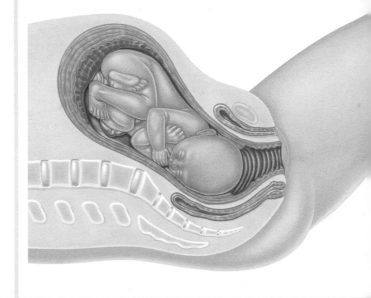

CONTRACTIONS BUILD IN INTENSITY
At the start of labor, the uterus begins to contract to push the baby's head into the cervix. Contractions become more regular until, at the end of the first stage of labor, the cervix is fully dilated.

JOURNEY DOWN THE BIRTH CANAL
Once the cervix is fully open, your baby starts to move out of the uterus into the birth canal. Your baby now turns toward your back with his chin on his chest, and your vagina stretches as he descends.

Birth is an incredible feat of nature, and takes you on a roller-coaster ride of emotional and physical highs and lows. No one knows exactly what triggers labor, but it is thought to be a hormonal reaction, possibly to signals from your baby's adrenal gland. Once labor starts, it follows a fairly predictable pattern of three stages: In the first stage your cervix dilates, in the second stage you push your baby out, and the third stage is when your placenta is delivered. The length of each stage varies between women. Typically, a first labor lasts around 17 hours.

Contractions start

The birth process begins with mild contractions that become increasingly frequent and more intense as the cervix opens (dilates) and thins out (effaces) to allow your baby to move into the birth canal. This first stage of labor is the longest of the three stages and is actually divided into two phases of its own: early labor and active labor. Signs of early labor can include pains in the back or abdomen, nausea, and a mucus-y vaginal discharge, which may be tinged

with blood (see p.277). This early phase can last for up to a day or so in a first labor—or even longer.

With the onset of active labor, contractions become more regular as the cervix dilates centimeter by centimeter until—at 10cm—it is fully open and wide enough for the birth of your baby's head. Contractions are felt higher in the abdomen and move down toward the pelvis and lower back as your baby is pushed downward, almost to the end of the birth canal. Labor usually speeds up as it progresses: It generally takes

"Being aware of how labor progresses and what is happening to your body and baby helps you cope better with the discomfort"

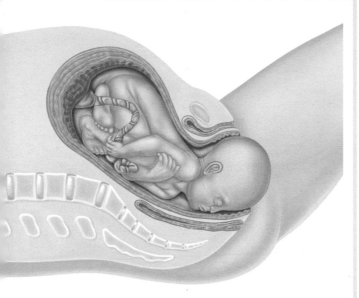

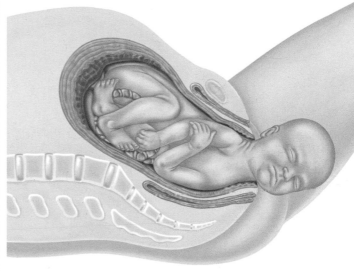

YOUR BABY'S HEAD "CROWNS"
As your baby passes down the vagina, he goes under the pubic bone and turns his head face down to negotiate the bend. Once his head can be seen at the vaginal opening, it is said to have "crowned."

THE MOMENT OF BIRTH
Your baby's head will emerge so that it is clear of the birth canal, and he will automatically turn his head to face one of your thighs to allow the rest of his body to be born more easily.

more time to go from being 1–2cm to 5–6cm dilated, than from 5–6cm to 10cm (fully dilated). Once you reach this stage, your baby can move further down the birth canal.

Pushing begins

During the second stage of labor, you push your baby out through your fully dilated cervix and into the world. Contractions tend to slow down now, although they become more intense.

As your baby presses down on the muscles of the pelvis, you'll feel an overwhelming urge to push or "bear down." Your doctor, nurse, or midwife will help to ensure that your baby isn't born too quickly. The second stage is usually a lot shorter than the first—often under two hours and sometimes even less.

As your baby journeys down the vagina, its flexible tissues allow him to pass through. He is helped by the fact that his skull bones are not yet fused together so they can overlap, making the skull smaller.

Your baby is born

Your caregiver will encourage you to use each contraction to push as hard as you can to get your baby's head out. You may feel intense burning pains as the vagina and vulva are stretched. Once his head is born, he turns to straighten his neck so that he's facing your side again. At this point, the doctor or midwife may support his head while the shoulders are born, one before the other, with his arms held close to his body. Once the shoulders are through, the rest of his body slides out quickly.

How your baby lies

Ideally your baby should be head down in your pelvis at the end of pregnancy to make labor easier, but some babies take up different positions. It's useful to know which way your baby lies and the implications for you.

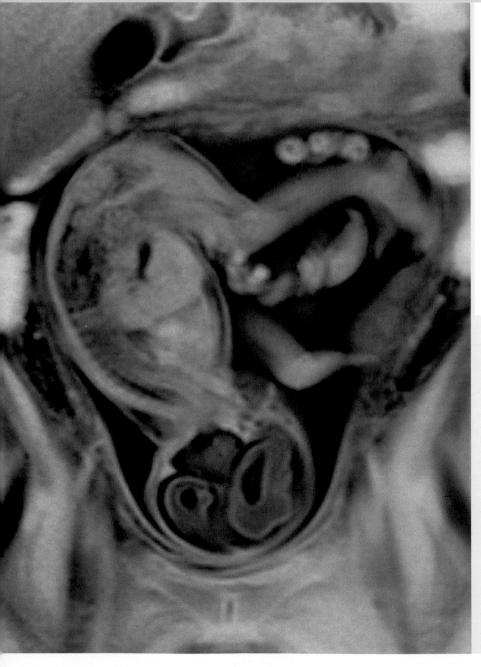

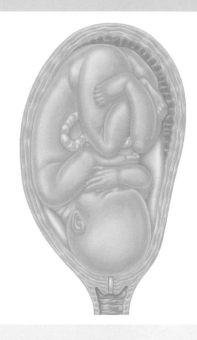

HEAD DOWN "POSTERIOR"
Some babies lie head down, but with the back of their head against the mother's spine. This is referred to as a "posterior" position, which can prolong labor and give the laboring mother a backache.

PRIME POSITION
The ultrasound (left) shows a baby lying head down in an "anterior" position, with the back of the head facing forward, toward the mother's abdomen. This is the best position for labor and birth.

"Some babies turn to a head-down position in the last month of pregnancy or just before birth, while others turn during labor"

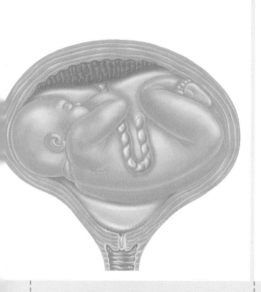

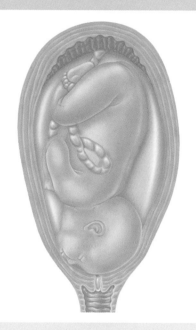

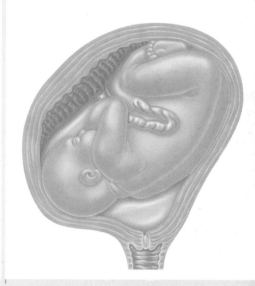

TRANSVERSE
The baby is lying horizontally in the uterus. Unless she turns prior to labor, a vaginal birth will not be possible.

BROW PRESENTATION
Occasionally, the head is tilted backward and the forehead presses on the cervix. This means a vaginal birth will be difficult.

OBLIQUE PRESENTATION
Here the baby is lying diagonally in the uterus. As with a transverse lie, a vaginal birth is unlikely.

The vast majority of babies (95 percent) turn around so that they are head down by the end of pregnancy in readiness for birth. This ensures that the baby's body is lined up to fit through the pelvis as easily as possible during the birth. This is often referred to as a cephalic or vertex position (or presentation). The other five percent of babies remain bottom-down, or "breech," or lie in a horizontal (transverse) or diagonal (oblique) position. How your baby is positioned when you reach full term may influence your birth plan.

Head down

The optimal position for labor and birth is a head-down, "anterior" (OA, or occipito-anterior) position, which means that the back of your baby's head faces toward your abdomen, with the crown (vertex) of her head pressing down on your cervix. This is by far the easiest position for delivering your baby; she will fit neatly in your pelvic cavity, with her chin tucked in closely toward her chest. These babies are born head-first, which is known as a vertex delivery.

FACING A DIFFERENT WAY
Head-down babies who are not in the anterior position may lie at a slightly different angle so they face another way. Around one in ten babies adopt a "posterior" (OP, or occipito-posterior) position for labor, which means that your baby's back is lying against your spine and she is facing forward, toward your abdomen. In this position, your baby has a tighter fit in the pelvis, and it is her forehead, rather than the crown of her head, that presses down on your cervix, which is less effective. This in turn

weakens your contractions, the cervix dilates more slowly, and labor tends to be longer.

Fortunately, most babies in a posterior position at the start of labor will turn to an anterior position during the course of labor because of the shape of the pelvic muscles and the mother's pushing.

Other head-down positions include a brow presentation, in which your baby's eyebrows are leading the way. More rarely, she may be in a "face" presentation, with her face pressing against your cervix. Both of these positions can lead to longer, more difficult labors, and a caesarean delivery may be necessary.

TRANSVERSE AND OBLIQUE

Some babies lie in a horizontal (transverse) or diagonal (oblique) position. You may be able to tell because your bump might feel especially firm and tight. If your baby is transverse, her head may be on your left or right, and her back may face upward—under your ribcage—or downward. It's not unusual for your baby to be in these positions earlier in pregnancy: She may be taking her time turning from breech to head down. However, if she is not head down by 36 or 37 weeks, your obstetrician will investigate the reason. For example, your baby may be unable to turn if you have a low-lying placenta (placenta previa— see p.386), or if your pelvis is smaller than usual—or small in relation to your baby's head. You will be observed closely and may need to check into the hospital in case labor starts while your baby is in one of these positions.

Breech babies

Many babies adopt a bottom-down breech position during pregnancy, but then turn naturally to adopt the best position for labor. If this happens late in pregnancy, you may feel something similar to an almighty somersault as your baby turns. However, the longer she remains breech, the less likely it is that she'll turn, as her growing size coupled with the confines of the uterus make it harder for her to do. If your baby is breech at 34 weeks, you will be offered a procedure to try to turn her (see below). Breech babies can be in one of three positions: a "complete," or flexed, breech, when both feet are crossed and the bottom sits in the pelvis; an "extended," or frank, breech, when the baby's hips are flexed, with the knees extended and feet by the head; or a "footling" breech, when one or both hips are extended and the feet are below the baby's bottom.

TURNING A BREECH BABY

If your baby is breech as you approach your due date, your doctor may offer to turn her with a procedure called an external cephalic version, or ECV. This involves manually massaging your abdomen to try to turn her from a head-up to a head-down position.

Its success depends on a number of factors, including whether you've had a baby before, if there's enough amniotic fluid around your baby, and whether your baby has engaged in the pelvis. You may be given medication during the procedure to relax the muscles of the uterus, which can help ease any discomfort you might feel. If a first

COMPLETE (FLEXED) BREECH
One of the most common types of breech presentation: Your baby's bottom is pressed against your pelvis with her feet tucked in.

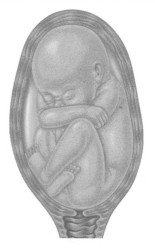

EXTENDED (FRANK) BREECH
Another common type of breech: Your baby has her legs fully extended. A vaginal delivery is most likely with this type.

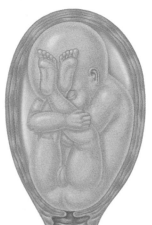
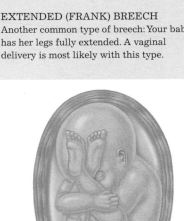

FOOTLING BREECH
A vaginal birth is unlikely with this type of breech and you will probably be scheduled for a caesarean delivery.

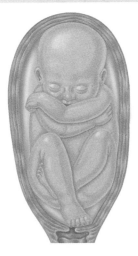

attempt is unsuccessful, your doctor may try again on a different day.

There are also techniques you can try at home to encourage your baby to turn. The first involves kneeling on your bed with your bottom in the air and hips flexed at slightly more than 90 degrees (keeping your thighs away from your bump). Your head, shoulders, and chest should be as flat as possible on the bed. Hold this for 15 minutes, every two hours during the day, for five days. One study found that 65 of 71 breech babies turned when their moms adopted this position. Another technique is to lie on your back with your hips raised on a pillow and hips and knees flexed. Slowly roll from side to side for 10 minutes three or four times a day. Avoid this though if you have suffered back, pelvic, or hip pain.

As well as at-home techniques, there is some respected research that suggests that acupuncture (see p.286) can help turn breech babies in the uterus.

If all attempts to turn your baby fail, your doctor will talk to you about your birth options. A vaginal birth may be possible depending on the exact position of your baby (see opposite), but this does require special expertise. Recent studies highlight an increased risk for mom and baby with breech births because the largest part of the baby's body, the head, is delivered last. You will probably be advised therefore to consider a caesarean to ensure her safe delivery.

DELIVERING A BREECH BABY

Most vaginal breech deliveries are of very premature babies, second twins, or to women who are found to have a breech baby in advanced labor. If you know that your baby is breech, your obstetrician will advise you whether it is possible—or safe—to deliver your baby vaginally. A natural labor is possible if your baby is not very small or large, your pelvis isn't unusually small, and your baby is in an extended or complete breech. While an extended breech is the best position for a vaginal breech delivery, a baby who is in a complete breech position (see opposite) can often be delivered naturally, too, as long as her bottom moves down and engages in the pelvis during labor.

A footling breech carries a greater risk of the umbilical cord falling out during labor, an emergency known as cord prolapse (see p.319).

Twin presentations

If you are carrying twins, their position is unlikely to change after 36 weeks due to lack of space in the uterus. Your doctor will assess their position and decide whether a vaginal birth is possible. Twins can be in the following positions:

• Vertex/vertex. If both babies are head down (vertex), you will be able to attempt a vaginal birth.

• Vertex/breech. This position makes the best use of space in the uterus, but is not ideal for delivery. If the first baby is head down and in a good position for delivery, your doctor will manipulate the breech twin into a vertex position after your first baby is born.
• Breech/vertex or breech/breech. If your first baby is breech (or both are breech), a caesarean will be advised.

• Oblique. If your first baby is in an oblique position, it's likely that a caesarean will be recommended.
• Vertex/transverse or transverse/transverse. If the first baby is head down (vertex) and the other horizontal, a vaginal delivery may be possible. If both babies are lying horizontally across your uterus, you'll need a caesarean to ensure that they are safely delivered.

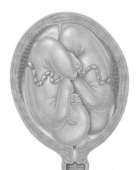

VERTEX/VERTEX
With both babies facing downward, a vaginal delivery may be possible.

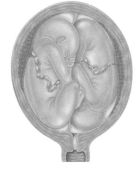

VERTEX/BREECH
In this presentation, the second twin may be turned head down after the first baby is born.

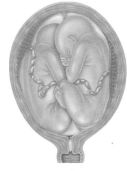

BREECH/BREECH
Both twins are in the breech presentation, with their bottoms in the lower part of the uterus.

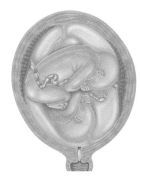

VERTEX/TRANSVERSE
One baby is in a head-down position, but the other lies horizontally across the uterus.

My baby is overdue

You may start to worry if your due date comes and goes with no sign of your baby. Remember, this date is simply an estimate: In reality just five percent of babies are born on their due date, with most born between 39 and 41 weeks.

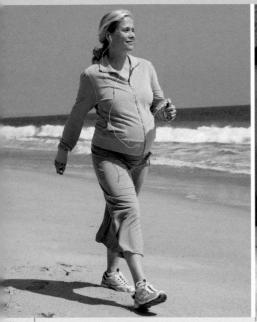

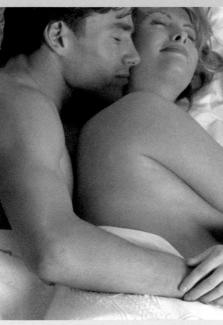

KEEPING ACTIVE
Movement and activity are often recommended to get labor going; being upright and moving around may encourage your baby to move down in the pelvis.

THE BENEFITS OF SEX
One of the more enjoyable ways to try to start labor is by having sex—although you may not be in the mood! Chemicals in sperm are thought to trigger contractions, so it may be worth a try.

COMPLEMENTARY THERAPIES
Several complementary therapies purport to help labor get underway. Therapies such as acupressure and acupuncture target specific points believed to stimulate labor.

Your due date is partly based on an average gestation period, which is 280 days, or 40 weeks. However, each pregnancy is different, and many women take a couple more weeks before giving birth, while some deliver fully developed babies at 37 weeks. If your pregnancy is progressing well and your baby thriving, your doctor or midwife will usually be happy to allow more time after your due date to let nature take its course. Ask about your doctor's policy on when she will advise an induction of labor.

When should I worry?

Once you pass the 40-week mark, both you and your baby will be monitored more closely. Your baby's heart rate will be checked, and you may be offered an ultrasound to assess her size.

As you approach the 41- to 42-week mark, your doctor or midwife may decide to start the process of inducing labor. This involves kick-starting labor, either through intervention or with drugs (see pp.280–281). First, at around 41 weeks, you will be offered a membrane sweep (see p.281), which is an internal examination carried out by your doctor or midwife with the aim of triggering contractions. If a sweep doesn't work to get labor started, you will be scheduled for an induction at the hospital. This is done because the risk of stillbirth increases slightly after 42 weeks, so the aim is to ensure the safe delivery of your baby by this date.

What can I do myself?

There are several techniques you can try at home to attempt to kick-start labor. There's no proof—although plenty of anecdotal evidence—that these work, but some might be worth a try. . .

EXERCISE

Gentle exercise is thought to encourage your baby's head down into the pelvic cavity, and the pressure of the head on the cervix may help to start the process of labor. It has been suggested that walking on an uneven surface, for example, with one foot on the road and one on the kerb, can loosen the pelvic ligaments and nudge the baby down. Some women swear by a long walk in the countryside or a park. It is also thought that getting the adrenaline going may contribute to the start of labor.

NIPPLE STIMULATION

Stimulating your nipple area, either during sex or on your own, is thought to kick-start labor. The reason for this is that massaging the whole of your areola (the dark area around the nipple) as well as the nipple itself may encourage the release of oxytocin, a hormone that is involved in starting contractions. There is some evidence that this method is effective, with one study finding that 37 percent of women who tried this went into labor within the following 72 hours, compared with just 6 percent of those who did not try this method.

SEX

Sexual intercourse is a well-documented way to try to bring on labor. It's thought that the release of oxytocin that occurs during sex, as well as physical changes that occur during orgasm, may trigger contractions. Also, chemicals called prostaglandins, found in sperm, can act on the cervix, causing it to soften and hopefully dilate. Avoid sex if your water has broken (due to the risk of infection), you have a low-lying placenta (see p.386), or you have a history of vaginal bleeding.

SPICY FOODS

There is no evidence that eating spicy food works, but some women claim they have had success stimulating labor this way. It's thought that hot spices stimulate the gut and the bowel, which in turn could trigger contractions. However, the resulting heartburn or indigestion may not be worth it!

ACUPUNCTURE

Research suggests that acupuncture, which involves inserting thin needles at specific points on the body to stimulate organs and/or energy flow, is a safe and effective way to bring on labor. Choose a registered and reputable practitioner.

HOMEOPATHY

Certain homeopathic remedies, like raspberry leaf tea, are thought to encourage the onset of labor. Ask your ob/gyn whether it's safe or recommended to try a homeopathic treatment.

PINEAPPLE

This contains a chemical called bromelain, which not only eases the discomfort of heartburn, but is claimed can soften the cervix. There is limited evidence to support this, and one pineapple is unlikely to have enough bromelain to have any effect. However, eating a couple of pineapples will certainly stimulate your bowels.

CASTOR OIL

Drinking castor oil (mixed with orange juice or another hydrating fruit juice) has a long history of use in inducing labor and was used as far back as Ancient Egypt. It's a powerful laxative, stimulating the bowels, which may trigger contractions. However, this is definitely not recommended due to the possibility of severe diarrhea, which can lead to dehydration. One study of overdue women did find that almost 58 percent began active labor after a single dose, as opposed to 4.2 percent who had none, but all of the women who took it suffered from nausea.

Staying calm

If none of these strategies work, try not to get too stressed—stress is unlikely to encourage labor. If labor doesn't start naturally, make the most of this time to rest before the start of your life with a new baby. It may help to turn off your phone, or ask friends or family to avoid daily calls to check on your progress.

What did—and didn't—work for us

I tried almost every method going, but none of them worked for me. I did take up knitting, too, which helped the time go by and took my mind off the waiting! MG

I took long walks, and walked up several flights of stairs, but all that did was give me some Braxton Hicks–like contractions, make me need to pee, and leave me short of breath. LJ

I tried acupuncture, homoeopathy, and reflexology to bring on labor. It's difficult to know what actually worked because I also ended up having two membrane sweeps (see p.281). However, just because you don't go into labor immediately after a treatment doesn't mean that it's not helping to encourage labor to start. Pre-labor may be underway without your being aware of it! TL

Am I in labor?

It is more difficult than you might think to pinpoint exactly when labor starts. It's helpful to know which signs may amount to little and which are really telling you that your baby is on its way.

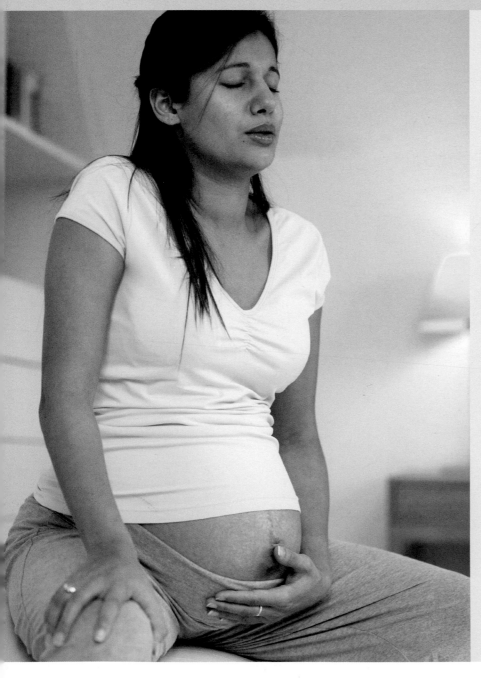

When you're close to your due date, you're aware of every twinge or suggestion of abdominal discomfort, wondering if this will be the start of something. The exact trigger for labor is unknown, but it's thought that hormones produced by your baby's adrenal gland encourage your placenta to release further hormones that cause your uterus to contract. Other signals are involved too, including the release of prostaglandins, which are also used to induce labor artificially (see p.281). When your uterus begins to contract, your cervix (neck of your womb) starts to open, or dilate (see p.294), and labor begins in earnest.

False labor

In the late stages of pregnancy, you may have Braxton Hicks contractions (see p.216), the practice contractions that prepare your uterus for action. In the days and hours prior to labor, these can be more uncomfortable and occur closer together, sometimes carrying on for hours. However, if the uterus is contracting, but there's no effacement or dilation of the cervix, this is known as "false labor." Braxton Hicks do encourage the baby's head to move down in the pelvis, but

INCREASING CONTRACTIONS
As you approach labor, you may experience more Braxton Hicks contractions. These differ from real contractions as they fade, rather than build up, and occur irregularly.

until contractions are strong, regular, develop a pattern, and occur closer together, you're unlikely to be in labor.

Approaching labor

The experience of labor varies between women, but as labor approaches, there are several signs and symptoms you may experience that tell you your body is preparing itself for the task ahead.

WATER BREAKING
Very few women find that their water breaks (when the amniotic sac breaks and leaks its fluid) before labor. The fluid can either gush or drip out, which can be confused with leaking urine. Usually the sac doesn't break until labor is established, and sometimes not until just before the birth. If your water breaks, it is a sign that labor is imminent and you should go to the hospital or call your doctor. If labor doesn't begin within 24 hours, there is a risk of developing an infection, so it's important that you take instruction from your doctor or midwife and go in for an assessment when asked.

Amniotic fluid should be clear. If it is smelly or blood-stained, contact your doctor or midwife at once. Contact them too if it's green, which suggests that your baby has passed meconium (see p.215), and is a sign that she may be distressed.

OTHER SIGNS AND SYMPTOMS
You may lose the mucus plug (a collection of mucus that plugs the cervix, which can be bloodstained and is known as a "bloody show"), as well as experience back and/or abdominal pain and feel queasy. Some women suffer diarrhea and even vomiting. This stage can take several days, so don't call your doctor yet.

ENGAGEMENT OF THE HEAD
You may experience "lightening," which describes how you feel when your baby's head drops down in the pelvis, or engages, and the pressure on the diaphragm, which may have made you breathless before, is alleviated. This can happen days or weeks before the birth, but some women feel it just before contractions start. You may need to go to the bathroom more often, as your baby puts pressure on the bladder.

FIRST CONTRACTIONS
As you approach early labor, contractions become uncomfortable and occur increasingly close together, although still irregularly. These differ from Braxton Hicks as they build up and begin to prepare the cervix for labor.

Symptoms you shouldn't ignore

Call your doctor or midwife if: Your water breaks; your baby moves less than usual; you have vaginal bleeding that is not associated with losing your mucus plug; you have a fever, changes in your vision, severe headaches, or abdominal pain; you feel an urge to push; or you feel like your baby's head is emerging.

How we knew we were in labor

My first baby was due in December, and a few days before my due date, it started snowing heavily. I woke up one morning at around 4am experiencing very strong contractions. As my husband went out to get the car ready, I shuffled down the stairs and into the car. We set off to brave the morning rush-hour traffic in the snow on our way to the hospital. I was absolutely convinced that this was the real thing since I was in so much pain. However, as the sun came out and the snow eventually stopped, so did my contractions. Needless to say we remained in the car, somewhat deflated, and drove back home. The very next night, things started off at exactly the same time—but this time it was the real thing! MG

After my membrane sweep, my contractions started right away, and things then progressed rapidly! I checked into the hospital, and when my midwife examined me at 11pm, I was 7cm dilated. I gave birth an hour later. There was no "bloody show" or gradual buildup of contractions. NK

I went into labor the evening before my daughter's due date. I didn't realize at first because the two signs I was waiting for—a bloody show and/or my water breaking—didn't happen. I started to feel contractions and took a bath, because I thought there were still hours or even days to go. At about 11:30pm, we went to the hospital and I was 8cm dilated. My baby was born two hours later. FF

At the end of my second pregnancy, strong contractions convinced me twice that I was starting labor, both prior to and on my son's due date. However, both times the contractions stopped within hours of starting, and it was three days later before I went into real labor and had my son. LJ

I was scheduled for a caesarean section because my son was breech, but the night before, my water broke. It took my husband and me a while to realize that it had happened—there wasn't much fluid at first—but on the drive to the hospital, water was pouring out! I had mild pains and was in active labor by the time I reached the hospital. VB

What does my baby feel?

There's so much to think about in the days before labor, but one thing that you may well be concerned about is what your baby is experiencing, and how the process of childbirth will affect him.

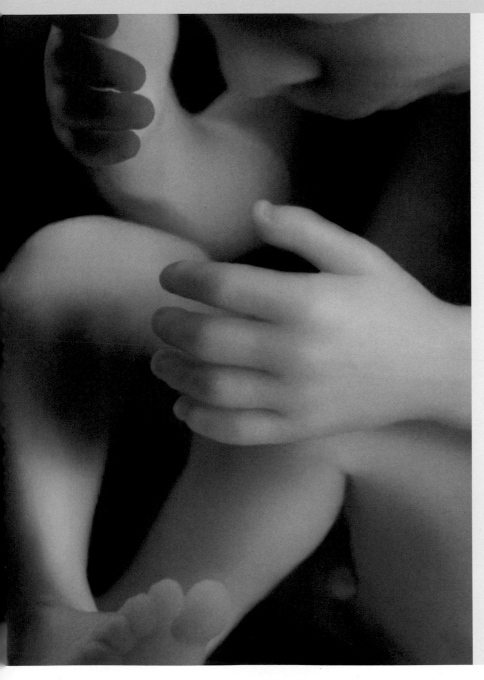

It is believed that your unborn baby can hear from as early as 16 weeks of pregnancy, and even responds to different sounds outside the uterus. Your baby will be familiar with your voice, and probably that of your partner, and will find it soothing. Many experts suggest talking to your baby regularly in the weeks leading up to the birth, and beginning to establish a rapport. Your baby will be able to hear your voice throughout labor, and you can continue to talk to him, soothe him, and encourage him throughout the contractions. Although he is likely to be in a semi-conscious state (see opposite), your reassurance will undoubtedly make the experience more pleasurable.

How your baby sees and breathes

Sight is the least developed of your baby's senses when he is born, and he will rely most heavily on auditory stimulation during the early days, as well as being reassured through touch. Your baby's eyes will have been open from

GETTING READY TO MOVE OUT
No one knows for certain what a baby feels during labor, but it is unlikely that they experience pain anything like that of a laboring mother. Most experts believe that the sensation babies have is akin to being gradually squeezed through a tight space, twisting and turning as they go.

about the 26th week of pregnancy, and studies have found that shining a bright light on your abdomen from 37 weeks will encourage your baby's heart rate to speed up, and he may even turn toward the source of light.

Chances are, though, that your baby will have his eyes closed as your contractions push him against your cervix and out into the world, and he will probably be shocked initially by the bright light when he emerges. Hold him close to your breast, and give your baby some time to adjust to his strange new surroundings.

Throughout pregnancy, your baby receives oxygen from your placenta through the umbilical cord. During the birth, he will continue to be nourished in the same way. Interestingly, his lungs are filled with fluid that helps them mature while in the uterus. During labor this fluid is dried up to help the lungs expand and fill with air once the umbilical cord—and your baby's oxygen supply—are cut.

Your baby's chest moves in the uterus as if he is breathing, but there is actually no air going in and out of his lungs. These breathing movements are a sign of well-being—a form of practice breathing—and are often used in the assessment of your baby's health during an ultrasound.

Does he feel pain?

There is very good research to suggest that babies can feel pain when they are in the uterus. Ultrasound observations of behavior in utero show that babies appear to react to needles that intrude into the uterus with a mixture of shock, withdrawal, and aggression.

However, don't be alarmed by this. The birth experience is a natural one, and therefore not painful for your baby. Women in labor experience pain when

What does "fetal distress" mean?

When your uterus contracts during labor, blood is squeezed out of the placenta, returning during the "relaxation" phase between contractions. This ensures that your baby has a constant supply of oxygenated blood. What's more, babies are designed for labor, with red blood cells that hold on to oxygen for long periods of time.

In some cases, blood flow to and/or from the placenta is not at an optimal level during labor, and babies can become distressed. There are a number of reasons for this—for example, a compressed umbilical cord, a failing placenta, or an infection.

When babies become distressed, it is known as "fetal distress," and this is identified in a number of ways. For example, babies who are distressed are more likely to pass meconium (a baby's first dark-greenish bowel movement) in the uterus; their heart-rate patterns (see p.293) can also indicate signs of distress by becoming accelerated or slowing down unexpectedly. Another sign of fetal distress is the baby moving excessively. During labor your doctor or midwife may have to extract a tiny sample of blood from your baby's scalp to measure oxygen levels, which will confirm whether or not he is distressed.

In most cases, distress means that your baby will have to be delivered as quickly as possible. If he is close to being born, forceps or a vacuum may be used to extract him (see pp.310–311); if your labor has not progressed very far, a caesarean will probably be necessary. For more information on pregnancy complications, see pp.384–387.

the muscles of the uterus contract and become starved of oxygen; however, babies are designed to cope with the process of labor; the red blood cells in their circulation can retain oxygen for longer periods of time. It's thought that babies experience something akin to a feeling of being squeezed or gently compressed, but do not feel anything like what their mothers feel during labor.

A great deal of research has been undertaken into the subject of what babies feel during labor and birth. It is now believed that because of the chemical environment within the uterus, babies are in a constant state of semi-consciousness, and never actually experience true wakefulness until they are born. Also, because of the warm amniotic fluid, they are lulled by and protected from even the strongest maternal contractions. Even if your water breaks before labor, there will be enough fluid remaining to cushion your baby, and he will not experience discomfort during labor.

"During labor, babies experience something akin to a feeling of being squeezed or gently compressed"

Induction

If you are one to two weeks past your due date and haven't gone into labor, an induction may be advised. Usually, there will be an attempt to trigger contractions naturally first; if this doesn't work you will probably be induced in the hospital.

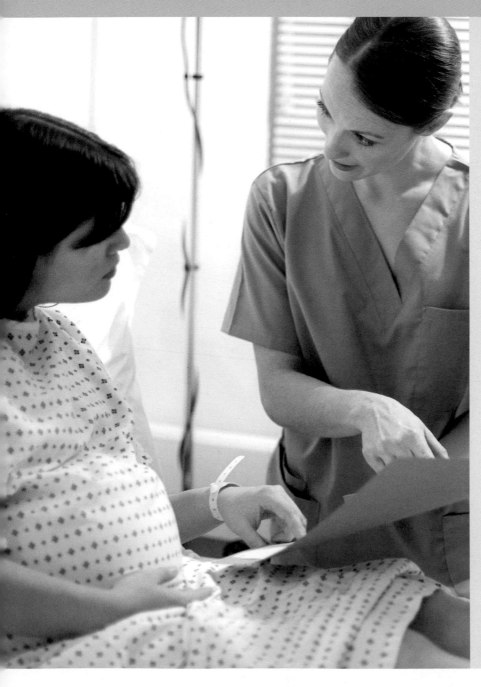

Most women don't like the idea of induction because they would prefer labor to happen naturally, and have often heard (or read online) that an induced labor is more painful than a normal one. However, it is recommended for sound reasons, the main one being that after 42 weeks, the placenta—the source of your baby's nutrition—becomes less efficient. This means that your baby might not be getting sufficient oxygen and nourishment, so for the sake of her health, she needs to be born soon.

Induction might also be advised earlier in pregnancy if you have preeclampsia (see pp.386–387) or a pregnancy condition such as gestational diabetes (see p.385); if your baby is not growing well; if you have unexplained bleeding; or if your water has broken but you haven't gone into labor naturally. The aim of inducing labor is to allow you to deliver your baby naturally and safely.

On the plus side, knowing that you're going to be induced ends the frustration of waiting, which most women find very tiresome after their due date comes and goes. There's no concrete evidence to suggest that induced labor is any more painful than natural labor, but with medical induction contractions may start more quickly and so might feel intense at

KEEPING YOU INFORMED
Your doctor or midwife will talk to you about your progress during each stage of an induction and will keep you fully informed of their plans.

first. Induction works in most cases, and you can expect to have a normal labor and delivery in the day or so afterward. There are several methods used to induce labor, which may be given on their own, in combination, or following on from each other, depending on the success or failure of a particular method.

The natural approach

Prior to a medical induction, your doctor or midwife may try to get contractions started by giving you a "membrane sweep," which means that she will try to separate the membranes around your baby from your cervix. This encourages the release of prostaglandins, the hormones that help to trigger labor. To do this, she'll need to insert a finger into your cervix to stretch it, and sweep around inside. Some women liken this to a normal vaginal examination; others find it more uncomfortable, so you may want to check whether pain relief is available to take the edge off any discomfort. If the procedure is successful, labor usually starts within 48 hours.

Medical induction

If a membrane sweep hasn't worked, the next step is to try to ensure that the cervix is soft and dilated enough for labor to begin. If your cervix is still thick/and or closed, you'll be offered a vaginal gel or another preparation containing the natural chemical prostaglandin, which is placed at the top of your vagina, to soften it artificially and trigger contractions.

A vaginal gel is given several hours to work; if nothing happens, you may be offered a second dose after about six hours. Prostaglandin is usually given in

the hospital, often in the evening with the aim that you rest overnight while it takes effect and feel refreshed in the morning if contractions start. Your baby's heart rate will be monitored before and after giving you prostaglandin to see how she copes with any contractions. Once this has been done, getting up and walking around can help labor progress, or get things started if you haven't had any contractions yet.

BREAKING YOUR WATER

Once your cervix starts to soften and open, or dilate, your doctor or midwife may decide to break your water—the membranes that hold the amniotic fluid surrounding your baby. This is called an amniotomy, or the artificial rupture of membranes (ARM). Some women find the procedure slightly uncomfortable, although many say they hardly noticed that it had been done.

A slim hook will be inserted into your cervix to rupture the amniotic sac, or something called an amnicot, which is a glove with a small pricked end on one finger, may be used. As the sac breaks, there may be a gush of water, or just some dripping or leaking. When your water has broken, more prostaglandins are released, which will hopefully encourage the cervix to dilate more and contractions to follow.

GIVING OXYTOCIN

If gels and an amniotomy fail to bring on labor, the next step is to offer a synthetic form of the hormone oxytocin, which in a natural labor stimulates the uterus to contract. Sometimes this is done at the same time as an amniotomy. Oxytocin is fed directly into your bloodstream via an intravenous drip. One of the concerns women have about oxytocin is that it can bring on strong, fairly frequent contractions that aren't usual at the outset of labor, which may feel more

painful because the body hasn't had a gradual buildup and time to adjust to the pain. This can happen, but you will be given a small dose at first, which will be increased gradually. Try to remain calm, practice your breathing and relaxation techniques, and remain as active as you can. Sometimes, if contractions stop and start, or are a little ineffective, you may be given oxytocin for much of the first stage of labor.

Your baby also has to adapt quickly to sudden contractions. For this reason, once you've been given oxytocin you will be monitored continuously so that your baby's heartbeat and your contractions can be checked to ensure that your baby and uterus are responding well.

When induction doesn't work

Inductions aren't always successful. If this is the case with you, try not to become downhearted or feel like it's your fault. Sometimes, for no apparent reason, babies simply are reluctant to be born naturally, which can happen even to women who have had successful natural births in the past. If your cervix fails to respond to induction procedures, it is called a failed induction. Or the cervix may open part-way and then fail to go further, called an "arrest of dilatation."

If induction fails, another induction may be planned or a caesarean will be performed. A caesarean may not be the type of birth you had anticipated, but your doctor or midwife will suggest it for the best reasons, namely for the well-being of both you and your baby. Repeated attempts to bring on labor can exhaust you and distress your baby—a caesarean is performed to ensure that your baby is delivered as safely as possible for you both.

Coping with pain

Most women worry about how they will handle the pain of childbirth. Everyone experiences it differently, but the better prepared you are, with strategies to cope and a positive mental attitude, the less anxious you will feel.

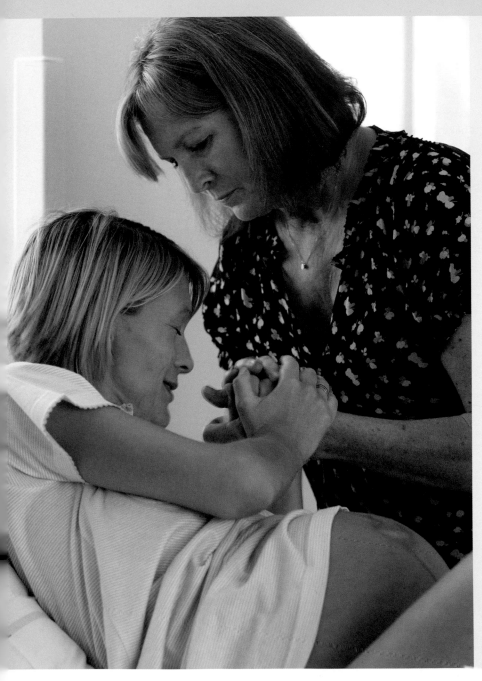

Pain during labor is caused mainly by the muscles in your uterus contracting, but also by the pressure of your baby's head against your cervix. Contractions are usually felt as cramping in the abdomen, groin, and back. Some women also experience pain in their sides or thighs. In addition, the baby's head can put uncomfortable pressure on your bladder and bowels, and pain is likely as he stretches and moves down the birth canal on his way to be born.

The experience of pain during labor differs widely between women, and even between pregnancies. Some report cramping similar to period pain that can be managed using breathing techniques. Others experience pain in strong waves that can seem overwhelming and drive them to seek medical pain relief.

The most effective way to make labor more comfortable is to avoid feeling stressed. There's plenty of research to show that women who cope best with labor are not those with a higher pain threshold—but those who approach it with less tension and fear. This makes scientific sense. During labor, the body releases its own natural painkillers, called endorphins. If you are stressed, however, your body produces stress hormones, which completely override the

A SUPPORTIVE PARTNER
Whether it's your partner, mom, or a doula, having someone with you throughout labor to offer encouragement and support can help you to cope with the intensity of contractions.

"Understanding how pain can build, peak, and decline through labor can help you plan your pain relief accordingly"

feel-good effects of endorphins. Also, if your body goes into stress mode, blood is diverted away from organs; this means that your uterus attempts its work with less oxygen, which increases pain.

The progress of pain

Being aware of the peaks and troughs of pain can help you to manage your labor. Although it's hard to predict the intensity of pain, since it depends on factors such as your baby's position and your ability to relax, there are particular types of pain relief that are appropriate for certain stages of labor.

EARLY FIRST STAGE
The early first stage of labor (see p.294), when your cervix begins to dilate, is usually the longest, averaging eight hours. At this point, contractions are mild, sometimes described as being like severe menstrual or gas pains, with cramps and backache. The pain peaks during contractions, and you can relax between them. Many women find breathing techniques helpful in this early stage, and some find that massage is helpful. Still others seek medication to lessen the pain.

ACTIVE FIRST STAGE
As your cervix dilates further, your contractions become longer, stronger,

and closer together. There may be greater pressure in your back and an intense tightening in the pubic area. When contractions are close together, less oxygen reaches the uterine muscles, making this stage much more painful. Some women have severe back pain that radiates down the thighs. You may be happy to continue using natural pain-relief methods or taking analgesics. Some women find this stage hard to cope with and request an epidural (see p.290).

TRANSITION
As your cervix opens the last couple of centimeters to allow your baby's head to enter the birth canal, you may feel severe pain that radiates across the abdomen and into the back and legs. Powerful contractions occur close together as your body becomes ready to push (see p.298). If you haven't had an epidural, it's too late to get one when you're just about fully dilated. If you have an epidural already in place, it can be topped up.

SECOND STAGE
In the pushing phase, which ends with the birth, you will feel different sensations. Contractions are accompanied by an urge to bear down, caused by the head pressing down on the pelvic floor and rectum. Pain can be extreme, but often women feel it is more productive because they now have some control over labor as they push out the baby. A stinging or burning sensation occurs as the head stretches the vagina. It's important to keep breathing.

THIRD STAGE
A series of short, efficient contractions accompanies the delivery of the placenta. If you opt for a managed third stage with drugs (see p.304), you can expect a fairly painless, quick delivery. If you want to deliver the placenta naturally, it can take up to an hour with mild contractions. Most women find this a bit uncomfortable, but are so involved with their baby it often goes unnoticed, and there's usually no need for pain relief.

Dealing with labor pain

Moms who are prepared for the pain seem to find that it isn't as bad as they imagined it might be, and are able to cope using breathing exercises and other natural methods of pain relief.

• Take things one step at a time and just focus on the fact that, after nine long months, your baby will soon be here.

• Try not to tense up and fight your contractions—just relax and let them wash over you, telling yourself all the time that you can handle them.

• Most women describe giving birth as the most amazing thing they've ever done—and they go back and do it again (and again), so it can't be all bad.

Natural pain relief

Many women wish to have a natural birth with a minimum of intervention, or to use natural methods alongside medical pain relief. There are plenty of drug-free ways to encourage the process of labor and ease pain and discomfort.

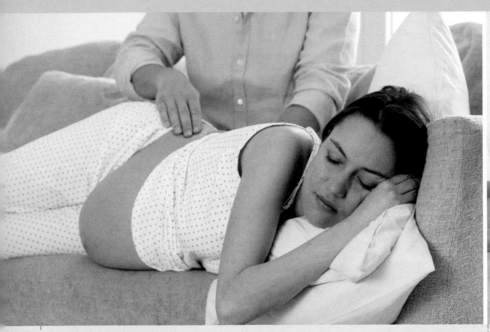

A SOOTHING MASSAGE
Some women find a lower-back massage extremely helpful in labor. Applying pressure with the heels of the hands, using the thumbs in a circular motion, or other practiced techniques can all help relieve tension.

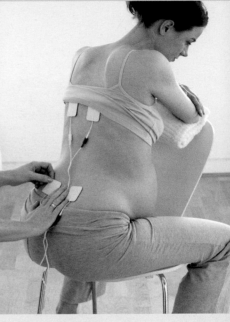

PAIN RELIEF WITH TENS
This is a helpful method of pain relief in early labor and, once the pads are in place, it allows you to remain active and mobile.

Although there are various medical methods for relieving labor pain, they can have side effects for you and your baby, so you may wish to consider natural pain-relief methods first. The most important thing to remember is to try to stay active. Many studies have shown that this approach results in shorter, easier labors, because you're using gravity to help your baby to emerge. Moving around during the first stage of labor can help to encourage your baby down into the birth canal and open your pelvis. It also encourages the release of endorphins. Even if you can't manage to walk, it's a good idea to rock and sway in rhythm with your breathing.

Try to change your position every 30 minutes or so. Use any labor aids available, such as a birthing ball, which you can lean on for support or bounce on to encourage regular contractions. Certain positions are recommended for each stage (see p.295 and p.298); you may find that you naturally adopt them.

Whatever you do, try to avoid lying flat on your back—this can restrict the blood flow to your baby.

Another thing to consider is your birth team. Being surrounded by encouraging people will lift your spirits and help you to feel more optimistic. Anxiety can not only slow down labor, but also creates more pain, so it is very important to have the support you need.

Popular methods

There are a few tried-and-true methods of relieving pain naturally that many women have found extremely effective.

"Some women will find labor bearable without pain relief, but most will need help at some point . . . luckily there are plenty of options"

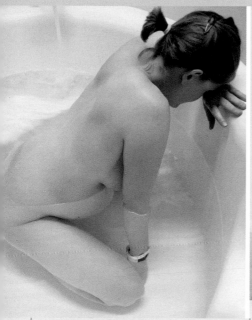

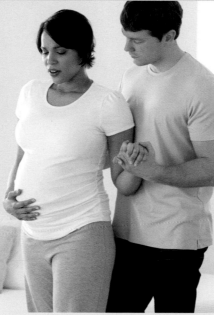

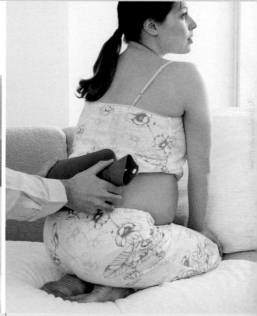

THE BENEFITS OF WATER
Immersing yourself in warm water can be immensely soothing. You may find movement easier, too, since the water aids buoyancy.

MOVING AROUND
Getting up and walking around between contractions is thought to speed up labor as gravity helps your baby to move downward.

USING WARMTH
Having someone hold a warm pack to your back may be soothing, as the warmth helps to relax tense muscles.

MASSAGE

Some women find massage beneficial in labor. The power of touch is well documented, and many women find that nurturing strokes lift their mood and increase their confidence in their ability to deal with the pain. Massage also stimulates the circulation, which brings oxygenated blood to the tissues around the uterus and encourages relaxation. Some women find a lower-back massage eases discomfort, while others find that having their shoulders, hands, or feet massaged is enough. Guide your partner, and ideally get him to practice different strokes before labor. Aromatherapy oils enhance massage, but essential oils should be avoided during pregnancy, labor, and delivery unless your doctor gives you the go-ahead, because they may have unknown effects on your baby. If given permission, use sparingly, adding a few drops to a carrier oil.

TENS

A TENS (transcutaneous electrical nerve stimulation) machine, used mainly in early labor, aims to relieve pain by stimulating the body to produce its own pain-relieving substances—encephalins and endorphins—and by blocking pain signals. Pads attached to wires are put on the back, and a small electrical current is passed through the skin and along nerve pathways to suppress pain signals to the brain. It takes about 30 minutes to work. Some women find it helpful, while others find it ineffective and don't enjoy the tingling sensation. You should begin to use it as soon as contractions start.

You can remain active while using TENS; there are no side effects for you or your baby, you can increase the voltage if needed, and it can be used alongside analgesic pain relief. The downside is that you can't wear the pads in water, and stopping and starting can reduce its overall effectiveness. Check in advance if the hospital supplies TENS machines, or whether you will need to rent one.

BREATHING

The importance of focused breathing in labor should not be underestimated. Using breathing techniques helps to ensure that your body and tissues have a good supply of oxygenated blood, which will help your body to work more efficiently in labor, in turn reducing pain and helping you relax.

Many prenatal classes teach breathing techniques, and it is worth practicing them at home prior to labor. There are specific breathing techniques to use during each stage of labor.

WATER

Whether you choose to spend time in a bath, shower, or birthing pool, you can benefit from the effects of warm water.

Research has found that warm water on the lower back (which contains the part of the spinal cord that receives nerve signals from the lower abdominal region) reduces tension and in turn labor pain. There is also evidence that women have a more relaxed and comfortable labor in water (see p.307), and that each stage is shorter. Water soothes and physically supports you, putting less strain on your back and legs. Adding a cup of sea salt to your bath at home will help prevent your skin from becoming waterlogged and wrinkly, and you can use scented candles around the bath to increase relaxation. Keep a bottle of cool water by the tub to sip, since sitting in warm water for long periods of time can dehydrate you.

HEAT AND COLD

Warmth has been used for centuries as a way to ease pain and promote relaxation. Try using a hot water bottle wrapped in a towel or a wheat bag (a cloth bag filled with wheat husks that you can warm in a microwave). Ice packs alternating with a hot water bottle or warm cloth can be applied to your neck,

back, shoulders, and lower abdomen to relieve pain and tension. Warmth will open up the blood vessels, allowing a flow of oxygenated blood, and cold will both be refreshing and ease tightness and discomfort.

Alternative therapies

There is a huge range of alternative therapies designed to relax you and help with various pains or ailments. Many of these can be used to reduce labor pain.

ACUPUNCTURE AND ACUPRESSURE

These two disciplines of Chinese medicine have a proven track record of both easing the pain of labor and encouraging a shorter first stage. Acupuncture works on the premise that there are channels in the body through which energy flows; blockages in energy can occur, and it's thought that by inserting thin needles into the skin at

Ways to relax

Think in advance about how you might relax in labor to help you approach the event with less anxiety.

• Learning yoga helps you use breathing techniques in labor, encourages deep relaxation, and improves focus.

• Using breathing techniques, where you focus on slowing down your breath, and listening to relaxing music undoubtedly helps some women.

• Every woman is different. Some women want their partner just to be there to help, but not to touch them, while others want physical support. Essentially, having

a responsive birth partner who will see to your needs can help you feel in control and more relaxed.

• A child's kneeling position is relaxing, with your knees wide apart, hips drawn to your heels, and forehead rested.

• Make sure you ask for information: The more you know about what's happening, the more relaxed you'll feel.

SWITCHING OFF
Distracting yourself between contractions, perhaps by zoning out to favorite tunes, or flicking through magazines, can reduce frustration and conserve energy for later on.

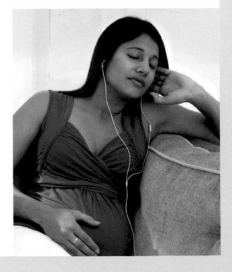

specific points, the flow of "chi" or energy can be restored. You will normally visit an acupuncturist in advance of labor, and then may need to arrange for him or her to visit you during labor.

Acupressure involves applying pressure to energy points, and can be done during labor by a therapist or by your birth partner. There are acupressure points on your hands and legs that are thought to help the cervix dilate, while points on the upper and lower back, feet, and shins can help to relieve pain.

HOMEOPATHY

This uses remedies prepared from very diluted natural substances that are thought to stimulate the body's own defenses. There is plenty of anecdotal evidence that homeopathy is helpful, but this has not been proven by studies. Homeopathic remedies are considered controversial within the medical community, and your doctor may tell you to avoid such treatments, since the effect of homeopathic remedies on your baby is unknown. If your obstetrician gives you the go-ahead to use homeopathy during your labor, consult with a certified homeopath ahead of time to find out which treatments might meet your individual needs during your upcoming labor and delivery. Ontario is the only province that currently regulates homeopathy. To find a homeopath in your area, visit the Canadian Society of Homeopaths at www.csoh.ca.

REFLEXOLOGY

The manipulation of reflex energy points on your hands and feet is thought to encourage relaxation and offer pain relief. There is also interesting research that suggests that women who have regular reflexology treatments during pregnancy have shorter labors.

During labor, specific points can be worked on to stimulate or calm your contractions, depending on what is required, and also to regulate them. If you wish to use reflexology in labor, arrange for your birth partner to get a few tips from a registered practitioner in advance; otherwise you will need to arrange to have a therapist present.

A good basic technique is having your second and third toes (the first toe being your big toe) squeezed firmly, released, and then squeezed again, which is believed to directly affect the uterus.

HYPNOBIRTHING

Hypnotherapy works by bypassing the conscious part of the brain, allowing the subconscious to take over. HypnoBirthing combines self-hypnosis with breathing and relaxation techniques and is an increasingly popular way to manage labor. If you decide to use this technique, you will need to attend classes for several weeks before the birth to learn the self-hypnosis techniques. These can include positive visualization, which helps you to form positive images of a pleasant, productive experience. Some women arrange to have a hypnotherapist with them in the delivery room.

> "Focusing on your excitement about meeting your baby, rather than your fear of and anxiety about labor, can give you a mental boost"

What worked for us

I had a nice long bath before going to the hospital to be induced, since I was starting to have mild backache, and it definitely relaxed me. The only medical pain relief I used was nitrous oxide, partly because my labor was so quick. NK

First and foremost, I used breathing techniques, and worked hard to stay positive. I also used a TENS machine and vocalized deep, low sounds, all of which helped to keep me focused and calm throughout the labor. TL

Aromatherapy and massage worked best for me. I used them during the pregnancy to remain calm and relaxed, and also had my birth partner give me a massage during the labor itself. MG

I found that it made a world of difference to go through most of my labor standing upright, since lying down made my contractions more intense and painful. I also found that concentrating on getting through the peak of each individual contraction, rather than thinking about how much more time was left, made labor a lot more manageable. LJ

Medical pain relief

If labor is more painful than anticipated, or your baby is in a difficult position, you may want medical pain relief in addition to, or instead of, natural methods. Most drugs offer quick and effective relief and are safe for you and your baby.

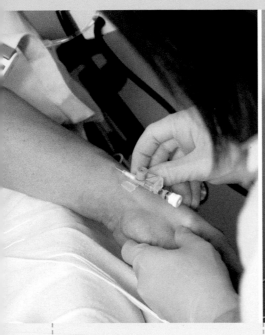

FAST-ACTING RELIEF
Pain-relieving drugs given intravenously take effect within minutes, although you may be confined to bed for a while.

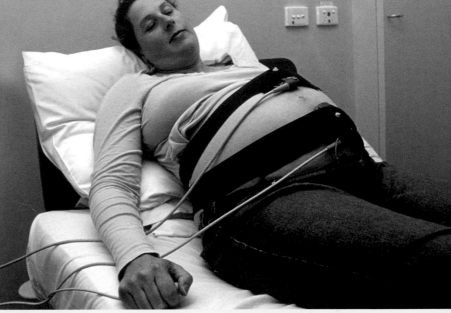

BEING IN CONTROL
Some hospitals have equipment that allows you to control your pain relief. A device called a PCA (patient-controlled analgesic) works with intravenous pain relief, giving you controlled doses at the click of a button.

There are times when natural pain relief may not be enough to help you deal with the intensity of contractions, particularly if labor is induced or your baby is in a position that prolongs labor or makes it more painful for you. There are two groups of pain-relieving drugs: analgesics, which dull the perception of pain; and anesthesia, which numbs pain.

Local anesthetic, known as nerve block, is injected during labor to numb the nerves that supply a particular area. Epidurals and spinal blocks numb sensation in the abdomen and back to reduce the pain of contractions; a pudendal block numbs feeling in the vagina and perineum and may be used in an assisted delivery (see pp.310–311).

Opioids

Pain-killing injections involve a group of drugs known as opioids, which are part of the narcotics family. Many studies have assessed the efficacy of these drugs, which are similar to morphine, in labor. They work by sedating the brain, causing drowsiness (narcotic literally means sleep-inducing). The drugs attach to receptors in your brain or nerves and block the transmission of pain.

The drugs are injected into the muscle of your thigh or buttocks. Occasionally they are given intravenously, and you may even be able to administer them yourself. They take about 20 minutes to work, and work for up to 3 hours.

PROS
Opioids are very effective when women are in extreme pain and are becoming exhausted by a long labor. Small doses

can encourage you to rest and recoup your energy, and relieve the pain of contractions. They can be administered by either a doctor or a registered midwife (if prescribed), which means that you may be able to have them at a home birth. Some opioids may produce feelings of euphoria, which many women find beneficial in labor.

CONS

Many women say that opioids make them feel nauseated or dizzy; others report feeling out of control after taking them, and therefore out of touch with how their labor is progressing.

Opioids cross the placenta, which can affect your baby's breathing and make him sleepy if given too close to the actual birth. This can mean that he takes longer to establish feeding and may need help with breathing after the birth. Doctors avoid administering opioids within 2–4 hours of a baby's expected delivery. If they are given too close to birth, your baby will be given antidote medication.

In too large doses, opioids can also be dangerous for you and affect your own breathing.

Tranquilizers

Although tranquilizers don't relieve pain, doctors sometimes administer them to women during labor if the situation warrants it. Occasionally, women even ask for a tranquilizer when they're admitted to the hospital to give birth. They can help you relax and relieve anxiety, which may make labor more bearable if you are frightened by the concept of labor. Tranquilizers can be given orally, intravenously, or intramuscularly (injected into a large muscle like the thigh).

PROS

If you are very anxious or nervous about getting through labor or experiencing intense pain from contractions, tranquilizers can help you relax for several hours during the early stages of your labor, making the experience easier to endure.

CONS

Tranquilizers aren't for everyone, because they can make you feel drowsy or out of control. Sometimes, it's difficult for a woman to fully remember her labor experience after the fact, particularly if she's given a very high dose of tranquilizers, which could even cause her to doze a little between contractions. Tranquilizers also affect the baby, decreasing his activity level before and after the birth.

"You can always try starting with natural techniques, move on to opioids if you want something stronger, then epidurals or spinal blocks if you need them"

Using pain relief effectively

Your doctor is there to help you with whichever form of pain relief you choose to try. So if you have any concerns at all, don't hesitate to ask. However there are a few tried and true ways to make sure that you're getting the best from each method.

• Before you decide to have any opioid drug, ask your doctor or nurse how far your cervix has dilated. If you are further along than you thought, you may decide to continue without it.

• If you definitely plan to have an epidural, check with your doctor or nurse to find out when it is allowed. At a certain point—usually around 7cm—it is considered too late in labor to administer one.

• If you are small-framed or are aware that, in your everyday life, medication affects you very quickly or powerfully, ask for a smaller dose to start off with, which can be topped up if it isn't having the desired effect.

• Although they're not available everywhere, walking epidurals are a good choice for those who want epidural pain relief but don't want to lose the ability to get up and move around.

• If you would like an epidural but also really want to feel your baby being born, ask your doctor or midwife if it's possible to let the epidural wear off before you give birth. Being able to feel your contractions can make it easier to push effectively.

Epidurals

An epidural is a type of local anesthetic, which means that it works directly on the area of the pain. It is the most commonly used and effective local pain relief for labor. Epidurals should only be offered if you are in established or active labor (see pp.295–296), not at the first sign of pain, since it's important to check that contractions are regular.

A fine, hollow needle is inserted into the space between two vertebrae in the lower back, and then passed into the epidural space—the space around the spinal cord protected by the spiny vertebrae. Once the needle is in place, a hollow tube is passed through it. A local anesthetic is injected through the needle and into the tube. The needle is then removed and the end of the tube is attached to your back with tape. Once the tube is in position, you will not be aware of it. The anesthetic can then be topped up through the tube as needed, usually every 1–2 hours.

You can also be given a continuous infusion, which feeds the epidural anesthesia directly into your back. In some cases, you may be given a pump to top yourself up when necessary, which is known as patient-controlled epidural analgesia, or PCEA. Although the long needle used and the prospect of having anesthesia directly injected into your spine can be alarming, epidurals are safe, simple, and effective.

The usual combination of drugs used is the local anesthetic and an opioid painkiller.

PROS

Epidurals provide complete pain relief in 90 percent of cases; 10 percent of women have some residual pain, but their level of discomfort is much improved. Once an epidural is in place, if you need medical intervention, such as forceps or caesarean delivery, it can often simply be topped up, avoiding the need for general anesthesia.

CONS

Unless you have a mobile epidural (see right), you won't be able to move around and you will lose feeling or experience intense heaviness in your legs, which can slow down labor. Also, you will be unable to bathe or relax in water.

You may need to have a catheter (a tube running into your bladder to allow the release of urine), which can make the urinary tract a little sore afterward. Some women worry that there's a risk of long-lasting backache, numbness, and even paralysis; however, there is no evidence to support this. You can suffer from headaches or low blood pressure during and after an epidural, but there are very few other symptoms, and your baby should not be affected.

Studies have shown that women who have epidurals have longer labors, and are more likely to need an assisted delivery with forceps or a vacuum. However, there is no evidence that you are more likely to need a caesarean.

Mobile epidural

You may be offered a weaker epidural, known as a "mobile," "walking," or "ambulatory" epidural, that allows you

---

PREPARING FOR AN EPIDURAL
A local anesthetic will be injected into your back first so you don't feel pain when the actual epidural needle is inserted. You will need to remain as still as possible while the anesthesiologist sets up the epidural.

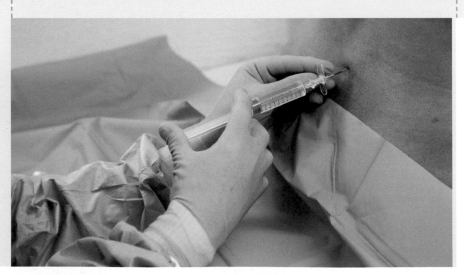

THE PASSAGE OF THE ANESTHETIC
Local anesthetic is fed through a hollow tube placed in the epidural space—the area between the vertebrae and the spinal cord.

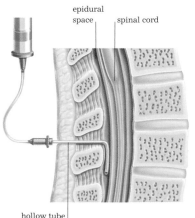

epidural space · spinal cord

hollow tube

to retain feeling in your legs. This provides very good pain relief, but you will need extra monitoring and support to ensure that you move around safely. The same combination of drugs used in a traditional low-dose epidural is used, but in smaller quantities.

Not all hospitals offer this type of epidural, since it requires additional trained support staff. The benefits, effects, side effects, and drawbacks are exactly the same as with a normal epidural, but it's worth noting that although you can stand up, you may not feel able to be quite as active as you would like. For example, some women can only manage to maneuver themselves between the bed and a chair or to the bathroom with a great deal of support from their partner.

Spinal block

Also known as "spinals," these involve having drugs injected directly into the fluid of your spinal column, which tends to work more quickly than epidurals. Spinals are a one-time injection, and cannot be topped up, since no epidural or spinal catheter is left in place.

This type of anesthesia is mainly used for caesareans and other procedures that are not expected to take longer than an hour or so. Like an epidural, a spinal block may also decrease your blood pressure, which in turn may lower your baby's heart rate and affect your ability to push. Side effects can include itching, tingling, nausea, and lightheadedness.

COMBINED SPINAL EPIDURAL (CSE)
As the name suggests, this is simply a combination of an epidural and a spinal block, in which you will be given a low dose of pain-relieving medication via an injection into your spinal fluid, and your anesthesiologist will then insert an

epidural catheter into your back so that the medication can be topped up: When the effects of the spinal epidural begin to wear off, medication will be passed through the catheter and into your spine to provide continuous pain relief. The side effects of a CSE are the same as those for a spinal block.

PUDENDAL BLOCK
This type of fast-acting local anesthetic is sometimes used before carrying out an assisted delivery (see pp.310–311). It involves injecting the vaginal area with a local anesthetic to numb the vagina

and perineum, the area between the vagina and the anus.

GENERAL ANESTHESIA
Occasionally, an emergency caesarean is carried out under general anesthesia, which means you are put to sleep. This may be necessary if, for example, other types of anesthetic haven't been successful, or if the mother's or baby's health is under threat and the operation needs to be carried out swiftly. Your partner will not be able to stay with you, but you should wake about 10 minutes after the surgery.

What really worked for us

When I had my son, 13 years ago, a "walking" epidural was a rarity and was only offered in a handful of specialist hospitals. I happened to be in one of them, and had a low-dose combined spinal epidural. I was then filmed by the anesthesiologist walking down the hospital corridor while I was five centimeters dilated! MG

I chose opioids via a PCA controller. With the push of a button, I could trigger a pre-programmed dose of the drug myself. Having this control was so empowering and such a comfort that, in the end, I actually used less than I'd expected to need. CH

My labors went incredibly smoothly and well, so I was able to continue with my plan to have my babies naturally. But some labors are much longer than planned or involve additional intervention and/or pain. Be ready to follow medical advice if your doctor (or your partner) considers it necessary. My doctor told me to consider natural childbirth like running a marathon. If you think, "Maybe I'll finish; maybe I won't," chances are good that you won't get there on your own. Instead, decide in advance whether you have the determination, set your mind to

it, and then just be ready to adjust and accommodate unforeseen circumstances. LJ

One of my moms said, "For my second baby, who was posterior like my first, an anesthesiologist was unavailable to set up an epidural. In complete frustration, I ended up walking around the hospital grounds . . . only to find that this not only took my mind off the proceedings, but also speeded up my labor to the degree that my baby was born just a couple of hours later. I hardly noticed the pain!" NK

A woman I oversaw said, "Opioids made me feel nauseated and a little 'drunk,' which was an uncomfortable feeling when I wanted to be aware of what was going on. I also didn't like the idea of doing anything that could restrict my movement or make the baby drowsy, so I decided to grit my teeth and see out my labor naturally. I used a birthing ball, bouncing almost ferociously when the contractions were at their worst, and this not only relieved pain, but jiggled my baby into a better position for birth. The labor was much shorter than anticipated, and I felt like I was in control for most of the time." MG

Monitoring during labor

Although babies are designed to handle the stress of labor, your nurse will monitor your baby's heartbeat often to ensure that it is regular and to pick up any changes that suggest she might be having difficulties.

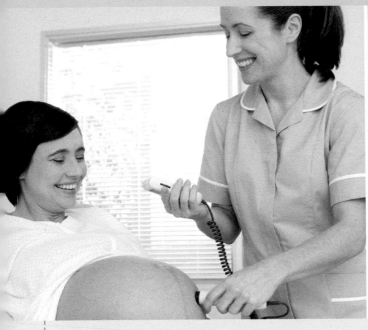

INTERMITTENT MONITORING
For a straightforward labor, a handheld monitoring device called a Doppler fetal monitor will be used to listen to your baby's heartbeat at regular intervals, leaving you free to move around at other times.

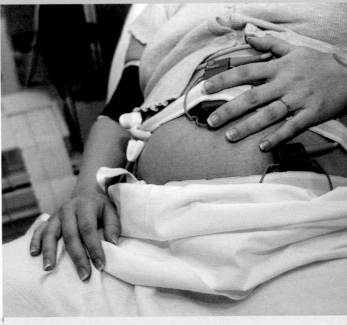

CONTINUOUS MONITORING
If there are any concerns about you or your baby, an electronic fetal monitor may be used to continuously track your baby's heartbeat and your contractions.

In labor, your baby's heart rate may drop a little during contractions due to the pressure on her head as it descends into your pelvis. This is normal, and her heart rate should recover after each contraction. Monitoring involves checking her heart rate to ensure that this pattern occurs. If your labor is progressing well, your baby's heart rate will be measured intermittently; if there are any concerns, it will be monitored constantly, known as electronic fetal monitoring, and the strength and frequency of your contractions will also be measured.

Intermittent monitoring

If your pregnancy has been progressing normally and there are no complications, it is unnecessary to monitor your baby's heart rate on a continuous basis. Being attached to a fetal heart-rate monitor (see opposite) is restrictive, and stops you from being as mobile as you may want during labor, so many women wish to avoid this. Instead you will have intermittent monitoring, which involves checking your baby's heart rate every 15 minutes or so in the first stage of labor, increasing to once every five minutes, or after each contraction, for a full one minute in the second stage of labor. The nurse or midwife listens to the baby's heartbeat using a hand-held device known as a Doppler fetal heart monitor, which is simply pressed against your abdomen.

If your nurse or midwife has any concerns regarding the heart rate after a contraction, she may recommend continuous monitoring (see opposite).

Sometimes, because of your baby's activity or the way she is lying, it is hard to pick up her heart rate through your abdomen. Or the monitor may pick up your heart rate instead, which is much slower. The average baby's heart rate at full term is between 110 and 160 beats per minute, whereas an adult heart rate is between 60 and 80 beats per minute.

If your baby's heartbeat is too high (above 160), which suggests that your baby may be distressed, or too low (below 110), continuous monitoring may be used, or a scalp electrode attached to your baby's head to monitor her heart rate this way. If it is difficult to locate the heartbeat, an ultrasound may be performed.

Continuous monitoring

There are a number of situations when continuous monitoring may be necessary. These include if your baby is overdue or your labor is premature; if you have had vaginal bleeding in pregnancy; if you're having twins or other multiples; if you've had a previous caesarean; if you have epidural anesthesia or an induced labor, if you've leaked meconium-stained amniotic fluid (see p.277); or if you have had a very long labor. There are many other reasons, and your nurse will explain why it is necessary at the time.

Try not to panic if continuous monitoring is suggested. In most cases your baby will be absolutely fine, and this is simply a precaution. Equally, don't be alarmed if the machine suggests that your baby is in distress. There are very good studies showing that an abnormal reading is not necessarily a clear indication of problems. To avoid unnecessary intervention on the basis of an unclear set of results, doctors will

sometimes take a small drop of your baby's blood from a pin prick on her scalp to measure oxygen levels. This is called a fetal blood sample (FBS). The majority of FBSs are normal, which is very reassuring in labor.

ELECTRONIC FETAL MONITORING

This is a form of continuous monitoring that tracks your contractions and your baby's heartbeat throughout labor. Two plastic pads are secured to the abdomen, with wires attached that are linked to a machine that measures both your baby's well-being and the progress you are making with your labor. A Doppler fetal monitor notes the rate of your baby's heartbeat, and another device measures the strength and frequency of your contractions.

SCALP ELECTRODES

A fetal scalp electrode is a tiny clip that is attached to your baby's head to obtain an accurate heart-rate reading. A wire attached to the electrode comes out of the vagina and is attached to a monitoring device. The electrode obtains

the reading by picking up the electrical impulses of the heart.

Although some women find the procedure scary, the risks to your baby are very small, and it leaves only a little scratch. It may be used for twins or triplets, if the signal from the electronic monitor isn't good, or if an earlier reading suggests fetal distress. Your nurse or doctor should explain clearly the reasons for carrying out the procedure before they go ahead with it.

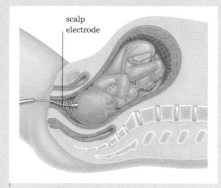

scalp electrode

PLACING A SCALP ELECTRODE
If your doctor wishes to keep a closer eye on the baby's heartbeat, an electrode may be placed on her head. It is attached with care during a vaginal examination.

What is in your chart?

Your doctor and nurses should refer to your chart for data and graphs that convey what's taken place during your labor. Various graphs are shown, recording your heart rate, temperature, and blood pressure, as well as your baby's heart rate, details of your contractions and how far your cervix has dilated, and how far the baby's head has descended in your pelvis. Some studies show that they help to make labor safer for you and your baby.

The graphs show the expected "norm" for factors such as the dilatation of your cervix, according to whether or not you have had a baby before. Your

doctor can then check your details against the expected progress to assess your labor. The results will be plotted on the different graphs at regular intervals in labor, making it easy for doctors and medical staff to see instantly how your labor is progressing, how you and your baby are doing, and whether any intervention is needed.

It also includes the results of any urine tests you've had, and other information, such as which drugs you've been given and when, and whether IV fluids have been given. Nurses joining you mid-labor can pick up seamlessly on your care because of your chart.

First stage of labor

During the first stage of labor, known as "dilatation," contractions cause your baby to press against the cervix, causing it to soften and dilate. This stage ends when your cervix is reaching full dilation and you are getting ready to push.

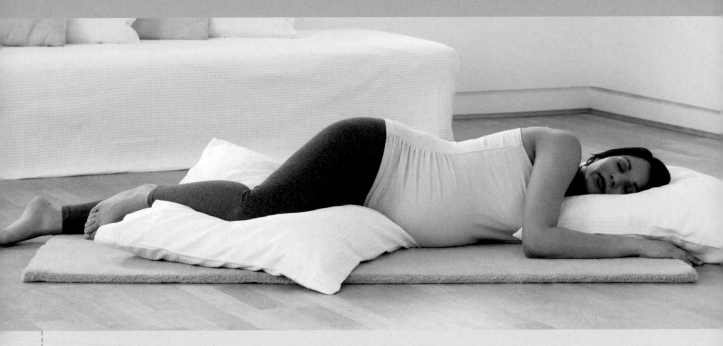

RESTING IN THE EARLY STAGE
The first stage of labor can take a long time, and you may get tired. If you'd like to rest or sleep between contractions, try lying down on a couple of pillows. Placing a pillow between your knees helps to support your bump and keeps you on your side.

The first stage of labor, when your cervix softens and dilates to 10 centimeters (yes, really) so that your baby can squeeze out, is generally the longest and most difficult. Typically for a first pregnancy it can last for at least 12 hours, sometimes longer. There are two phases in this stage: the early or latent phase, which takes you up until you are around 2–4cm dilated; then the active or established phase, which ends when you are fully dilated at 10cm and ready to push.

The early phase

When contractions start in early labor, they are generally mild to moderate. Some women describe them as feeling like "trapped gas," others describe backache or period-like cramps. Normally at this stage you'll be able to talk through contractions, and they'll be irregular, possibly 5–20 minutes apart, with each lasting 30–50 seconds. Sometimes these irregular contractions continue for days, perhaps stopping for a while and starting again; but typically for first-time moms, this phase lasts for about six to eight hours.

Your contractions will gradually become more frequent and increasingly uncomfortable during the early phase of the first stage. However, there is a slow progression toward these more intense contractions, which means that your body can adapt to and get used to the pain over a period of time.

"Stay focused and remind yourself that every single contraction brings you one step closer to the birth of your baby"

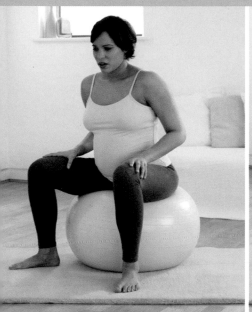

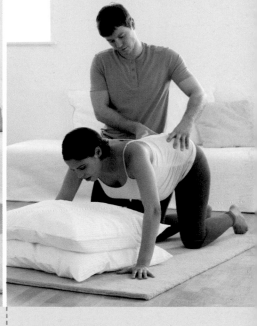

BIRTHING BALL
Sitting on a birthing ball is an excellent way to take the weight off your feet but still remain in an upright position.

USING A CHAIR
You can sit backward on a chair, using the back rest to lean on. This is a good position if you'd like to use a TENS machine.

BACK MASSAGE
Getting onto all fours helps to bring your baby into a good position for birth. It also allows your birth partner to massage you.

HOW TO DEAL WITH EARLY LABOR

It can take hours, or even days, for your cervix to dilate those first few centimeters and for contractions to build up, so try to be as patient as you can. Find ways to relax and zone out—and sleep or take naps when you can. Alternating periods of rest with some gentle activity can help distract you, and may help things to get moving. Taking a warm bath or shower can help you de-stress and soothe backache, and massages may take the edge off any

discomfort. This period of waiting for labor to build up is the perfect time to eat some light, nutritious snacks, which will help to keep you going now and in the hours and days ahead. Once your contractions become stronger and start to form a recognizable pattern, it's a good idea to start timing them and to call your doctor or midwife to let her know you're having contractions. She can let you know if it's time to head to the hospital right now or if you should continue waiting at home, monitoring your condition. If your contractions are

still far apart, she may ask you to call again when they are closer together. If you feel disheartened that it's taking so long for labor to start in earnest, reassure yourself that when you enter the active phase, it will speed up enormously.

Active labor

If this is your first baby, once your contractions are coming more frequently and in a fairly established pattern—say every five minutes or so, with each lasting 50–60 seconds—this is the time to head to the hospital. Second and subsequent babies tend to arrive more quickly, so you may have less time before the delivery. If this is your second baby, wait until your contractions are 10 minutes apart and lasting about 50–60 seconds each, before heading in. There are circumstances when you will need to go to the hospital sooner. These include going into premature labor (before 37 weeks); experiencing noticeably fewer movements from your baby; having vaginal bleeding; or if your water breaks, particularly if the fluid contains meconium, blood, or mucus. As well as being stronger and more painful, the nature of your contractions will alter during this phase. You will start to feel them higher in the abdomen, and then the pain will sweep downward as your uterine muscles tighten and push your baby down into the pelvis so that his head presses on your cervix.

ARRIVING AT THE HOSPITAL
Once you've checked in at the hospital, you may be admitted to a labor and delivery room right away if it is obvious that you're in active labor. Otherwise, you will be checked by a nurse in a different room. She will observe your contractions and do an internal check with her fingers to see how far your cervix has dilated before she confirms that you're in active labor. When active labor is confirmed, you will be given a labor room, and a nurse and your doctor or midwife will keep an eye on your progress, regularly checking how far your cervix has dilated, and recording changes on your chart. How quickly your cervix opens depends on factors such as the position of your baby, the efficiency of your contractions, and how far you are into the first stage. It's generally thought that labor is progressing at a normal rate if your cervix opens 1cm per hour once it's more than 3cm dilated, although it can dilate much more quickly.

DEALING WITH ACTIVE LABOR
Despite the greater intensity of your contractions, you can continue to use breathing techniques to help you focus and stay calm, as well as other methods such as TENS or water (see pp.285–286). However, you may find now that you want medication, such as opioids, which block the transmission of pain, and you might request an epidural (see p.290). Your doctor will time opioids carefully, since they cross the placenta and cause drowsiness in your baby if given up to two to three hours before the birth.

How the cervix changes

During pregnancy, your cervix (the neck of the womb) remains closed and lengthens and thickens to protect your baby. However, for your baby to be born, the cervix needs to shorten and soften (a process known as effacement) and open up (dilate). At the start of labor, the cervix begins to efface in response to contractions: Its long neck shortens, and it becomes generally softer. The degree to which your cervix has effaced is measured as a percentage, so at 0 percent it is thick and hard, and at 100 percent it is soft and thin. Your cervix needs to efface before it can effectively open up, or dilate.

Contractions in early and active labor dilate the cervix to allow your baby to pass through. The degree of dilation is measured in centimeters. In first labors, the cervix dilates an average of 1cm an hour, but this may be faster in subsequent labors. When you are fully dilated, at 10cm, you will feel a strong urge to bear down and can then start to push your baby out.

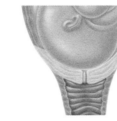

THE END OF PREGNANCY
As labor approaches, your cervix is still as firm and thick as it was during pregnancy.

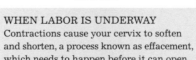

WHEN LABOR IS UNDERWAY
Contractions cause your cervix to soften and shorten, a process known as effacement, which needs to happen before it can open.

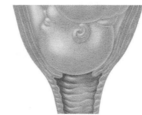

2CM DILATED
Once the cervix is sufficiently softened, it starts to open up, or dilate, so that your baby can eventually pass through.

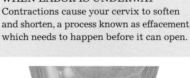

6CM DILATED
As contractions intensify and become more regular, your cervix starts to open up more rapidly. You are in active labor now.

This is a good time to adopt positions that encourage the descent of your baby and increase your comfort (see below).

YOUR BABY'S PROGRESS

When your doctor or midwife checks your progress, you may hear her mention your "station." This refers to where your baby's head is in your pelvis. The stations are levels in the pelvis that are described as between -3 and +3, with -3 being the first level, which means your baby's head has just entered the narrow part of your pelvis. When the top of his head (or another part of his body, if he is breech) is about halfway down the pelvis (at the level of bony prominences known as the ischial spines), he is at 0 station. Once the station is a positive number, the head is moving down the pelvis, and when it reaches +3, the head is crowning (see pp.301–302). With a first baby, the head is often deep in the pelvis before labor starts, and is at station -1, 0, or even +1. Women who've had previous babies often don't engage until the start of labor.

THE BEST POSITIONS

Staying as mobile as possible and adopting upright positions to help the force of gravity increases the effectiveness of your contractions and helps labor progress. This is borne out by a recent study, which found that women who walk, sit, stand, or kneel—rather than lie down—have a shorter first stage and were less likely to ask for an epidural.

If you experience pressure in your back during contractions, leaning forward—either over a bean bag, your partner's lap, or a birthing ball—can help alleviate the discomfort. Your partner can also massage your lower back in this position if you find it helpful. Some women find that rocking their hips in rhythm with their breathing while leaning forward also helps enormously. Sitting astride a birthing ball can be very comfortable and can encourage the descent of your baby's head. Between contractions, try walking around, then stop and get into a comfortable position for the next contraction.

YOUR PARTNER'S SUPPORT

This is crucial now. If progress is slow, your birth partner needs to be patient, positive, and encouraging, and allow you to progress at your own speed.

On the other hand, you may feel shocked and slightly out of control when active labor starts. Your birth partner needs to be aware of the techniques that can help you relax, and he or she can help you put into practice the techniques you learned together at prenatal classes. Many women feel unaccountably angry and irritated in labor. This is normal, too, and the result of the stress you are under, the hormones circulating in your body, and your heightened emotional state.

Your partner can help by being calm and ready to do whatever you need, whether that is massaging your back, helping you into a different position, offering you sips of water or even light snacks, helping you take natural remedies, distracting you, or simply leaving you alone for a few moments.

Throughout, your birth partner can discuss your progress with the doctor, nurse, or midwife, and check your birth plan to ensure that things are working as you'd hoped. If you need to make changes, your birth partner can speak on your behalf, and make decisions if you feel too frustrated or distracted to do so yourself.

What we wish we had known

I wished I'd understood that each labor would be different. I expected my second one to be like the first, maybe a little quicker, so I ended up getting the timing wrong. I went into the hospital too early, which I think slowed things down because I was less active. CH

Anything can happen in labor, so it's a good idea to try to be open minded, with no fixed expectations. TL

I was fortunate that, as a physician, I was comfortable in a hospital. I had seen plenty of labors and deliveries, so I knew more about what to expect than most. Yet the thing I think helps new moms approach labor confidently is reminding them that this is their experience and their baby. While it's definitely important to have a healthy respect for hospital staff and doctors, I have seen too many women go to the hospital feeling completely helpless—as if they have no say in what's going on and simply need to do everything they're told. This completely out-of-control feeling does nothing to instill confidence. LJ

As a midwife, I knew that most first-time births take an average of 12 hours, and was well prepared for that, with relaxing music, a game of Scrabble, and a packed lunch for my husband. I didn't consider that I might be one of those rare moms-to-be who miss out on the slow build-up to established labor and end up delivering in under three hours! It was a bit of a shock for me, my husband, and my baby daughter. NK

One of my moms said, "I wish I'd known how important it is to be active. My first labor was horrifically long, with most of it spent on my back, hooked up to an epidural. Second time around, I had a nurse who encouraged me to walk around, which not only took my mind off things, but speeded up labor. Despite having a posterior baby, I had no need for any medical pain relief." NK

Dealing with transition

The last part of the first stage of labor, when you still need to dilate fully to 10cm before you can push, is called transition. Many women describe this as the toughest part of labor, although thankfully, it's usually the shortest.

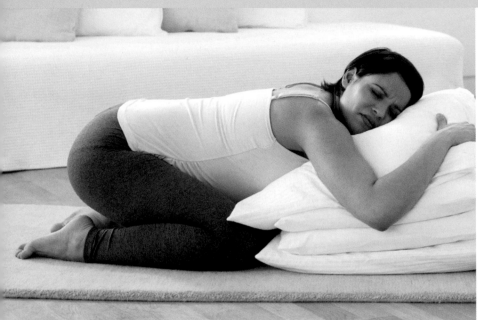

TRANSITION POSITION
Kneeling and leaning forward onto a pile of pillows or cushions with your bottom raised can be a helpful position for transition, because it relieves backache and can help you resist the urge to bear down.

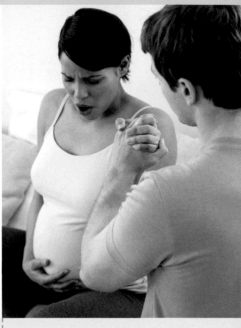

A HELPING HAND
Your partner's support may be most needed now, especially if the intensity of contractions makes you feel discouraged.

Transition, so called because it marks the shift to the second stage of labor, can trigger a number of physical and emotional symptoms that can be difficult to deal with. They are thought to be caused by a peak in hormone levels, and it helps to be prepared for them— because even if you're not feeling exhausted from a long first stage, they can seem overwhelming.

Typically, transition lasts anywhere from about 15 to about 60 minutes, so just try to keep focused on the fact that your baby will be arriving very soon.

Physically, contractions may take on a new momentum now, lasting up to 90 seconds and occurring every 2 minutes, leaving little time to rest in between. They may even "double-peak," coming one after the other without a break. You may shake, shiver, or tremble; experience cold or hot flashes; feel nauseated or vomit; or suffer from inexplicable hiccups or burping.

It's not unusual to feel rectal pressure; if you urgently need to open your bowels, this can be a sign that your baby has descended further into your pelvis. Some

women begin to spontaneously bear down at this point (though your doctor will tell you not to push until she is sure your cervix is ready) and sometimes there's a lot of bloody discharge.

How you may feel

Transition can make you feel agitated and out of control. This is the point when most women report screaming or shouting at their partners, or feeling very needy and vulnerable. You might feel that you

"Transition can make you feel very agitated, panicky, and out of control . . . Try to take one contraction at a time and focus on your baby being born"

cannot go on any longer or, if you haven't had pain relief so far, that you can't keep going without it. However, with the birth so near, your doctor will be unwilling to give you opioids at this stage due to the risk of drowsiness in your baby. Try to take one contraction at a time and focus on your baby being born.

A brief respite

While many women experience some or all of the above, others experience a sense of calm at this point, as contractions seem to slow down, or even stop, before the second stage kicks off. This is fondly referred to as the "rest and be thankful" part of labor, as your body is given restorative time before undertaking the effort of pushing. If this is the case, have a few sips of water and try to rest before your contractions start up again.

For many women, the transition phase is the period when encouragement and support from their birth partner is most important. Your partner may need to help you to change position, keep you warm (or cool), and, most importantly, reassure you as much as possible.

Some birth partners feel alarmed and worried by your distress, but it's important that they remain calm and understand that this is a normal part of childbirth.

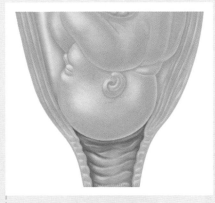

FULLY DILATED
By the end of the transition period, your cervix will have opened up fully, at 10cm, and the head will soon start to crown as you enter the pushing stage of labor.

How your birth partner can help

Every woman responds differently to the transition phase. Your birth partner can help by trying to figure out what you need, and remaining patient if you can't seem to settle on anything in particular.

• A massage may help, or you may want support to move onto all fours (see p.300). Your birth partner can place a cool cloth on your forehead, play some soothing or uplifting music, offer encouragement, and remain positive. Together you can visualize your baby moving downward with each contraction.

• Some birth partners feel alarmed at this point, and worried by your distress, but it's very important to keep calm, even

(and especially) if you are very upset—it's not unusual for women to cry during transition and vent their emotions—and it won't help if they can see that their birth partner is getting ruffled by this.

• Your birth partner should keep giving you plenty of support, even if you are expressing your pain by swearing and shouting, or if you're ignoring him and saying nothing.

• As you learn that you're in transition, your birth partner can remind you that you will see your baby very soon. This knowledge can hold you together as the storm of contractions takes over. Express your pain however feels natural—

swearing and shouting, or saying nothing. Anything is acceptable now.

• Make sure your birth partner is aware that you won't be able to take in complex information, so any advice or suggestions need to be clear and brief.

• The best way for both you and your partner to cope is to be aware of what's happening. Ask your doctor or midwife in advance to let you know what's going on, so you don't feel shocked or disheartened.

• Your birth partner should not leave you at this stage. You need the reassurance that he is there to speak up for you if you're too busy focusing on contractions.

Second stage of labor

The second stage begins when your cervix is fully dilated at 10cm, and you can start to push your baby out. Even if you're tired after a long labor, the prospect of seeing your baby for the first time can give you a renewed sense of purpose.

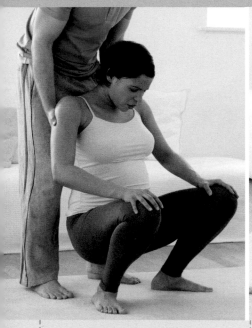

SUPPORTED SQUAT
Squatting down with the support of your birth partner helps open up your pelvis during the second stage.

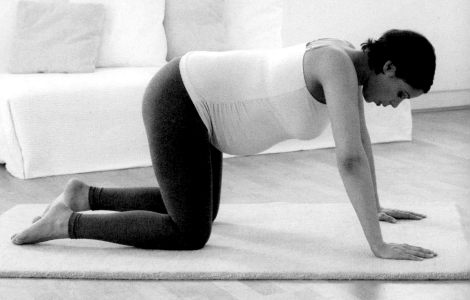

RESTING BETWEEN CONTRACTIONS
It's a good idea to rest and recover your energy between contractions. Staying in an all-fours position can help to ease the pressure of your baby's head on your rectum and lessen the pushing sensation.

The second stage of labor can take anywhere from 30 minutes to 2 hours: typically 1–2 hours for a first labor, and 45 minutes or under for a subsequent labor. Some women find this stage easier to deal with because they can actively work with their contractions to push the baby out. Others find the effort of prolonged pushing very difficult and tiring. Contractions usually become stronger now, although they may be a little less frequent, occurring every 2–4 minutes. In some cases, they may even stop for a short while as your uterus

adjusts (to become snug around your baby again). If you had an epidural, this can lengthen the second stage, and your contractions may be more sluggish. As a result, you may be advised to wait before pushing to give the contractions time to move the baby down into the pelvis.

When to push

For some women, pushing comes naturally. You may experience an overwhelming desire to push—which

feels something like an uncontrollable bowel movement—and you'll simply bear down, using your pelvic floor muscles to move your baby downward. The urge to push comes from the pressure of your baby's head on the nerves that signal the need for a bowel movement. Try not to tighten the muscles in your buttocks to prevent a bowel movement; doing so can slow things down and prevent an efficient delivery. It is natural to have a small bowel movement in labor, and your caregiver will discreetly take care of it, possibly without you even knowing.

If you're not sure when to push, your doctor or midwife will guide you and tell you when your baby moves into the correct position. With each contraction, you will need to concentrate on pushing deep down into the pelvic area and bottom. It can help to put your chin on your chest and to bear down for as long as possible during a contraction, during which time you may need to take several steady breaths.

You may feel like grunting and making noises when you bear down, or you may prefer to breathe deeply and quietly. Your caregivers will offer suggestions on how to control your breathing during this stage to help lessen your discomfort and help the natural process of encouraging your baby to move downward.

Alternatively, some women prefer to exhale during a contraction to help them remain as relaxed as possible and focus on pushing into the bottom. You can try both techniques to find out which works best for you. Just remember to avoid holding your breath for longer than necessary, because this lessens the amount of oxygen available to you and your baby.

Second stage positions

It's a good idea to use the force of gravity to help your baby move downward into the pelvis. Research has found that women who give birth in an upright position or on all-fours have less pain during labor and birth, shorter labors and pushing times, fewer incidences of shoulder dystocia (when the baby's shoulders get stuck in the pelvis, see p.319), and fewer perineal tears.

What's more, adopting an all-fours position allows the pelvis to open an extra centimeter or two, which gives adequate room for even a large baby to pass through.

At the beginning of this stage, you can sit leaning onto the back of a birthing chair or stool, or sit on a birthing ball or even the toilet, which allows you to squat. Many women are too tired to adopt this position without help, so your nurse and partner may need to support you. They can also support you in a kneeling position with your knees open wide, which opens up your pelvis.

Another good position is lying on your left side while your nurse or partner holds your right leg upward with every push. As well as reducing the pressure on your rectum, in this position, a mirror can be held up to show your baby's progress, which can be enormously motivating. There's also some evidence to suggest that lying on your side can reduce the risk of your perineum tearing.

You might also find it helpful to use props while kneeling and leaning forward, such as pillows, a bean bag, a birthing ball, or a large cushion.

Coping with the second stage

Discuss the best positions with your doctor or midwife before you start pushing. The idea is to push when your baby is low enough in your pelvis and, given time, your contractions should automatically move her into the correct position. Don't worry if you don't feel an urge to push; your doctor can guide you.

• Many women are exhausted by this stage, so encouragement is imperative. Allow your birth partner, nurse, and doctor to direct your pushing and rest whenever you can. Sips of cold water in between pushes, and a cold washcloth on your forehead will help to both soothe you and encourage you to carry on.

• Strong emotions of excitement, expectation, or anxiety may be rippling through you, along with the physical sensations of this stage. Accept your feelings, but try to keep a focus on the advice and instructions you are receiving; they are vital to getting your baby out and into your arms.

• Make sounds—keeping them low and deep—and imagine the sound traveling down and out of the body like a letter "J." Try making a loud "G" sound, and imagine the sound is coming from the hip area and that there is a lot of power behind the sound to help push the baby out. Use your partner for support by putting your arms around your partner's neck or waist and leaning on him and rocking. Or try kneeling on a large pillow on the floor, resting your upper body on the seat of a chair or bed.

Your baby's descent

As your contractions and pushing continue, your baby starts to descend further down into the pelvis, ready to emerge through the birth canal. You may feel pain and discomfort and experience a stinging sensation as the head puts pressure on your rectum, and the mouth of your vagina and your perineum slowly stretch to accommodate him.

CROWNING
As your baby continues to move downward, his head will eventually become visible through the mouth of the vagina at the peak of each contraction, known as "crowning."

At first the head will slip backward a little after each push, but finally it will remain in the opening of the vagina. If you wish, your nurse can hold a mirror so that you can see the top of your baby's head as it crowns, or you can reach down to touch the head as the walls of your vagina draw up.

As your baby's head crowns, you will be instructed to pant rather than push to prevent the head from delivering too quickly, which can cause tearing in your vagina and perineum (see p.311). You can slow things down by leaning back and attempting to go limp, making a conscious effort to breathe deeply and relax the muscles of your pelvic floor.

At this point it is important to follow the cues from your medical team, who will literally coach you from the sidelines, encouraging you to bear down and push with some contractions as your baby moves downward.

Your birth partner's support

Your birth partner's role is particularly important during the second stage of labor, and he or she can become actively involved in the final stages of delivering your baby. Your partner needs to be both emotionally supportive and encouraging, maintaining eye contact with you to help you to keep going. He or she can verbally coach you to push when your doctor signals, and tell you to relax between contractions and when things need to slow down. You may want your partner to massage you between contractions to help you relax. Encouraging you by keeping you informed about progress will also help to keep you motivated.

Your birth partner can support you and help you maintain an upright position. He or she can also help you reach down to touch your baby's head once it crowns, or hold a mirror to let you see what's happening.

Part of your birth partner's role is to ensure that your labor follows your birth plan as closely as possible, and guiding the doctor to handle your baby as you wish can help to ensure that things go according to plan. Finally, your partner may choose to cut your baby's umbilical cord (see opposite), which can be a moving experience for him or her.

Your baby is born

Eventually, under your caregiver's guidance, your baby's head will be pushed out. Your doctor will check the position of the umbilical cord and ensure that it isn't wrapped around the baby's neck. If it is, she will lift it gently away from the neck and over the head.

Once the head has been delivered, your baby will begin to turn to work his shoulders through your pelvis. You'll be encouraged to work with your contractions to push out his shoulders, which should take just a few more contractions. Once his shoulders emerge, his body will follow quickly afterward—sometimes simply sliding out once his shoulders are released. As your baby comes out, you will feel a gush of water as the rest of the amniotic fluid empties from your uterus.

After the delivery, your baby will be placed directly on your chest, if you wish, to enable skin-to-skin contact.

CROWNING
When the top of your baby's head can be fully seen at the entrance to your vagina, your baby is said to have "crowned." You may experience a burning, stinging sensation, which some call "the ring of fire."

FIRST CRY
At last, your baby has arrived! He will probably emerge covered in blood and vernix and, as he utters his first cry, you may feel overwhelming relief that labor is over and he is safely delivered.

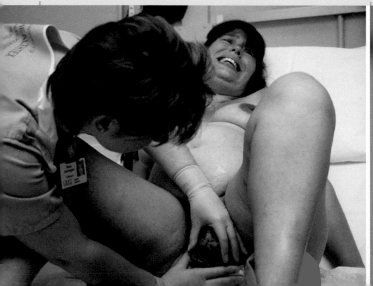

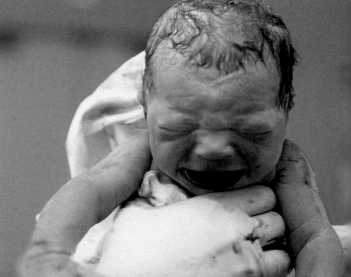

First contact

Immediate skin-to-skin contact with your baby is believed to encourage bonding between you. Early skin-to-skin contact has also been shown to help initiate breastfeeding, since the emotional and hormonal reflexes that you experience play an important role in ensuring that the milk that is being produced starts to flow.

One review of 17 studies found that skin-to-skin contact between mother and baby after birth had many benefits, including improving the success rate of breastfeeding as well as its duration; helping to maintain a normal temperature in the baby; encouraging stable blood-sugar levels; reducing crying; and improving the process of bonding. One study found that premature babies held skin-to-skin had greater head growth than babies held in a traditional way. What's more, the overall physical and emotional health of new moms is believed to be positively influenced with skin-to-skin contact.

Placing your baby on your chest with his skin against yours also stimulates his "rooting reflex," which means he will instinctively move his head and open his mouth in search of food. This can help greatly with breastfeeding, since your baby will actively seek out your nipple when he feels his mouth or cheek in contact with your skin.

Cutting the cord

After your baby's birth, the umbilical cord may be left to pulsate for several minutes before it is cut. This means that your baby receives more placental blood, which boosts his oxygen supply and blood volume.

Your birth partner may be nominated to cut the cord, which will be done under the guidance of the doctor or midwife. It is normally clamped in two places and then cut with scissors in between the two clamps. If you've arranged to have stem cells collected (see p.305), the collection will be undertaken at this stage too.

"Holding your baby skin-to-skin helps him make the difficult transition from the inside of your body to coping with the outside world"

CLOSE CONTACT
Wrapping your baby in a blanket and holding him skin-to-skin right after the birth has many proven benefits, helping to keep your baby warm, encourage breastfeeding, and, not least, start the process of bonding for both of you.

CUTTING THE CORD
After the birth, your baby's umbilical cord will be clamped and then cut, releasing your baby from the placenta that nourished him for the last nine months.

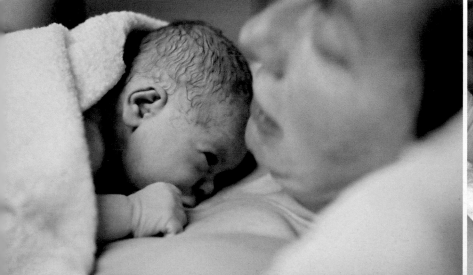

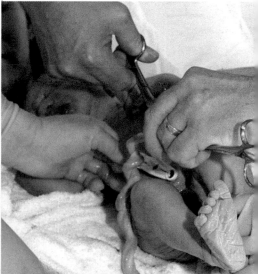

Third stage of labor

Labor isn't quite over once your baby is born and the cord is cut. As your uterus begins to shrink back to its normal size, you'll deliver the placenta that nourished your baby during pregnancy. This is a largely painless stage of labor.

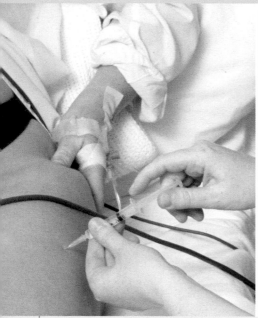

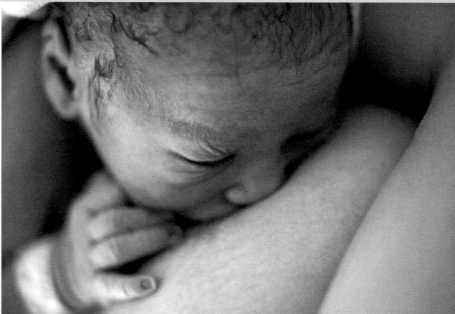

DELIVERING THE PLACENTA
An injection of a synthetic version of the hormone oxytocin into your thigh speeds up the delivery of the placenta.

YOUR BABY'S FIRST FEED
As you hold your baby next to your skin after the birth, she will instinctively move toward your breast and "root" around for her very first breastfeed.

The third stage begins when your baby is born and ends when the placenta and membranes are delivered. The placenta's delivery can be speeded up with drugs, known as a managed third stage, or it can be delivered naturally. You can discuss this with your doctor and state in advance which you'd prefer, although there are times when a managed third stage is advised. These include if you had a long labor, you had a stressful delivery with a big baby or twins, you suffer from anemia, or you have had a retained placenta (see p.320) in the past.

Managed third stage

This involves having an injection of oxytocin shortly after delivering your baby or around the time your baby's shoulders are being delivered, if your doctor feels that it's needed. The injection may be given into your thigh or intravenously.

A few minutes after your baby is born, your doctor will look for signs that your placenta has separated from your uterus, normally signaled by a gush of blood and a lengthening of the umbilical cord. At this point she will gently pull on the cord while pressing down on your abdomen, to assist the delivery of the placenta. This usually happens around between five and thirty minutes after your baby is born.

Using drugs during the third stage encourages a quick and efficient delivery of your placenta, and may reduce the risk of an excessive loss of blood after the birth, known as a postpartum hemorrhage (see p.321). It also means that this stage of labor occurs without you having to do much work. If the idea of a managed third stage appeals to you, ask your doctor her opinion about giving patients oxytocin injections to help speed along the delivery of the placenta and whether she does this for patients.

Natural third stage

More common is a natural or "physiological" third stage, which involves delivering the placenta without the aid of any drugs. In most cases, a natural third stage takes around 20 to 60 minutes.

As your uterus starts to shrink, the placenta becomes detached from the wall and is forced down toward your cervix and out through the birth canal with the help of mild contractions. You may feel mild discomfort, but most women are so involved with their new baby, they hardly notice this process. Giving your baby a breastfeed and holding her against your skin can encourage a natural third stage, since contact and nursing triggers the release of oxytocin, which in turn brings on contractions.

If the process is slow, you may be asked to adopt a position to help make the delivery more efficient, such as squatting or kneeling. It can also help to empty your bladder, since a full bladder may be preventing your placenta from being expelled.

Your blood loss is likely to be higher with a natural third stage. If your doctor is at all worried, she can decide at any stage to advise you to take medication to help speed up the delivery of the placenta. She is likely to advise you to do this anyway if the third stage takes longer than 60 minutes, since this increases the risk of you having a postpartum hemorrhage and a retained placenta.

Stem-cell collection

The blood in your baby's umbilical cord is rich with cells known as stem cells, which have the ability to change into other types of cells. When your baby is born, these cells migrate to her bone marrow soon after birth, and transform themselves into various blood-making cells. It's now known that stem cells can be used to treat a wide range of conditions, especially those that involve the destruction or malfunction of healthy cells, such as in leukemia. Potentially, diseased cells can be cured by introducing fresh stem cells to the relevant site.

For this reason, you can now arrange to harvest and store your baby's umbilical cord blood, which contains these stem cells, in a blood bank, either to help your baby should she become ill in the future, or to aid the treatment of others. This stored cord blood would be a perfect match in the event that your baby needed a transplant. You will need to pay for the processing and storage.

Harvesting the blood involves clamping the cord as early as possible and withdrawing the blood. Some experts are against this practice, as your baby may not get quite as much of this oxygen-rich blood as she might if there was no interruption to the third stage, and clamping took place a little later.

If you do wish to harvest your baby's stem cells, you'll need to discuss this with your doctor in advance and sign up with a cord blood bank. You must bring the cord blood storage kit you've been mailed to the hospital.

Now that labor is over

If you have had an episiotomy (see p.311) or tearing of your perineum, the affected area will now be cleaned and stitched. In most cases, the stitches are administered under a local anesthetic, injected at the site, and are designed to dissolve after a few days. This process can be a little uncomfortable, so you may be given a suppository for pain relief immediately after you've been stitched, and painkillers and anti-inflammatory medication may be recommended.

Depending on the length of your labor, and any medication you had, your initial feeling may be one of exhaustion, although it's normal for adrenaline to kick in with the excitement of holding your baby. You may also feel shivery or jittery, and even faint. This is caused by the stress hormones that have flooded your body, and a natural drop in blood sugar. Eating something as soon as possible will help you to feel calmer and more alert.

You may be amazed by the rush of emotions that you'll experience in the first few moments of motherhood. New moms often find themselves feeling a mixture of love, pride, astonishment, achievement, shock, and relief—sometimes all at the same time!

You may find that one of your first emotions is worry—about whether your baby is healthy and has all the right parts, and if you are capable of parenting her properly. Try not to panic. You will need time to find your feet and get to know your new baby, but rest assured that you will soon relax into parenthood with the support of your partner, pediatrician, and family and friends.

Don't underestimate the physical toll of labor on your body and your emotions. It's perfectly normal to feel wobbly and tearful, and to experience mood swings, culminating in drifting off to sleep. Practically, it's helpful to have someone with you to be sure that you aren't in danger of losing your grip on your baby if you fall asleep, although you will likely be offered a bassinet for your baby.

Home and water births

Giving birth at home in familiar surroundings can make it easier to relax, which can help you to have a more efficient labor. Likewise, many women find the soothing effects of warm water incredibly beneficial during labor.

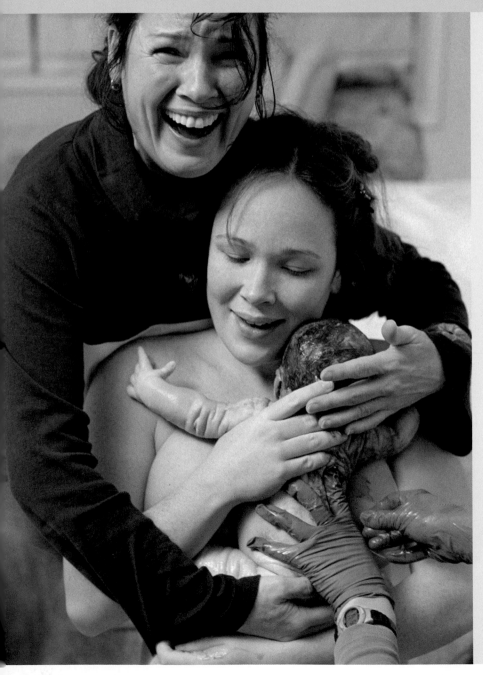

Studies show that labor is often shorter and less painful for women who choose to give birth at home and/or in water. Both types of birth have a good record of safety for low-risk pregnancies.

Having your baby at home

Giving birth at home gives you more control over your birth experience and avoids routine medical interventions that you would have to put up with in a hospital. Many women feel much more relaxed at home, which helps them to deal more easily with pain. You can have as many family members or friends as you like to share the experience with you in privacy and comfort. You may also find you move around more, which can speed up labor.

It's thought, too, that staying in one place helps labor, since changing your environment, for example if you leave home to go to the hospital, interrupts the production of labor hormones. Furthermore, there is a significantly lower postpartum infection rate for home births compared to hospital ones.

A NATURAL BIRTH
Couples planning a home birth sometimes combine it with a water birth, renting and setting up a birthing pool in advance. Giving birth under water under a midwife's care is a safe way to deliver your baby and can be a gentle introduction to the world for him.

WHAT YOU'LL NEED

Your midwife will let you know what you need to get ready ahead of time. Usually her list will include the following:

• Plastic sheets to protect your bed, floor, or sofa. Disposable bed mats (used for bedwetting or incontinence) work well too. You'll also need old towels or sheets to lay on top.

• Candles, music, calming artwork, bean bags, or anything else you want to create a comfortable environment.

• Natural pain-relief remedies, such as massage oils.

• A hot-water bottle or heated pad.

• Light snacks for you and your partner.

• A clean towel and blanket to dry your baby and keep him warm after the birth.

• A plastic container for the placenta.

• Your birth plan: If you have a midwife you don't know, this will help her familiarize herself with your wishes.

• A hospital bag for you and your baby —just in case.

PAIN RELIEF

You can use natural methods of pain relief (see pp.284–287)—including a water birth if you rent a pool, see right—or massages from your birth partner. Your midwife may be able to offer prescription pain relief. (Check this out in advance.)

WHAT HAPPENS

Once you're having regular contractions, call your midwife. She will arrive with her home-birth pack (unless she has dropped it off already), which includes a blood pressure monitor, equipment to monitor your baby, oxygen and equipment for an emergency, and any other tools she needs.

Throughout labor, your midwife will check your cervix to see how far it is dilating, monitor your blood pressure and temperature, and keep tabs on your baby's heart rate. Before the delivery, a second midwife may arrive, so that one midwife can care for you while the second midwife looks after your baby.

After you deliver the placenta (see pp.304–305), your midwife can stitch minor tears or an episiotomy cut (see p.311), although more serious tears will need to be treated at the hospital. After the birth, your midwife will check you and your baby, help you to establish breastfeeding, and encourage you to rest while she clears up.

If, at any stage, your midwife is worried about you or your baby, she will arrange for you to be transferred to the hospital, probably by ambulance. Also, you can change your mind at any stage of labor, or before, and ask to go to the hospital, and if you want an epidural you'll need to do this. One in six women who plan a home birth is transferred to the hospital.

Giving birth in water

You can have a water birth at a birthing center or possibly a hospital, depending on the facilities, or at home, in which case you'll need to rent a pool. If you want a home water birth, check in advance that your midwife is used to delivering babies in water. Also, if you rent a tub, it needs to be big and deep enough to sit in easily; your faucet adaptor must fit the water outlet; and your floor must be strong enough to support the weight of a full tub with occupants. There should be space all around the tub for your midwife, too.

You can choose to both labor and give birth in the pool, or to use the pool for pain relief during labor and then get out to deliver your baby.

WHAT YOU'LL NEED

• Have a sieve ready so that clots, mucus, feces, or vomit (all of which are normal) can be removed as soon as possible.

• Have a spray bottle of water and cool drinking water nearby—you can become hot and thirsty in the warm water.

PAIN RELIEF

You can use the breathing techniques you learned in prenatal classes, gentle massages from your birth partner, or homeopathic remedies, if they're pre-approved by your doctor. You won't be able to use a TENS machine or to have pain relief that requires injection.

WHAT HAPPENS?

Once you are in the pool, find a position in which you feel most comfortable. You can use inflatables for support, or a folded towel or rubber mat to protect your knees if you're kneeling.

The water will be kept between 93–98.6°F (34–37°C). Your midwife will monitor your baby's heartbeat regularly with a waterproof fetal monitor. If possible, she will check how far you're dilated while you're in the water, or, if this proves tricky, will look when you get out to use the bathroom, and she will take your temperature and blood pressure regularly.

When your baby is born, your bottom and your baby's head will be under water. Once your baby is completely delivered, your midwife will lift him to the surface and hand him to you. You can put him to your breast right away, keeping his head above water.

Some midwives will let you deliver the placenta in the pool, but you may be asked to get out if yours needs to assess your blood loss. Your partner can have warm, clean towels ready to wrap around you and your baby.

You will be asked to leave the pool if any intervention is needed. If you are at home, you may need to be taken to the hospital if there is a problem.

When labor fails to progress

Although labor is a natural event and entirely straightforward for the majority of women, it can sometimes slow down or stop—and medical intervention may be needed to ensure the safe delivery of your baby.

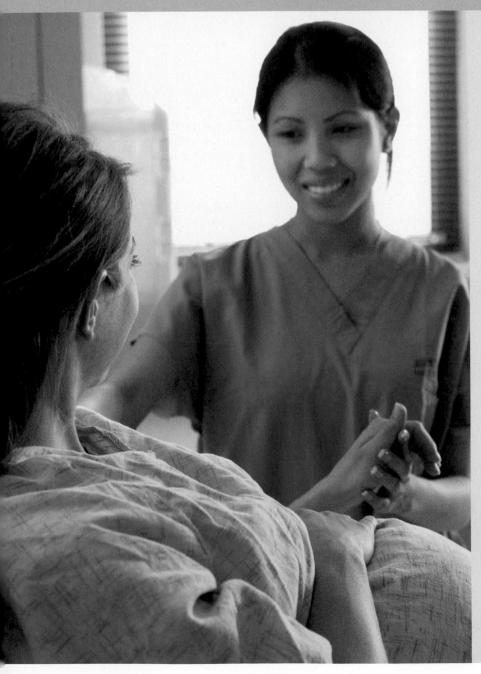

It used to be standard practice to set a time limit on how long labor should be allowed to go on before medical intervention was deemed necessary. Today, though, practice has changed, and women are left to labor for much longer—while being monitored regularly to ensure that mother and baby are doing well—before a labor is considered abnormally slow.

Medical intervention is only thought necessary if you are exhausted or your baby is showing signs of distress, or when it is otherwise clear that things are not progressing as they should. Speak to your doctor or midwife if you are concerned.

Common causes of slow labor

Slow progress in labor can have several causes, including weak and inefficient contractions, the position of the baby, or an overlarge baby.

A stall in the progress of labor is known as "dystocia." This can sometimes occur as a result of anxiety or dehydration, but is more common in

COPING WITH STOPS AND STARTS
You may feel frustrated and concerned if labor comes to a halt. Your doctor will talk to you about your progress and discuss what might happen next.

obese women, those over 40 years old, in pregnancies over 41 weeks, and in women less than five feet (150cm) tall.

Dystocia usually happens during the first stage of labor, although it does sometimes occur in the second stage. If all steps to get your contractions going or to move your baby manually into a better position fail, an assisted delivery (see p.310) or caesarean (see p.316) will need to be considered.

YOUR BABY'S POSITION

The ideal position for your baby during labor is with the back of her head facing your front, known as an anterior position (see pp.270–271). If your baby is in a posterior position, with the back of her head facing your back, this can make labor very uncomfortable, with pressure put on your back.

Labor can be prolonged as the baby finds it hard to rotate and move down in the pelvis. In addition, cervical dilation is more difficult, because the relatively wide forehead (rather than the crown of the head) presses against the cervix. Also, posterior babies sometimes try to turn to the anterior position during labor, which means that they don't press down on the cervix for long enough to encourage it to dilate.

A bottom-down breech baby may slow dilatation. When the baby's head presses firmly against your cervix, it signals the release of oxytocin, the hormone that stimulates contractions. When the bottom or feet are the presenting part, the pressure is less effective.

INEFFECTIVE CONTRACTIONS

This is more common in a first pregnancy, possibly because your body, unused to labor, hasn't responded properly to the start of labor. If it's thought that your contractions are weak, the membranes surrounding the amniotic sac may be broken to speed things up (see p.281) and put more pressure on the cervix.

You may also be offered a drip of an artificial form of the hormone oxytocin, which stimulates the uterus to contract.

WHEN YOUR BABY IS TOO LARGE

Occasionally, the baby's head is too big to fit through the mother's pelvis, which is referred to as "cephalo-pelvic disproportion" (CPD). Although this may be suspected during pregnancy, there is no accurate way to measure it prior to labor, and the situation may only become clear when your labor simply doesn't proceed as expected and within safe time frames.

If your baby's head has already moved down into your pelvis, a vaginal delivery may still be possible. However, your labor will be closely monitored by your doctor and nurses, and a caesarean delivery may be necessary if there are signs of distress or labor doesn't progress as expected.

THE CERVIX

Occasionally, the cervix doesn't dilate adequately despite good contractions and your baby being in the ideal position. Previous surgery on the cervix or a fibroid in the lower part of the uterus might cause this.

Coping with delays and intervention

It is only natural to feel disappointed if you had high expectations of achieving a natural birth, and labor doesn't go as you had planned. For some women, having a caesarean may feel like the ultimate failure. What you must remember is that the main goal is to have a baby; however this is achieved, it is still an overwhelming and significant event in your life. Be positive and logical, and don't let disappointment tarnish your happy experience. MG

The most important outcome ultimately is the safe delivery of a healthy baby, by whatever means are necessary. Bear this in mind when you draft your birth plan, and try to prepare for the unexpected as well, so it isn't such a shock if and when it occurs. Ensuring the healthy delivery of your baby by caesarean is far from failure; you have understood the need for medical intervention and are providing for your baby's well-being. NK

You can't "try" harder to speed up your labor any more than you can control the birth itself. Try to remember that labor is not a test that you can pass or fail; it is an experience that you are

going through, with an ultimate goal in mind. If you achieve the goal—with a healthy baby at the end of it all— you have succeeded. CH

I didn't experience any major delays myself, but a good friend was really disappointed that she labored for hours in a birthing pool (to the point where the midwife could see her baby's head), only for her contractions to slow down. It turned out that her baby's progress had been impeded by a full-to-bursting bladder—she'd forgotten all about going to the bathroom. So the midwife had to get her out of the pool, drain her bladder using a catheter, and give her intravenous oxytocin to get her contractions going again. Her baby was born with a bit more pushing a couple of hours later. FF

I was disappointed when attempts to turn my breech baby didn't work and so I needed a caesarean section. Ultimately, I realized that this was safer for my baby, and the delivery was still a wonderful experience. VB

Assisted delivery

Sometimes a vaginal delivery needs assistance with a vacuum or forceps. This can happen if you are exhausted after a long labor, or if the second stage doesn't run smoothly and you need extra help to deliver your baby.

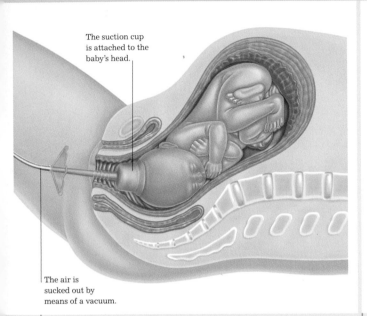

The suction cup is attached to the baby's head.

The air is sucked out by means of a vacuum.

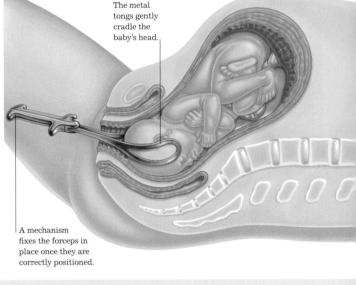

The metal tongs gently cradle the baby's head.

A mechanism fixes the forceps in place once they are correctly positioned.

ATTACHING A VACUUM SUCTION CUP
Once the suction cup has been attached to your baby's head, he will be gently pulled down the birth canal. Using a vacuum allows the baby to turn around in the birth canal if necessary.

USING FORCEPS
The metal tongs are placed gently on either side of your baby's head, and he is guided out during contractions. Different types of forceps are used depending on the position of your baby's head.

If the end of the second stage of labor becomes difficult or prolonged, your doctor or midwife may suggest assisting the delivery with a vacuum suction cup or forceps. This intervention will be made only if absolutely necessary, and can avoid the need for an emergency caesarean. However, your cervix must be fully dilated before an assisted delivery can be considered; otherwise a caesarean will probably be the only option for you.

The method used will depend partly on the experience of the doctor or midwife carrying out the procedure, but mainly on the position of the baby, your ability to push, and the urgency of the delivery. Be reassured that babies are delivered safely with both methods.

Why intervene?

There are a number of situations when an assisted birth may be suggested to ensure the safe delivery of your baby. These include the following:
• You are absolutely exhausted (perhaps after a very long labor) and don't have enough energy to continue pushing.
• Your contractions are too weak to help push your baby out.
• Your baby is in an awkward position.
• Your baby is suffering some distress, and his heartbeat is becoming irregular.
• Your labor is premature.
• Your baby is breech (see pp.272–273).
• You've had an epidural and are finding it difficult to feel how and when to push during contractions.

You will be asked to lie on the bed with your feet in stirrups so that the doctor or midwife can access your baby as easily as possible. Because an assisted vaginal delivery can be painful, you will usually be offered some type of pain relief, such as a local anesthetic, or sometimes an epidural or spinal block (see pp.290–291).

USING A VACUUM

A vacuum is a type of suction cup that fits onto your baby's head and then gently pulls him out. This method is often chosen if you still have energy to push and your contractions are strong enough. The cup is positioned onto your baby's head, and the air is extracted with the vacuum. Once in place, during your next contraction you'll be encouraged to push, while your doctor pulls. Your baby's head should be delivered in the next three contractions. The cup is removed right after the birth.

PROS AND CONS

Vacuum births are very safe as long as you are at least 34 weeks pregnant. Before this time, your baby's head may be too fragile to cope with the suction. Some women prefer this method because they think it is less traumatic for the baby and it doesn't always require an episiotomy (see below), which is usually necessary with a forceps delivery. You may experience some discomfort after the procedure, but any bruising, tearing, or swelling should go down within a week.

On the downside, a vacuum delivery can cause temporary swelling to your baby's head, which can take up to six weeks to disappear. Sometimes, the vacuum doesn't attach properly during the procedure and forceps are required. Occasionally a caesarean has to be performed if the vacuum fails.

USING FORCEPS

Forceps may be a better choice if your pushing is not effective. These large, stainless-steel tongs curve around your baby's head to help move him down the birth canal. Your doctor or midwife will usually need to enlarge your vaginal opening with an episiotomy.

The forceps are opened and put gently around your baby's head, then held in place. As with the vacuum, you'll be asked to push with contractions while the doctor pulls.

PROS AND CONS

Forceps have a good success rate and pose little risk to your baby, although he may have some bruising on his face—but this usually disappears within 24–48 hours. You may be uncomfortable for a while afterward.

Perineal tears and episiotomies

It is common to experience some tearing during labor, especially if your baby is large or in an awkward position. The likelihood increases further if your baby is delivered by forceps or vacuum and you haven't had an episiotomy. Tears are classified into degrees—first, second, and third—according to how deep they are. A first-degree tear is a small tear to the skin of the vagina; a second-degree tear affects the vagina and the perineal muscles, the muscular area between your vagina and back passage known as the perineum; and a third-degree tear extends further to the muscles around the anus.

When a tear occurs, it will need to be examined and its extent, or degree, identified, so that it can be stitched appropriately. Once your baby has crowned (see pp.301–302), you may be offered an episiotomy—a small cut in the perineum—to widen the vaginal opening, prevent a tear, and ease the delivery.

Your doctor may decide that an episiotomy is necessary if your baby is in distress and needs to be delivered quickly. Or she may think that you are in danger

of severe tearing if a controlled cut isn't made. However, most midwives will try to avoid episiotomies if possible, because they can cause a degree of pain and can take a while to heal.

You can avoid the need for an episiotomy by practicing pelvic floor exercises during pregnancy (see p.192) to strengthen the muscles used for pushing. You can also massage your perineum with vitamin E oil in the third trimester, gently stretching out the area inside the vagina. Furthermore, adopting different positions during the second stage of labor—in particular, getting into an all-fours position—can help the descent of your baby's head and avoid a bad tear or the need for an episiotomy.

Episiotomies and large tears will require stitching afterward, but smaller ones can be left to heal naturally. A local anesthetic is administered before stitching, so you shouldn't experience any pain while this is done. A third-degree tear needs to be stitched by an experienced practitioner, under general anesthesia and possibly in an operating

room. You may also need laxatives and antibiotics following this procedure to ensure complete healing.

After the birth, you will probably experience some discomfort and itching as the site heals. Taking painkillers and pouring warm water over your perineum as you urinate can help to ease the discomfort. Most tears feel better after a few weeks, although episiotomies can take a week or so longer to heal.

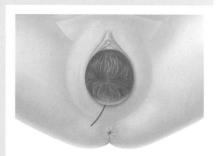

EPISIOTOMY INCISION
A surgical cut in the perineum is sometimes necessary to aid delivery.

Multiple births

If you're carrying twins or more, your birth options can be limited, depending on your babies' positions. Be assured, though, that you will be attended by a team of experts who are there to ensure the safe delivery of your babies.

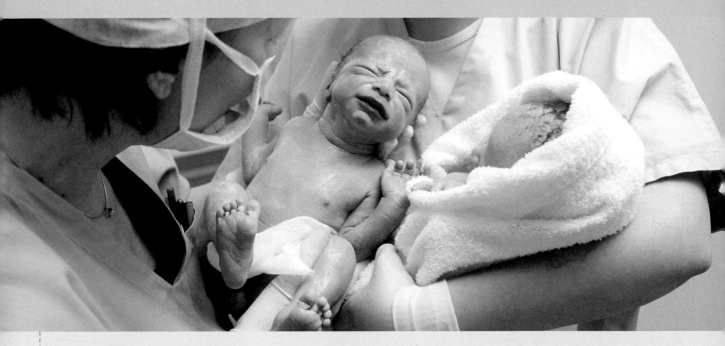

EXTRA SUPPORT
A dedicated birth team will be on hand to ensure that the delivery of your babies runs safely and smoothly for you all, and that your babies receive any necessary care and attention promptly after the birth.

If you're expecting twins, you will be closely monitored toward the end of your pregnancy to check the position of the babies and how they're growing.

A vaginal delivery will only be recommended if the leading baby is in a head-down (cephalic) position (see p.273). This is because if the first baby is breech, the risk of a lack of oxygen in labor to this baby is increased. The position of the second baby isn't as important, since he can be turned to face head-down or delivered in a breech position.

If you have three or more babies, you will need a caesarean, regardless of how they are positioned. If your twins aren't in the right position or you have triplets or more, a caesarean will be scheduled in advance. Multiple pregnancies increase the risk of premature labor, because the uterus stretches to a greater degree much earlier than it would with a single baby. Also, the function of the placenta deteriorates earlier in pregnancy. For these reasons, a caesarean with twins will be carried out by around 38 weeks, and with triplets by about 34 weeks.

If labor is early

If you go into labor before 34 weeks but your membranes are intact, your babies' heart rates are stable, and there are no signs of infection or any other problems, your doctor may attempt to delay the delivery to give your babies' lungs more time to develop.

"Don't be alarmed to find yourself attended by a team of medical specialists when delivering multiples . . . take heart that you are in the safest possible hands"

This is done by giving you medication to try to halt contractions for a while, so that you can be given a corticosteroid injection to speed up the development of your babies' lungs (see p.315). If this doesn't succeed and you were already planning a caesarean, you may be taken into surgery right away. If you were planning to deliver naturally, you may still be able to.

You can expect to be attended by your obstetrician, labor and delivery nurses, a doula (if applicable), a pediatrician or neonatologist (to ensure that your babies receive any necessary treatment after the birth), an anesthesiologist (in case a caesarean is necessary), and other medical support staff. Try not to let this worry you. The professionals are there as a precaution, and you can be assured that both you and your babies are in safe hands. Try not to be distracted by them, and focus instead on the actual birth.

Delivering twins vaginally

A twin vaginal delivery is done under controlled circumstances, often in a room equipped to deal with emergency procedures so that help is at hand if an assisted delivery or caesarean is required. You may be advised to have an epidural, in case special maneuvers are necessary to get your second twin out. A fetal scalp electrode (see p.293) will be placed on the first twin's head; the second twin will be monitored through your abdomen.

DELIVERING THE FIRST TWIN

Your first baby may be delivered normally, or a vacuum or forceps (see pp.310–311) may be used to keep things moving swiftly so that the second baby can be attended to as soon as possible. The first baby's cord will be clamped and cut, but the placenta will usually be left in your uterus until your second baby has been born.

DELIVERING THE SECOND TWIN

After your first baby has been delivered, the position of your second baby will determine how much intervention is needed for her birth. However, it is unusual for one baby to be delivered vaginally, and the other by caesarean. It's common for second babies to be delivered within an hour of the first.

Once your first baby is born your uterus may suddenly relax, allowing the second twin to move around more and, potentially, take up a transverse or other difficult position, making delivery trickier. To avoid this, you may be offered oxytocin (see p.281) to encourage your uterus to contract. Your doctor may examine your abdomen and hold it firmly to keep the second twin in the best position and prevent her from moving away from the birth canal. The position will be checked with an ultrasound.

If all is well as your contractions continue, the second twin will descend into the birth canal either head first or bottom down. If her amniotic sac hasn't already ruptured spontaneously, it will be ruptured artificially by your doctor (see p.281) and the delivery will then continue as normal.

If, despite every effort to keep her head or bottom down, a second twin turns into a transverse position, the doctor may try to reach into the uterus via the vagina to take hold of a foot and deliver her feet first. This is called a "breech extraction" and is a very skilled technique that is undertaken only by the most experienced obstetricians.

After the births

If your babies are full term (which for twins is around 37 weeks), they may not need special care. Before this time, they are more likely to need to stay in a neonatal intensive care unit (see p.336) because they may require ventilators or incubators to help them breathe and thrive until they have developed sufficiently to manage on their own. The average birth weight for twins is 5.5lb (2.5kg), and for triplets 4lb (1.8kg).

Following a vaginal delivery of twins, a managed third stage (see p.304) is usually suggested because your placenta is larger and the uterus often doesn't contract efficiently after delivery, which means you have a slightly higher risk of bleeding after the birth. You may also require medication to help prevent further bleeding later on.

Premature birth

Around 15 percent of babies are born prematurely—before 37 weeks. It can be worrying going into labor weeks before your due date, but you will receive additional care and monitoring to help ensure the safe delivery of your baby.

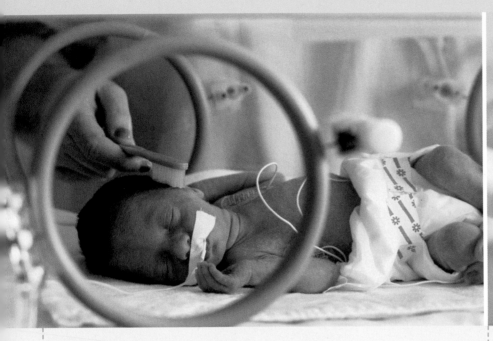

STAYING CLOSE BY
Being close by will help your tiny baby to thrive. The staff in the NICU will show you ways to touch him gently and enjoy contact with him, and will encourage you to talk and sing to him.

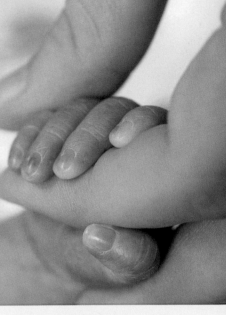

LOVING TOUCH
Stroking, touching, and holding your baby will comfort him and help him to recognize your smell and presence.

Significant improvements in the treatment and care of premature babies means that the outlook for tiny babies has never been better, and, nowadays, the vast majority of babies born after 30 weeks do well after birth, often with no long-lasting complications. However, the earlier a baby is born and the lower his birth weight, the greater the risk of short- and long-term problems.

In about 40 percent of cases, the cause of premature labor is unclear. However, there are risk factors, which include a multiple pregnancy; preeclampsia (see pp.386-387); prenatal hemorrhaging; diabetes; infection; cervical weakness; and abnormalities in your baby.

When labor starts early

Contractions are not a reliable sign of premature labor; many women have intense Braxton Hicks contractions (see p.216). If, however, contractions do not stop and start, and are increasingly close together, you may be in labor. If your membranes rupture and you lose amniotic fluid, labor is even more likely.

If you have any of these signs well before your due date, call your doctor for an immediate assessment. Try not to panic: Most women with early contractions do not go on to deliver early, and the contractions stop spontaneously, known as a threatened pre-term labor.

A test called the "fetal fibronectin test" may be done to help assess if you're in labor. Fibronectin is a protein produced by your baby's membranes that, once released, can be a signal that labor has begun. A negative result means you are not in labor and probably have at least a week or two before the birth. If it's positive, labor isn't definite, but steps may be taken to protect your baby in the event that the birth is imminent.

SLOWING THINGS DOWN
Once your cervix begins to dilate, nothing can be done to halt your labor. You will probably be given drugs known as "tocolytics" to slow labor down, giving your baby a little more time in the uterus (usually about 48 hours) so that steroids can be given to help mature your baby's lungs. These are injected into your system, which then transfers them to your baby, but they need to be given at least 24 hours before the delivery to be effective.

Your baby's immune system will be significantly less mature than that of a full-term baby, so you may also be offered antibiotics to lessen the risk of your baby acquiring a bacterial infection during the birth.

You'll be transferred to a hospital with a neonatal intensive care unit (NICU) (see p.336), where your baby will be cared for after the birth. This is routine, and almost always necessary for babies under 34 weeks, since they need special care until they're strong enough to breathe and feed alone. If you have time, it's a good idea to familiarize yourself with the unit when you're transferred— meeting the staff and understanding how your baby will be cared for is reassuring. If you are unable to visit yourself, your birth partner could go on your behalf. Your pediatrician (or one assigned by the hospital) will visit you to discuss the likely outcome for your baby.

Outlook for early babies

Babies born after 34 weeks have a lower risk of complications because their systems are almost mature. Before this time, there is an increased risk of

problems, but many can be dealt with by the specialist teams. Risks include breathing problems, hypothermia, low blood sugar, jaundice (see p.334), infections, and eye problems.

Your baby may be very small (sometimes weighing as little as 1.1lb/500g) and will be born with a large amount of lanugo—the down-like body hair that is normally shed as a baby approaches full term. He'll also have more vernix, the wax-like substance that protects his skin in the uterus. If he is born before 36 weeks, his sucking reflex won't be mature, and he'll probably need to be fed breast milk through a tube. He will not have acquired the layers of fat that come in the final weeks of pregnancy, so he may look thin, and his veins may be visible through his skin.

Seeing your baby hooked up to monitors and tubes can be alarming, but take comfort from the fact that they are helping him feed, breathe, and grow. In many cases, premature babies do well, and, after being assisted in the first days or weeks, soon gain weight and feed and breathe independently.

Treatment for premature babies

The prognosis for premature babies is better than ever, because medical advances have contributed to massive improvements in treatment and care. The statistics are encouraging, with a survival rate of up to 90 percent for babies born around 28 weeks.

NUMBER OF WEEKS	POSSIBLE PROBLEMS	TREATMENT
Pre-28 weeks	Low muscle tone; can't suck, swallow, and breathe at the same time; very low birth weight (less than 2.2lb/1kg).	Need intravenous feeding through an IV; need oxygen and assistance to breathe with a tube; high risk of complications.
28–31 weeks	90 to 95 percent survive. Risk of serious disabilities if birth weight is less than 3.3lb (1.5kg).	Most require oxygen and medical assistance to help them breathe; some fed intravenously, although others may be able to be fed breast milk or formula through a tube placed into their nose or stomach.
32–33 weeks	More than 95 percent survive; some can breathe on their own, and others may just need extra oxygen.	Those with breathing difficulties will require tube feeding, but others may be breast- or bottle-fed. Slightly increased risk of learning or behavioral problems.
34–36 weeks	Almost as likely as a full-term baby to survive. Higher risk of mild health problems, including feeding and breathing difficulties.	Most can be breast- or bottle-fed, but some may need tube feeding. At 35 weeks, the weight of the brain is only 60 percent of that of full-term babies.

Caesarean section

Nearly one third of babies born in Canada are delivered by caesarean section, which involves making a cut in the abdomen and uterus to deliver the baby. This is done if it's considered the safest option for both you and your baby.

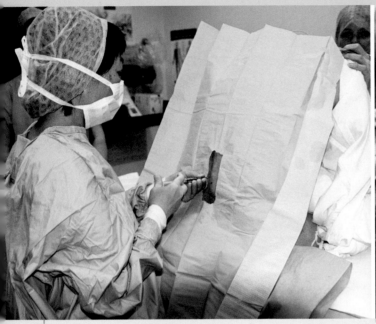

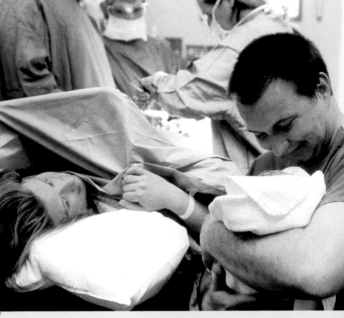

PREPARING FOR THE PROCEDURE
You will be held steady while a needle is inserted in your back; then you will be given either a spinal block or an epidural. Once the team is certain that the anesthetic has worked, the operation will begin.

OVER TO YOU
While you're being stitched, your baby will be wrapped in a blanket and you and your partner will be able to hold her for the first time. Your partner can support her next to your head while you greet her.

A caesarean delivery is advised if it's thought that a vaginal birth could put you or your baby at risk. It's a safe method of delivery, although because it's a major operation, your recovery may be longer. The procedure can be planned in advance, known as an elective caesarean, which will be done before your due date, or is carried out as an emergency in labor. This happens if your baby is thought to be in distress during labor, or your labor is failing to progress (see p.308) and a caesarean delivery is considered the safest option for you both.

Types of caesarean

Caesareans are planned in advance for a number of reasons. You may need to schedule one if there is an obstruction to a vaginal delivery, such as a low-lying placenta that covers the cervix (see p.386); you have preeclamsia (see pp.386–387) or diabetes (see p.385), which increase the risks during birth; you have an infection that could be passed to your baby; or you've had a previous caesarean,

since there's a risk the scar could rupture in a vaginal birth. Also, if you had a previous stillbirth, a caesarean may be suggested for emotional reasons.

A caesarean may also be planned if the position of your baby or twins makes it a safer option; if your baby has a condition called intra-uterine growth restriction (IUGR), where growth slows or ceases in the uterus (see p.388); if she is too big to fit through your pelvis, known as cephalo-pelvic disproportion (see p.309); or if a known abnormality may make birth difficult.

"Once you've been given an anesthetic and prepared for surgery, the actual delivery of your baby will happen swiftly, usually in around 10 minutes"

Emotional and physical considerations are also taken into account. For example, some women want a caesarean because of a previous traumatic vaginal birth. It's worth noting, though, that a caesarean is a major operation, so the risks should be carefully considered. When possible, elective caesareans are usually scheduled for 39 weeks or later, because there is good evidence to suggest that delaying the delivery as long as possible reduces your baby's risk of respiratory problems.

Emergency caesareans are carried out if unexpected complications arise with you and/or your baby in pregnancy or labor, putting one or both of you at risk. This can be the case if labor stops or doesn't progress, despite medical intervention (see p.280); the umbilical cord prolapses (see p.319) or becomes compressed, affecting the baby's oxygen supply, or your baby shows signs of distress. An emergency caesarean may also be done in late pregnancy if the placenta comes away from the uterine wall too early, known as placental abruption (see p.386).

Caesareans are safe for you and your baby. There are, however, risks associated with any surgery, which you will be told about before the operation. These include increased bleeding and infection (antibiotics are routinely offered to avoid infection). There's a small risk of a bladder or bowel injury and a blood clot (which is unlikely if you're generally healthy, and you will be given medication to prevent clots). There's also the risk that you will react to the medication.

The operation

You will be prepared for surgery and given an anesthetic. This is usually an epidural or a spinal block (see pp.290–291), both of which block out pain below your chest and allow you to stay awake, which means your partner can be with you.

Occasionally a general anesthetic is used, although this usually happens only in emergency situations when your baby needs to be delivered instantly and there is no time to hook up an epidural. The operation usually takes about 45 minutes.

Your birth partner will usually be asked to wear a surgical mask and possibly surgeon's scrubs. A screen is placed across your abdomen, so neither you nor your partner will see the incision and delivery. Throughout the operation, your heart rate, breathing, and blood pressure will be monitored.

You will be given an oxygen mask, or a tube may be inserted into your nose to provide oxygen during the operation. You will also have a catheter inserted into your bladder through your urethra, and an intravenous drip placed in your arm (to deliver fluids).

DELIVERING YOUR BABY

A horizontal cut, called a "bikini cut," will be made in your abdomen, just above your pubic bone. In emergencies, or if your baby is in a tricky position, your doctor may choose to use a vertical cut, between your belly button and pubic bone, to get your baby out more quickly,

but this is rare. The doctor will gently separate your abdominal muscles so that he or she can get to your uterus, and will then make another incision in the uterus, which can also be horizontal or vertical.

Your baby will be lifted out, which can feel like a tugging sensation, and as your baby emerges, the umbilical cord will be clamped and cut. If you wish, your birth partner may be able to do this.

You can usually hold your baby while the placenta and membranes are removed and you are stitched up. You'll be given pain relief (which won't harm your baby if you plan to breastfeed), so that you won't feel undue discomfort when the anesthetic wears off.

Your recovery

You may feel itchy, nauseated, and sore, all normal reactions to surgery and anesthetics. If a general anesthetic was used, you may also feel cold, groggy, confused, and even frightened. You will usually stay in the hospital for about four days, and will probably need to stay in bed for at least 12 hours. You may feel discomfort for a few days, but your pain relief will be topped up to counter this.

Some babies born by caesarean experience breathing difficulties, known as "transient tachypnoea," since they've missed out on the process of labor, which encourages fluid to clear from the lungs. However, most babies are fine in a day or two.

When labor doesn't go as planned

Unexpected complications can arise at any stage of labor. Being aware of this and of how different situations are handled helps you deal with any eventuality and reassures you that steps will be taken to deliver your baby safely.

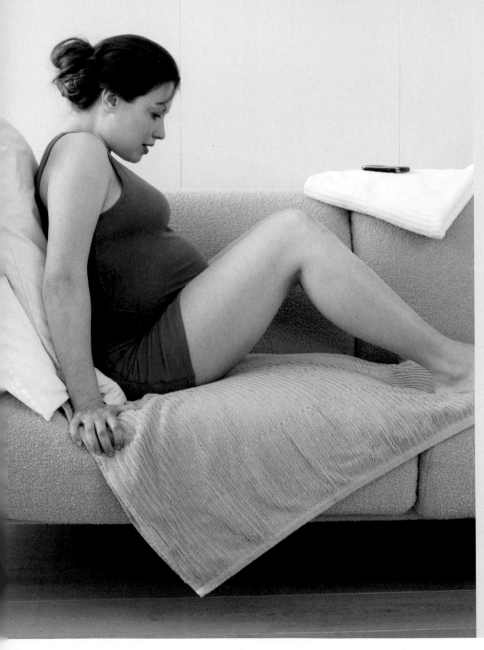

Women commonly feel traumatized, and even guilty, after a difficult birth. Or you may feel shocked if your baby was born very quickly. If you feel any of these things, ask for reassurance and support from your doctor, midwife, or partner.

Fast labor

A rapid labor that lasts less than two hours from the first contraction to giving birth is called a "precipitate labor." This is a rare occurrence that happens in just 2 percent of pregnancies. It's unknown why some women have fast labors, but they're more common with second or subsequent babies.

A very quick labor can be a traumatic experience for mothers, since they have little time to acclimate to the labor process. As a consequence, labor can be very painful, because there's no time for your body's natural painkillers (endorphins) to build up. On the other hand, some women have little discomfort, and are simply shocked by the situation. However, in most cases, the delivery is normal, with little or no intervention required, and without complications for mother or baby. Having an idea of what to do can help you feel more in control.

A SUDDEN ARRIVAL

If you feel your baby coming and there's no time to get to the hospital, a safe position for delivery is sitting on a soft surface with your knees drawn up. It's a good idea to have a towel nearby to wrap your baby in.

WHAT TO DO

If you experience sudden contractions that are intense and very close together, or any urge to push, do not attempt to get to the hospital on your own. Call your ob/gyn's office; they're likely to tell you to call 911 for an ambulance.

Wash your hands, and if you have someone with you, ask them to put trash bags or a plastic cloth and newspapers down, with clean towels on top. If you're on your own, leave the door unlocked so that the paramedics can get in. Call someone who can come over quickly to help you, for example a friend or neighbor. Keep a cordless phone or your cell phone near you.

If you feel a strong urge to push before help arrives, breathe calmly, or pant or blow, to slow down the delivery of the head, but don't keep your legs together or resist the urge to push; doing so could hurt the baby. Once you feel the head, or your partner can see it, start to push. When the head is out, make sure the cord isn't around the neck; if it is, gently lift it over the baby's head. You will have more contractions as you deliver the body.

AFTER THE BIRTH

Once your baby has been born, dry him and wrap him in a clean towel, and put him on your chest so that he stays warm. You can rub him firmly with a towel to encourage him to cry, which kick-starts the process of breathing. Your baby may also be surprised by a quick birth, but your heartbeat, warmth, and voice will be reassuring.

Soon after your baby is born, you may feel some more contractions, which is your uterus expelling the placenta. Don't pull on the cord if the placenta doesn't deliver on its own. Once the placenta emerges, place it into a bag or bucket if you'd rather not look at it. At this point, you should have your baby in your arms, still attached to the cord, which is attached to the placenta. Don't attempt to cut the cord yourself. The paramedics will do this when they arrive.

Cord prolapse

This is an emergency situation affecting around 1 in 200 pregnancies. It occurs when the umbilical cord prolapses out of the cervix into the birth canal. The baby may then compress the cord, reducing his blood flow, which in turn compromises or cuts off the baby's oxygen supply. An immediate delivery is needed to prevent the lack of oxygen to your baby from causing serious problems.

WHY DOES IT HAPPEN?

Cord prolapse is most likely when a baby is lying in a transverse or breech position (see pp.272) or his head is high in the uterus when your water breaks. It's more likely in a premature labor, with twins, or if there's too much amniotic fluid around your baby, a condition known as polyhydramnios (see p.166).

Sometimes there is little warning of this complication, but it may be diagnosed when your water breaks or in a vaginal examination, and sometimes when the baby's heart rate slows down, which can indicate he isn't getting enough oxygen. Occasionally it's obvious that something is wrong—you may feel the cord in your vagina, or even see it emerge.

If a prolapse occurs, you'll be admitted to the hospital. The cord needs to be kept warm and moist so that it continues to pulsate and supply oxygen. Usually, the doctor puts her hand in your vagina to hold and support the cord. If the head has moved into the vagina, your doctor may gently insert a hand and lift the head to stop it from squeezing the cord. A catheter may be put in your bladder to fill it with fluid, which helps to move the head away from the cord.

DELIVERING YOUR BABY

Unless the cervix is fully dilated and it's possible to deliver your baby vaginally within minutes, you will be given an emergency caesarean under general anesthesia. The doctor will continue to hold the cord, positioning herself on your gurney as you go into surgery, and only releasing it after the delivery.

There is usually no long-term harm. Very occasionally, babies suffer oxygen deprivation that can cause brain damage or, rarely, death. This is why it's vital to call 911 if you have symptoms.

Shoulder dystocia

This happens when the baby's head has been delivered, but the shoulder becomes wedged behind the pelvic bone so that the rest of the body gets stuck. This is potentially very dangerous because the umbilical cord may be compressed, reducing or preventing the flow of oxygenated blood, and your baby can't start breathing because his chest is compressed in your pelvis.

It occurs in about 1 in 200 births and is impossible to predict, although there are a few risk factors, including large babies (over 10lb/4.5kg); diabetes in pregnancy; previous shoulder dystocia; and induction of labor.

WHAT WILL BE DONE

Urgent action is needed, and your doctor or midwife will call for help, because more than one person is needed to maneuver your baby's shoulders out.

The aim is to rotate your baby's shoulders in the birth canal. You will be asked to stop pushing, and will be repositioned, perhaps on all fours, or lying on your back with your legs up toward your abdomen. Your doctor will then press on your abdomen just above the pelvic bone to try to release the shoulder. It may also be necessary to perform an episiotomy (see p.311) to enlarge the vaginal opening so that your doctor or midwife can put their hands into the birth canal and free the shoulders.

About 10 percent of babies may suffer some nerve damage to the shoulder and arm, but this is usually temporary. In very rare cases, your baby's arm or shoulder may fracture, but it will be treated promptly and heal naturally. If you didn't have an episiotomy, you may have more significant vaginal tearing and may also experience heavy bleeding.

Scar rupture

After a previous caesarean section, most women who have a subsequent pregnancy can have a successful vaginal birth, which is known as vaginal birth after a caesarean (VBAC). However, occasionally the caesarean scar (the site of the original incision in the uterus) ruptures during labor, which is known as "uterine rupture."

This is more likely if you have had more than one previous caesarean; if medication, such as oxytocin, is used to induce labor before the cervix has had a chance to soften and dilate; or if the incision in your uterus is vertical, rather than horizontal, which is usually only undertaken in an emergency situation.

It is a dangerous situation that can lead to severe bleeding and a decrease in oxygen to your baby. The first warning sign of uterine rupture is usually a change in your baby's heart rate, indicating that your baby is distressed.

WHAT WILL BE DONE

If you're having a VBAC, your baby will be monitored for signs of fetal distress. If your uterus ruptures, you will need an emergency caesarean to deliver your baby as quickly as possible and repair the rupture. There is an increased risk of heavy bleeding, so you may need a blood transfusion, and there is also a risk of damage to your bladder.

In the worst-case scenario, if a rupture cannot be repaired, you may need a hysterectomy (which involves removing the uterus). Even if this is avoided, future pregnancies will be discouraged because of an increased risk of cerebral palsy if the baby loses oxygen.

Retained placenta

If all or part of the placenta or membranes remain in the uterus during the third stage of labor, it increases the risk of a postpartum hemorrhage (see opposite).

There are several reasons why this happens. It can occur if your uterus stops contracting or the contractions are not strong or efficient enough to encourage the placenta to separate from the wall of your uterus, known as "uterine atony." Your placenta may also become trapped, usually because your cervix closes before it can be expelled. Sometimes, part of the placenta remains attached to the uterus, known as "placenta accreta." Or the cord may snap while your doctor is encouraging the delivery of your placenta, leaving the placenta trapped inside the uterus.

CAREFUL MONITORING
It can be reassuring to know that you will be watched closely during labor if you are aiming for a vaginal birth after a previous caesarean, so that any problems are quickly spotted.

CHECKING YOUR UTERUS
If there are any concerns that fragments of the placenta remained in the uterus after the delivery, an ultrasound may be carried out to confirm or eliminate this possibility.

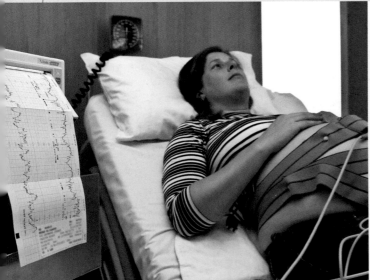

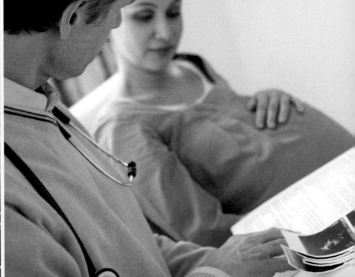

WHAT WILL BE DONE

If the delivery of the placenta takes longer than an hour for a natural delivery, or 30 minutes for a managed one (see p.304), you will be given an injection of oxytocin to encourage stronger, more efficient contractions to expel the placenta and reduce the risk of hemorrhaging.

Once the oxytocin takes effect, your doctor will gently pull on the umbilical cord to draw out the placenta from the uterus. You will also be encouraged to empty your bladder—or you may have a catheter inserted so that this can be done manually—because a full bladder can prevent your placenta from being delivered swiftly.

If these measures don't work, the placenta will be removed surgically to prevent infection and heavy bleeding. You'll be given an anesthetic—usually an epidural or spinal block—and will have a catheter inserted in your bladder. You'll also be offered antibiotics to reduce the chances of infection.

Although your placenta will be examined after the delivery, sometimes it won't be obvious to the doctor or midwife that part of it has been retained. If you have heavy bleeding after the birth (see right), you may be sent for an ultrasound to ensure that there are no fragments of placenta or membranes remaining. In this scenario, surgery will usually be carried out to remove them.

Postpartum hemorrhage

Once the placenta has been delivered, the site where it was attached to the lining of the uterus, known as the "placental bed," has to close off to prevent further blood loss. This usually happens naturally as your uterus contracts and clamps down after the delivery, shutting off the blood vessels. However, if you had a particularly long labor, or you delivered twins or more, this clamping action may not occur quite as efficiently.

If the vessels bleed, you may feel blood trickling or even building up inside your uterus. This is a potentially dangerous condition that can cause a drop in blood pressure, a raised pulse rate, dizziness, and shock. Losing a large amount of blood is known as a postpartum hemorrhage (PPH). Any heavy bleeding that you experience in the 24 hours after the birth is known as a primary postpartum hemorrhage.

WHAT WILL BE DONE

If you have heavy bleeding, your doctor will monitor you frequently, and you may be offered an injection of oxytocin or another drug to encourage the blood vessels to close. If you have lost a significant amount of blood, you will probably need a blood transfusion. In many cases, antibiotics, iron supplements, and intravenous fluid are sufficient follow-up treatment.

If parts of the placenta or membranes are retained in the uterus, you may experience heavy bleeding and/or infection later on. This type of bleeding is known as secondary postpartum hemorrhage. It is unusual, but to be on the safe side, it's important to always report any heavy bleeding after the birth; an operation may be needed to look inside the uterus.

When things go wrong

Try to remember that obstetricians and midwives have regular, ongoing training, to deal with emergencies. All labor and delivery wards are fully equipped with the necessary drugs and equipment. Try to relax and remember that you are in good hands. If things didn't go according to plan, you should be debriefed by the team who delivered your baby, and have all your questions answered. This is extremely important from an emotional point of view, since you may feel very shocked and even guilty that the birth you had anticipated could not take place. Understanding the reasons why things went wrong can help you to accept the situation, and move on. MG

Ask for a full set of medical notes for both you and your baby to be left with you to look at in your own time. Talk through any concerns you have with your doctor or midwife as soon as possible after the birth, when your worries are still fresh in your mind. Reassurance and an explanation of why intervention was necessary can help to put your mind at rest. Above all, try not to feel guilty. NK

During labor, ask your health professional or birth partner to tell you often what is happening, such as the stage you are at and what might come next. Fear grows when information is lacking and is easier to manage if you are updated. If the unexpected happens, try to stick to as much of the rest of your birth plan as you can. This way, you'll feel like you had some influence in your birth experience under difficult circumstances. CH

Few women plan or prepare for emergency situations. All too often, new mothers feel like they've failed because they didn't manage to deliver vaginally or naturally as they had envisioned. Try to bear in mind that your ultimate goal is to deliver a healthy baby; how you get there is simply a means to an end. LJ

After my first baby, I was so absorbed by him that I didn't notice that I was bleeding heavily. The team looking after me was wonderful. After some treatment, including a blood transfusion, I was much better. VB

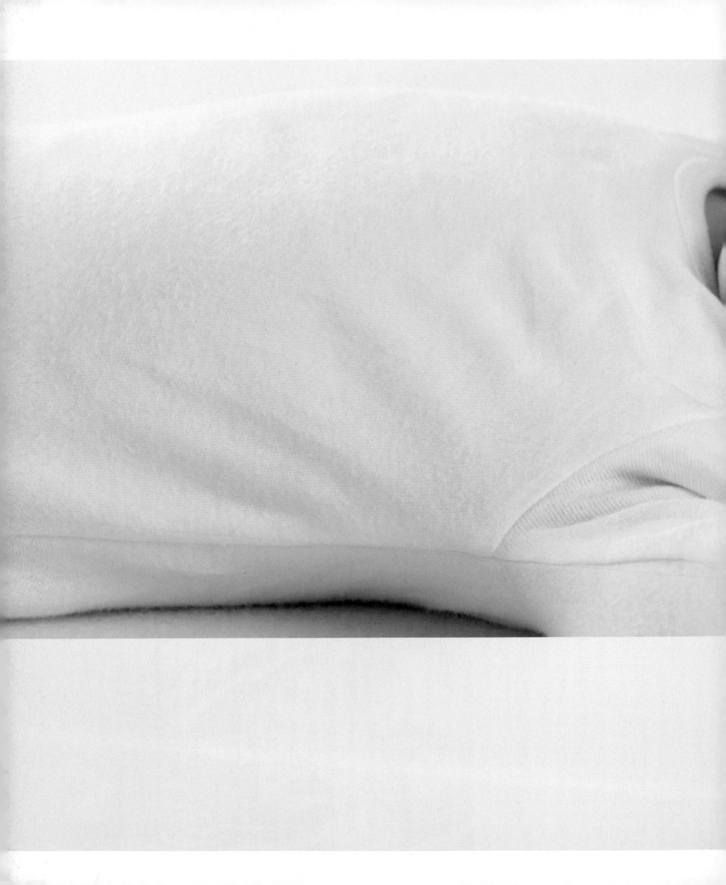

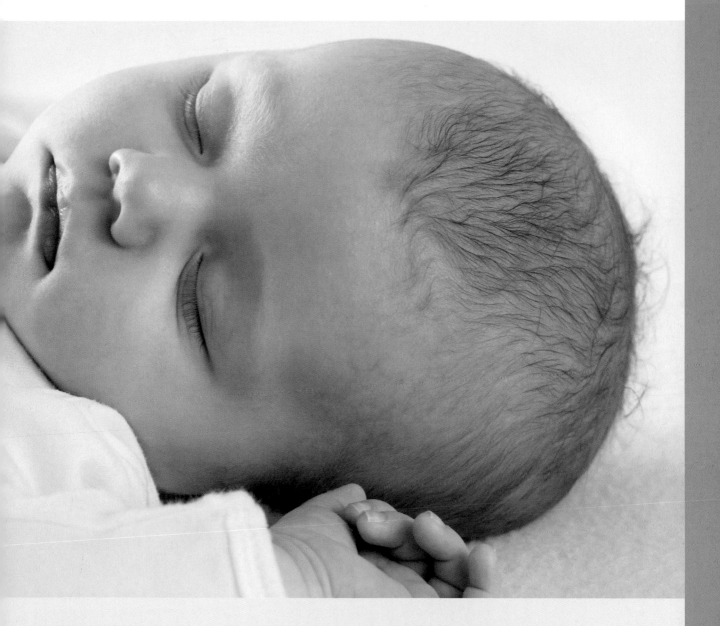

My new baby and me

From the moment your new baby is placed in your arms, your life will change for ever. This is it—she is here, and she is yours.

Meeting my baby

Nothing can quite prepare you for how it will feel to finally set eyes on your baby. This is the moment you've been waiting for—when you can see, touch, and hold her for the very first time, and begin your new life together.

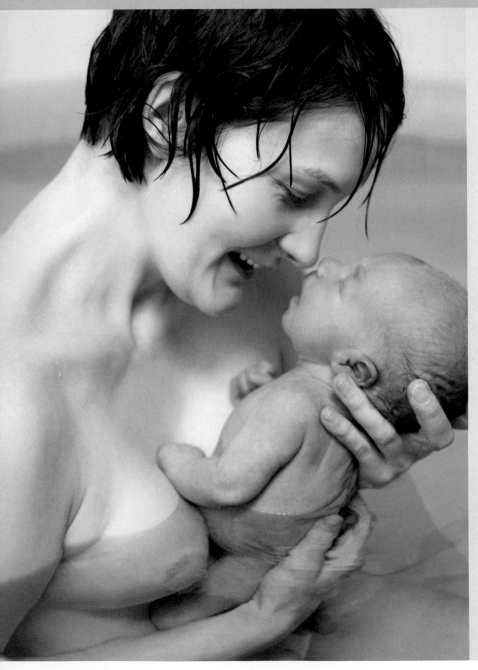

There are no hard-and-fast rules for how you will feel when you meet your new baby. You may feel an overwhelming sense of joy, love, or responsibility, and be re-energized now that she has been safely delivered. It's also very normal to feel so shocked and tired from labor that you can't process the incredible thing that's just happened, and you simply feel desperate for sleep. One thing is for sure—you, your partner, and your beautiful new baby are on the brink of a new life together.

Holding her close

If all is well with you and your baby, as soon as she is born she'll be placed on your chest for your first peek at her. She will recognize your voice from hearing it in the womb and be comforted by your close presence. If you can, hold her skin-to-skin; doing so has many benefits (see p.303), not least that it helps to kick start the bonding process, encourage breastfeeding, and keep your baby warm. Many of these benefits are also evident if your baby has skin-to-skin contact with her dad shortly after birth, so once you've enjoyed a cuddle, you can pass her over to your partner for his first hold

HOLDING YOUR BABY AT LAST
At first you may simply gaze in wonder at the new life you and your partner have created. Over these first few days and weeks, you will find it hard to take your eyes off her!

and a chance to start bonding with his new baby. It's not just your baby who benefits from skin-to-skin contact—it has been shown to have positive effects on your physical and emotional well-being, too.

If you don't manage this contact right away, perhaps because you had a difficult birth or a caesarean, don't fret—there will be plenty of time later to enjoy close cuddles. When you can, hold your baby next to your skin for a snuggle, or take off her onesie and blanket and give her her first breastfeed naked.

How you adapt

After your initial reaction, you are likely to go through a whole gamut of emotions in just a short period following your baby's arrival. You may feel incredibly elated one moment, overcome and tearful the next, and then hugely relieved that labor is over, before finally realizing you're completely exhausted. This is not at all surprising: You've been through a mentally and physically grueling experience and shouldn't underestimate how draining the process of labor can be on both body and mind.

You may feel strangely "empty" after the birth, which is a fairly common reaction. You've had an active little person inside you for the past nine months, so it's no wonder that there's a sense of loss for your bump and possibly even a feeling of anticlimax after such a long period of anticipation. However, you will soon find that spending time with and caring for your baby quickly dispels this sense of loss.

A team effort

In the precious first few hours of your newborn's life, you might feel a little nervous handing her over to anyone else to hold. However, your partner can provide an opportunity for you to have a bath or some much-needed rest, and watching him hold his baby and begin to bond with her can be magical in itself.

You may well find yourselves talking about who she looks like, or what you're going to call her if this is undecided. Or, if you're both too tired for that, you might simply enjoy this time alone to sit quietly together and look at her. Those first special hours, when it's just the three of you, are a wonderful time to start to get to know each other, celebrate your new family, and feel proud of the new life you've created together.

Your baby's Apgar score

About one minute after the birth, and again at five minutes, the doctor or midwife will assess your baby's health with a series of tests known as the Apgar score. This straightforward test simply observes your baby's movement, pulse, breathing, responses, and appearance. For each of these five categories the baby is given a score of 2, 1, or 0, so there's a maximum score of 10. It's common for the score to be below seven at one minute after the birth, as newborns often breathe erratically and have weak muscle tone or bluish hands and feet. By five minutes, about 90 percent of babies score seven or higher and require no medical help. If your baby's score is still low, this may simply mean that she needs a little bit of medical attention, for example some oxygen to assist her breathing at first.

Your doctor or midwife will explain exactly what your baby's score means. If it's lower, they will reassure you and advise you not to be overly anxious at this early stage. The following chart shows the Apgar guidelines used to give your baby her score.

APGAR SIGN	2	1	0
PULSE: your baby's heart rate	Above 100 beats per minute	Below 100 beats per minute	Absent
BREATHING: the rate and strength of your baby's breathing	Regular, a good cry	Slow or irregular breathing, weak cry	Absent
REFLEXES: how your baby responds to stimulation	Pulls away, sneezes, or coughs	Grimaces, making a facial movement only	Absent
ACTIVITY: your baby's muscle tone	Active, spontaneous movement	Arms and legs flexed with little movement	No movement, "floppy" tone
APPEARANCE: your baby's skin color	Normal color all over, including pink hands and feet	Normal color, but bluish hands and feet	Bluish-gray, or pale all over

My baby's appearance

You may have formed an idea of what your baby will look like, but the reality can be very different. She may have a few blemishes and look somewhat squashed after the rigors of labor and birth, but she will no doubt still seem perfect to you.

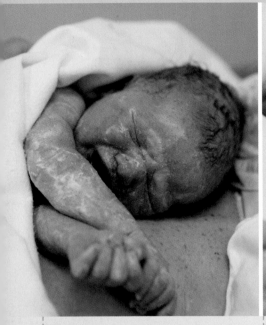

HOW YOUR BABY ARRIVES
Your baby will be lifted out looking a little bloody and may be covered in a waxy substance called vernix that coated her in the womb.

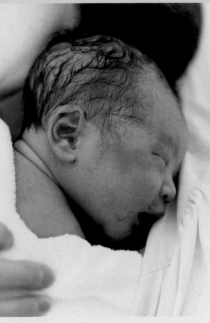

MISSHAPEN HEAD
The heads of newborns often have a pointy shape, because the bones in the skull overlap to fit through the birth canal.

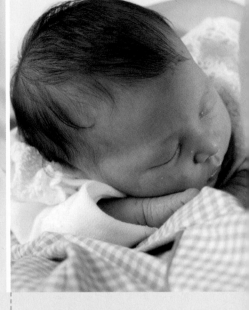

FULL HEAD OF HAIR
Some newborns arrive with an impressive head of hair, while others are bald. Newborn hair is often shed in the first few months.

The first time you lay eyes on your new baby may come as quite a shock. Even if you were expecting her to look a little squashed, you may be surprised at just how strange she looks! Curled up in the uterus for over nine months, floating in amniotic fluid, she is likely to enter the world looking a bit wrinkly. She will probably be covered in a whitish substance known as vernix—a waxy covering that prevented her skin from becoming waterlogged in the uterus—as well as amniotic fluid and some blood from the birth canal. To top it all off, if she passed meconium (her first green–black bowel movement, see p.215) during birth, she may be stained with it. Many babies, particularly premature ones, are covered in a downy hair called lanugo.

Your baby's body

Your newborn's head is disproportionately large at birth, making up a quarter of her body size; her belly is swollen, and her arms and legs are short. If you had a vaginal birth, her head may also seem a little elongated. This is because the plates in her skull don't fuse until after the birth; during delivery, they need to overlap in order to fit through the birth canal, hence the "pointy" head. Her breasts and genitals may be swollen (see p.223), which is perfectly normal and caused by your baby receiving a dose of your hormones before the birth. Any swelling should settle down within 24–48 hours.

YOUR BABY'S FACE
Most moms and dads try to look for family resemblances in their baby.

However, even if you do spot a familiar feature, some of her physical traits are simply a result of her newborn status. For example, babies' noses can be a bit flattened after a vaginal birth, and are often a little upturned to enable them to breathe easily while breastfeeding. Also, her eyes may be swollen from the pressure of squeezing through the birth canal, and their color may be fairly nondescript. Most caucasian babies are born with dark blue eyes, and it's not for at least six months, sometimes up to a year, that their true eye color is revealed. Black and Asian babies are usually born with dark gray or brown eyes that become darker brown or black.

YOUR BABY'S HEAD

On the top and at the back of your baby's head are soft areas called "fontanelles" (see p.223). These are where the bones of the skull haven't yet fused together; you may be surprised to see a pulse on the top fontanelle as you hold your baby. Although you need to be gentle around these areas, a mesh-like covering beneath the skin that protects your baby's brain means it's fine to stroke her head gently or wash her hair.

A LITTLE BRUISING

At birth, your baby's skin is likely to be pale (even in black babies) and delicate, which makes it susceptible to bruising. Since your baby's passage through the birth canal can be a battering experience, don't be too surprised or concerned if she has some bruises around her face or head, especially if you had a forceps or vacuum delivery. Your nurses will keep an eye on any bruises, since the breakdown of blood cells that causes bruising slightly increases your baby's risk of jaundice (see p.334).

SPOTS AND BUMPS

It's common for newborn babies to develop the odd rash or cluster of spots. Many babies develop small yellowish bumps, which can look like fluid-filled blisters or pimples, over their face, chest, and elsewhere on the body. This is called erythema toxicum, and usually appears about a day or two after the birth. It's perfectly harmless and will eventually clear, but in the meantime resist the temptation to pick at the spots; doing so could lead to an infection.

THE UMBILICAL STUMP

After the umbilical cord has been cut, a stump remains, which your doctor will seal with a plastic clip. A few days after your baby is born, the stump will turn black and then, between around seven and twenty-one days later, come away naturally—you'll probably find it in your baby's diaper one day.

Birthmarks on newborns

It's common for newborns to have birthmarks. Most are harmless and fade over time, although some are permanent.

The most common birthmarks are red "vascular" ones, which are caused by an abnormal growth of blood vessels. These include stork bites, port-wine stains, and strawberry hemangiomas.

Stork bites (also known as salmon patches or naevus simplex) are pale, pink-red patches that can appear on the eyelids, nape of the neck, forehead, or the nose and mouth. Caused by dilated blood vessels, they are completely harmless and, except sometimes for those on the back of the neck, usually fade after two years.

Port-wine stains (naevus flammeus) are pale, purplish patches that are present at birth or appear over time. They are permanent and can appear anywhere, but are harmless and usually left untreated.

Strawberry hemangiomas are red, raised patches caused by cells in the blood vessels developing too rapidly. They can be pimple sized or larger and are harmless, unless their position affects something such as your baby's line of sight. These may not appear until weeks after the birth, and usually fade within 10 years. Rarely, a mark may need to be removed if it's causing an obstruction.

Tan or dark-brown birthmarks are pigmented, resulting from pigment cells clustering. A "café-au-lait" mark is a harmless coffee-colored skin patch. Babies can have more than one patch, each often no more than about an inch across.

Dark-brown patches of skin, such as large moles, are known as congenital melanocytic naevi (CMNs). Small CMNs are usually harmless and often lighten, although they may become slightly hairy. If a CMN is large there is a slightly increased risk of skin cancer later in life, so it's important to consult your doctor about what changes you should look for.

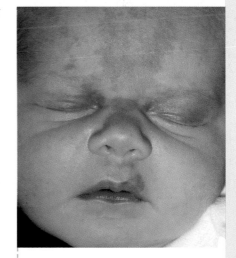

STORK MARK
These are the most common type of birthmark, appearing typically on the face and the back of the neck. Most fade over time, although some persist into adulthood.

Our first 12 hours

Your first day as a new family can be magical, but also unnerving—there's so much to take in, from the first feed to medical checks on both you and your baby. Knowing what to expect can make the whole experience less daunting.

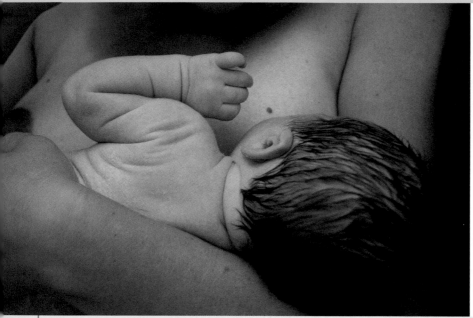

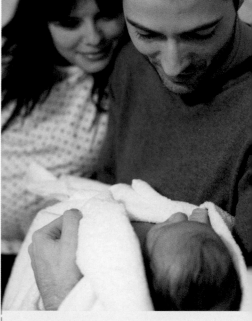

GETTING STARTED
Try to make your first feed skin-to-skin. Your baby isn't born knowing how to breastfeed, but she does have a "rooting" reflex that encourages her to search for your nipple when she feels skin against her cheek.

TIME FOR DAD
It's important that dad has time for a cuddle, too. Your baby will quickly learn to recognize the smells of the people closest to her.

Labor is over, and finally you're holding your baby, enjoying your very first cuddle. Once you've had a chance to say hello, your baby will be checked quickly and given an Apgar score (see p.325) and your doctor will stitch you if you had a tear (see opposite). You may be able to have a much-needed snack now, and then you and your partner can enjoy some quiet time getting to know your new arrival. If you had a caesarean, you will be moved to a recovery room and left alone for a while. In an hour or so, you and your baby will probably be moved to the maternity ward, where you can have a shower or freshen up. During your stay in the hospital, you will both have various checkups, and you will be given help with the practical care of your baby.

Your baby's first breastfeed

Shortly after the birth, as you hold your baby skin-to-skin, her rooting reflex (see p.344) will kick in and she will start nuzzling around, searching for your nipple. Your baby's first feed can help to shape your attitude to breastfeeding in the long term, so take your time and try to relax. Your nurse may help your baby to latch on this first time, and then you can simply concentrate on tuning in to your baby and allow her to follow her instincts. The first time your baby nurses, she may fall asleep at your breast or give up within minutes—or she may stay attached for up to an hour. At this stage, there are no rules to nursing—simply do whatever feels right for you both.

GO EASY ON YOURSELF

Breastfeeding may be among the most natural activities in the world, but it isn't always easy, and getting it right often takes practice. Don't hesitate to ask for help getting started—many birthing units have special lactation consultants to offer guidance. Take pressure off yourself by thinking of this first feed as bonding time, rather than essential nutrition for your newborn. Surprisingly, this first feed isn't likely to provide any more than half a teaspoon of food for your baby, which is fine because she is still well-nourished from her time in the uterus.

WHAT'S IN THE FIRST FEED?

Your first feed isn't fully fledged breastmilk—it's made up of a yellow, sticky substance called colostrum, which is rich in antibodies that help boost your baby's undeveloped immunity. It also helps your baby's waste systems start working, clearing out the fluids, mucus, and meconium that are inside her body.

or massage, your abdomen to encourage the uterus to contract and shrink back to its pre-pregnancy size.

Many women don't realize that after childbirth it takes a while for the uterus to settle down; while this is happening you may experience cramping, known as afterpains, which is likely to continue for several days (particularly as you breastfeed), and longer for subsequent babies, as your uterus shrinks back. You can take painkillers to ease the pains; the hospital will provide options that are safe if you're breastfeeding. Your doctor will palpate your abdomen again several times before you leave the hospital to make sure your uterus has contracted. By your six-week checkup, your uterus should be back to its usual size.

SLOWLY HEALING

If you had a tear or an episiotomy (see p.311) during the delivery, as soon as your baby has been handed to you, your doctor will begin the process of stitching

you up, using a local anesthetic to numb the area if necessary. You may feel some discomfort once the anesthetic has worn off, and find that it stings when you pass urine. Pouring lukewarm water over your vaginal area when you urinate can help to ease the stinging; you should find that it gets better within a few days.

You'll receive regular checkups over the next few days to ensure that the torn tissue is healing well. It's important to keep the area as clean as possible to reduce the risk of an infection; wash your hands with soap before and after using the bathroom. Pour warm water over your genitals a few times a day and, when you're ready, take a warm bath.

OTHER CHECKS FOR YOU

As soon as you've given birth, your doctor or nurse will check your pulse, blood pressure, and temperature to ensure they're returning to normal. If you were anemic during pregnancy, you may be asked to give a blood sample to

What's happening to your body?

You've been through hours of labor and possibly a major operation, so the nurses and doctors will need to keep an eye on you for the next few hours, making sure that your body is recovering and that you're in good shape following the birth. You will also be encouraged to start moving around to help your circulation and to get your bladder and bowels working again after the labor. If you had a caesarean, you will be encouraged to move your ankles and to get out of bed the following day.

CHECKING YOUR UTERUS

Once your placenta has been delivered (see pp.304–305), your doctor will palpate,

After giving birth

I had all three of my children naturally; afterward I didn't feel groggy, but as though I was on a "runner's high"—exhausted, but energized by pure adrenaline. Each time I felt relieved, proud, and in awe. Then, once the adrenaline rush was over, several hours in, I was pooped! I felt completely drained and knew it was time to get as much rest as the baby would allow. LJ

My first baby was born by caesarean and was covered in waxy vernix. My instinct was to rub it off, but my midwife told me to leave it to absorb naturally—apparently it's great for a baby's skin. The caesarean left me feeling shaky, and I was frustrated that I couldn't hold my baby properly for the first day. I was shocked by how ragged I felt in the following days, but then I started to recover, and after about five days felt as

though I was getting my strength back. One thing I hadn't expected was how I'd feel a sense of separation anxiety—this tiny baby who'd been part of me for nine months was now a living, breathing entity in her own right. I felt complete and unconditional love, and wanted to protect her in every way possible. TL

I can still remember with total clarity the first eye contact I had with my baby. All the tiredness and pain seemed to disappear and I had complete tunnel vision, locked onto looking at him and holding him against me. CH

Both my babies were delivered onto my chest before the cords were cut, even though I had caesareans. This made me feel more involved with the delivery. I was elated and recovered quickly with minimal pain relief. VB

check your iron levels. In some hospitals, you'll be asked to collect a urine sample the first time you go to the bathroom so that your doctor can check that your kidneys are functioning properly and you don't have an infection. Before you leave the hospital, you may also be asked if you've had a bowel movement.

BLEEDING

After the birth, you will have vaginal bleeding known as "lochia," which is a discharge containing tissue from the lining of the uterus. At the outset, this may be fairly heavy and bright red, but over the following 10 days or so (and in some cases up to four weeks), it should become lighter, both in quantity and color, until you're discharging only a yellowish mucus. If at any time you expel something more substantial, such as a lump of bloody tissue larger than a quarter, alert your doctor and, ideally, keep the tissue to show her. She will need to make sure there are no traces of placenta left in your uterus that need to be removed (see p.320).

My baby's first checkups

As well as the initial Apgar score, within the first 24 hours your baby's temperature may be checked and she will have a head-to-toe assessment to ensure that everything is in working order. These are routine checks, done to ensure that your baby doesn't need special care. You may also be asked how well your baby is nursing and whether she is urinating and passing meconium, her first green–black bowel movements (see p.350).

IN THE DELIVERY ROOM

Before you leave the delivery room, the nurse or doctor will weigh your baby and measure the circumference of her head and her length. She'll record these measurements and have the information sent along to your pediatrician's office, where it will become a part of her permanent medical records. When you show up at the pediatrician's office a few days later for your baby's first in-office

appointment, her medical records will already be there. If your baby weighs less than 5lb 8oz (2.5kg), she will be considered a "low birth weight," and your pediatric team will monitor her carefully once you're back at home to ensure that she gains weight and is developing properly.

THE FULL NEWBORN EXAMINATION

During the time that your baby is in the hospital with you, a hospital pediatrician will do a series of checks on your baby. As well as all the checks shown in the photographs below, the following will also be looked at:
- Your baby's skin will be examined and any birthmarks noted (see p.327).
- Her eyes will be looked at. The doctor will shine a light into your baby's eyes to check for "red eye," and confirm that there is no sign of cataracts.
- Your baby's genitals will be checked. These tend to be swollen at birth as a result of your hormones passing into your baby's system. If you've had a girl,

---

THE HEART AND LUNGS
Your baby's heart and lungs will be listened to with a stethoscope to ensure the heart is beating normally and she is breathing well, indicating that her lungs are healthy.

CHECKING THE HEAD
It's normal for a baby's head to be cone-shaped after birth; your pediatrician will make sure this is correcting itself, and look at the fontanelles, or "soft spots" (see p.327).

LOOKING AT THE FEET AND HANDS
Your baby's feet and ankles will be checked for signs of club foot (see p.388), and the doctor or midwife will look between the toes and fingers for any webbing.

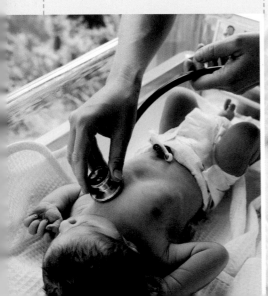

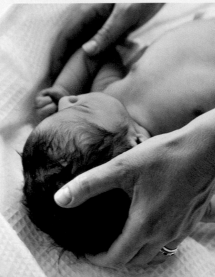

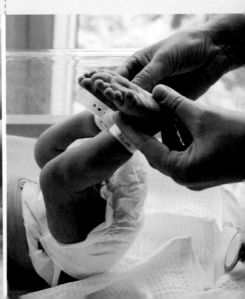

she will be checked for any vaginal discharge (again a result of your hormones); and, if you had a boy, that the hole is in the top of the penis, rather than the side, and that the testicles are fully descended.

• Your baby's reflexes will be tested. Your baby instinctively displays several newborn reflexes, including grasping, rooting, and sucking (see p.333). She will be stimulated to ensure that her reflexes are normal, and the doctor may even startle her gently to check her Moro reflex, which is when she flings out her arms and legs in response to stimuli.

Your baby will also be offered a screening test and a dose of vitamin K before going home (see right).

Newborn screening tests and vitamin K

After 24 hours and within the first two weeks of life, all Canadian babies have a blood test (from a heel prick) that tests for a number of hereditary conditions (see p.341). All of these conditions can be treated if diagnosed early. Which conditions are tested for depends on your province or territory, so check with your doctor or midwife on what is offered in your area. You can opt not to have your baby tested, if you prefer. All newborns are also tested for hearing loss before they go home from the hospital.

Your new baby will be offered a dose of vitamin K, typically by injection and in the first day of life. Vitamin K is essential to help the blood clot. Our bodies manufacture vitamin K in the intestine, and this function is undeveloped in newborns. This means that, very rarely, babies are born with a deficiency of the vitamin and a serious condition called hemorrhagic disease of the newborn (HDNB), also known as vitamin K deficiency bleeding (VKDB), which holds a very slight chance of internal bleeding.

The injection of vitamin K will help reduce the risk of bleeding within the brain after delivery. It's especially necessary for newborns who are being breastfed, because breast milk has barely any vitamin K in it. If you do not wish to have the vitamin K injected, you may have the option of giving your baby an oral dose. Speak to your doctor or midwife if you have any concerns.

Going home

If you had a straightforward delivery, your baby has been given a clean bill of health by the pediatrician, and you have been signed off by the doctor, you should be able to go home within two days if you wish. If you had a caesarean, you will need to stay in the hospital for about four days to start recovering.

If this is your first baby, you might feel uneasy about being left to care for her, but you'll have contact numbers and can call a doctor at any time. You'll also have regularly scheduled appointments at the pediatrician's office, including one on your baby's fourth or fifth day of life, so help and reassurance are not far away. If at any point you have a concern, call your doctor or pediatrician, who will almost always be able to put your mind at ease.

EXAMINING THE MOUTH
The roof of your baby's mouth will be felt to ensure she has a complete palate, and that her tongue moves freely and she isn't "tongue tied."

CHECKING THE HIPS
A doctor will bend and unbend her legs and open them wide to ensure there is no instability or "clicking" in the hips, which may be a sign of hip dysplasia.

LOOKING AT THE SPINE
The doctor will turn your baby over, suspending her over his or her palm, and check that there's no curvature in her spine and there are no abnormalities.

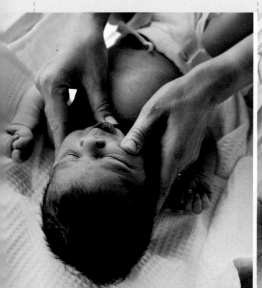

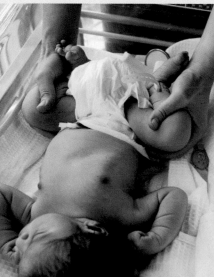

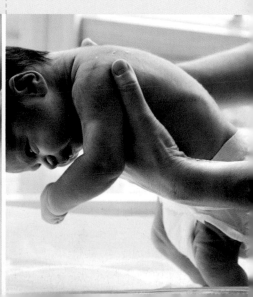

What my baby can do

Your newborn baby is amazing. After about 9 months curled up in your uterus, she has come into the world equipped with all her senses, as well as unique newborn reflexes that are essential for her survival.

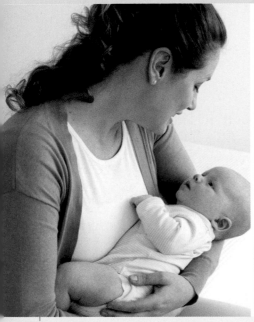

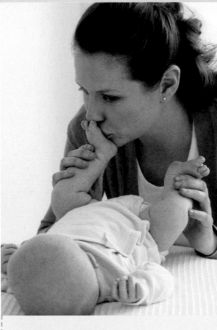

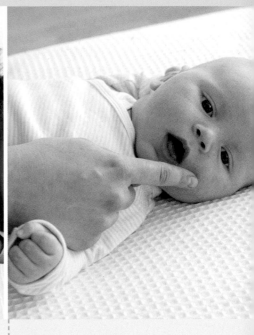

A LOVING GAZE
At birth, your baby focuses on objects about 12in (30cm) away from her face—so when you cradle her in your arms, she can focus on you.

STIMULATING TOUCH
Your baby responds positively to soothing touches, strokes, and kisses. Enjoying physical closeness will help you both connect.

ROOTING FOR FOOD
If you stroke your baby's cheek, she will turn her head in the direction of your touch and open her mouth, rooting for a nipple and food.

Your baby may seem tiny, fragile, and vulnerable at birth, but already she is well equipped to deal with the business of being alive. Not only is she born with the innate ability to search for food, she is also a fast learner and getting stronger and more savvy with every passing day.

Early senses

Your baby is born with a full set of senses, although some are more developed than others. At birth, her vision is a little fuzzy, but she can focus on objects and faces that are close by— about the distance from your breast to your face as you look down at her as she nurses. This means that one of the first things she will focus on is your face.

Her hearing has been well developed since about 28 weeks of pregnancy, and by birth is fully developed. Although she doesn't understand most of what she hears, she already knows the sound of your voice (she's been listening to you talk for weeks), and can respond to and be calmed by it. She also has a good sense of smell at birth: She quickly recognizes your scent and prefers the smell of your breast milk to that of other mothers. Researchers also believe that babies have a well-developed sense of taste even before the birth, and show a preference for sweet over bitter (your milk is slightly sweet) and an aversion to sour flavors.

One of your baby's most important senses is touch, which is well developed at birth. This is one of her main sources of communication, and your instinct will guide you to soothe your baby with gentle stroking and touching.

"Your baby's incredible journey of learning and discovery begins from the moment of birth— and there is already so much she can do"

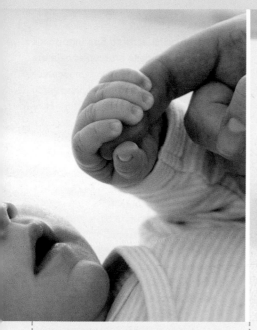

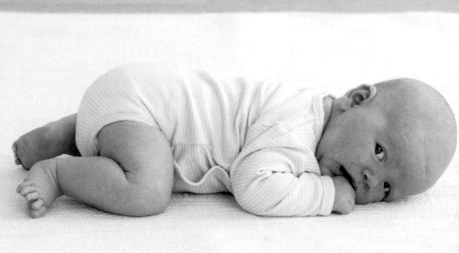

HOLDING ON TIGHT
Your baby's instinct to grasp something in her hand is great for encouraging bonding with siblings as she instantly holds their finger.

LEGS AT THE READY
In the early weeks, your baby has a crawling reflex: when you lay her down on her tummy, she'll automatically draw up her legs as if to crawl. Don't leave her on her tummy if she becomes distressed.

Newborn reflexes

After only an hour in the world, your baby's innate survival reflexes, designed to protect her in her first weeks, begin to show themselves. Testing these out can be a rewarding way to interact with your new baby.

• Research shows that skin-to-skin contact in the hours after birth has a profound effect on your baby's "rooting" reflex: When she feels your skin on hers, she is encouraged to turn her head and open her mouth in search of your nipple.

• One of your baby's most vital reflexes is her sucking one, which leads her to draw on anything put in her mouth (at this stage, a nipple or bottle). She loses this reflex at around two months of age.

• If you place your finger on your baby's palm, she will grasp it tightly, known as the palmar grasp; and if you tickle the sole of her foot, she will spread her toes, known as the plantar reflex. Both these reflexes will have gone by six months.

• If you "stand" her on a flat surface supporting her head, you'll see a stepping reflex, as she lifts one foot after the other in a walking motion—an instinctive response to the feeling of something underfoot, which fades after four months.

• Your baby has a "tonic neck," or fencing, reflex. If you lie her on her back and gently turn her head to one side, she'll automatically extend the leg and arm on that side, bending the opposite arm and leg to assume a "fencing" position.

• If she feels unsupported, or is startled by a loud noise, she'll display the startle, or "Moro," reflex—her arms and legs will splay out quickly and then she'll bring her fists into her chest to protect herself.

Common concerns in newborns

Becoming a new parent can be an anxious time as you take on responsibility for your tiny baby. Being aware of common conditions in newborns and how these are treated will help you feel less daunted if your baby has a problem.

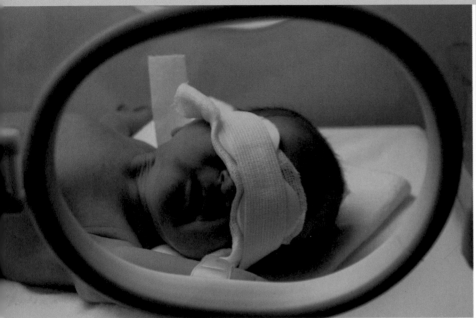

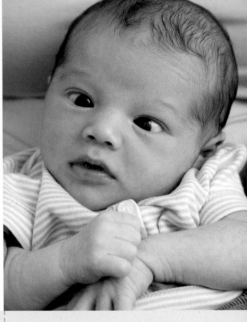

TREATING JAUNDICE:
If your baby's jaundice hasn't cleared after a couple of weeks, she may need phototherapy treatment at the hospital. She will be placed in a special crib where she will be exposed to ultraviolet light. During the treatment, her eyes will be covered to protect her retinas.

CROSSED EYES
A newborn's gaze is often misaligned, with the eyes appearing uncoordinated. This usually resolves itself in a matter of weeks or months as the eye muscles become stronger.

Some problems that occur in newborn babies are so common that hospital staff can seem almost dismissive about them. However, as a new parent, you will no doubt feel unsettled and anxious about any concerns there are with your baby, especially if something requires treatment, or means that you and your baby can't go home as soon as you would like. Take heart, though, that few of these problems have long-term consequences, and most are remedied over time with care and attention.

Jaundice

Between one half and one third of newborns develop neonatal jaundice, caused by an over-accumulation of a substance in the blood called bilirubin. This is produced by the body as it breaks down red blood cells, and is normally processed by the liver and passed to the gut so that it can pass out of the body in the stool. However, your baby's body has proportionately more red blood cells and these have a shorter lifespan; this puts

extra pressure on her immature liver, and she is less able to break down the red blood cells quickly enough. If bilirubin builds up in her blood, its yellow color begins to show through her skin—which is what we see as jaundice.

Jaundice is usually harmless and resolves itself in the first couple of weeks. Occasionally, however, bilirubin levels rise too high and cause a strain on your baby's liver, and she will need treatment. Your pediatrician will monitor your baby and arrange treatment if the jaundice becomes too severe or lasts longer than two weeks, which involves a short stay in the hospital while she receives phototherapy treatment. She will be placed in a special unit under an ultraviolet light to help metabolize bilirubin so that her body can expel it more quickly. She'll usually need to stay in the hospital for a day or so afterward to be sure that the bilirubin levels are under control.

Strabismus

This occurs when an imbalance in the eye muscles causes the eyes to look in different directions. It's common for a newborn's eyes to appear "crossed," turning inward or looking different ways, and if this is the case, you may worry that your baby has strabismus.

However, newborns have tiny folds of skin in the inner corners of the eyes that can make them appear slightly out of sync. Chances are that it's these folds giving the impression that her eyes are crossed. Bear in mind, too, that it takes up to three months for your baby to develop the muscle strength in her eyes to move them in the same direction, to the same degree, at the same time. Talk to your pediatrician to put your mind at rest. If problems persist, however, visit your pediatrician, who may refer your baby to an opthalmologist for assessment and, if necessary, treatment.

Umbilical hernia

Before your baby was born, a hole in the wall of her abdomen allowed blood vessels to run into the umbilical cord to nourish her. This hole usually closes up spontaneously after birth, but sometimes this doesn't happen, and when your baby cries or coughs, a tiny section of intestine is forced out of the hole, making the belly button bulge. This is an umbilical hernia, and although it sounds alarming, in most cases it is completely harmless and resolves itself within a matter of months; or for larger holes by the time your baby has reached the age of two. Tell your pediatrician if the bulge doesn't go away when your baby stops coughing or crying, or if you can't push it back in. They may suggest a simple operation to remedy this.

Heart murmur

After the birth, your baby's heart needs to make some adjustments in the way it works. In the uterus, babies' hearts beat differently, the two sides beating together.

After your baby's first breath, the two sides of her heart start to work separately.

Between four and forty-eight hours after your baby is born, a pediatrician will listen to your baby's heart using a stethoscope (see p.330) to check that the chambers of her heart are working properly, and are now alternately pumping blood in and out. If there's a rush of blood between pumps or an irregular rush during a heart pump, your baby may have a heart murmur.

Although this sounds alarming (it's your baby's heart, after all), heart murmurs occur in around half of all children and most are completely benign and usually sort themselves out without any treatment.

If your baby has been diagnosed with a heart murmur, your pediatrician will check her heart regularly. It's usually possible to tell what the exact problem is merely by the type of sound it creates, or with a simple ultrasound. If there's any other cause for concern, he or she will discuss this, explain what it means for your baby, and give you guidance on the appropriate course of action.

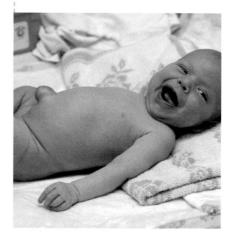

UMBILICAL HERNIA
A swollen belly button results when a small piece of intestine protrudes through the wall of your baby's abdomen, but this usually resolves itself in a matter of months.

Problems that affected our babies

My first baby had swallowed meconium during the birth. Although not inherently a problem, it did mean that he had problems nursing on his first day. In the end, the maternity staff gently suctioned his stomach contents and encouraged me to keep trying to breastfeed until he latched on. CH

My daughter developed mild jaundice shortly after she was born. It was a worrying time, but after about a week of being exposed to lots of natural light, she recovered on her own without any need for intervention. TL

With my second baby I was discharged from the hospital without a problem, but when we saw her doctor a few days later, he was worried about my daughter's excessive jaundice. We had to return to the hospital for her to be monitored. The jaundice resolved itself and all was well. MG

My special-care baby

Seeing your tiny baby in an incubator can be alarming, and you will be concerned about how vulnerable she seems. Rest assured, however, that all the equipment and attention means your baby is receiving the best possible care.

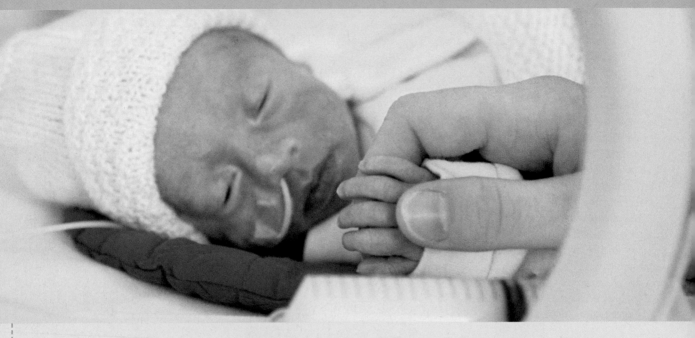

YOUR NOURISHING TOUCH
Even if you can't hold your tiny baby, there are many ways to let her know you're close by and to interact with her. Reaching through the incubator to hold her hand and stroke her helps her enjoy your touch and initiates the bonding process between you.

If your baby is premature—arriving before 37 weeks—or there are concerns about her health at birth, she may need to spend some time in a neonatal intensive care unit (NICU). These units can be intimidating places for parents, filled with incubators and tiny babies, but the expert care they provide is exactly what your baby needs to thrive.

Being told your baby needs special care can be confusing and frightening, so try to find out how the units work at your hospital before the birth. If you've gotten to know the system beforehand, you'll be better able to focus on how to help your baby. Many hospitals will show you the NICU when you take a tour of the labor and delivery wards during pregnancy. Although most moms won't

need to have their babies spend any time in the hospital's NICU, it's certainly reassuring to know that it's there, and to hear a bit about the types of high-tech treatments that babies receive there.

Why babies need special care

Your baby will go to a NICU if:
• She was born earlier than 37 weeks and needs help breathing, feeding, and maintaining her body temperature.
• The delivery was difficult and/or she swallowed meconium.
• She has a low birth weight (under 5lb 8oz/2.5kg).

- She needs observing because you take insulin for diabetes.
- She is very jaundiced (see p.334).
- She has a life-threatening condition, usually affecting her heart or circulation.
- She needs surgery, or has had surgery.

What's the equipment for?

Your baby will probably be in a special crib (or bassinet) called an incubator. This has built-in devices to measure her temperature, oxygen levels, heart rate, lung capacity, and brain activity. It provides oxygen, if necessary, and ensures that she is kept as free as possible from germs. There will also be monitors and cords around her incubator, and, if your baby isn't able to feed from the breast or bottle, she may have a feeding tube put in her mouth that passes into her stomach. If you don't understand why your baby is attached to something, ask a neonatal nurse to explain what it's for and how it's helping her, to reassure you.

How can I help?

You may feel at a loss as to how you can help your baby while she's in the NICU. There are, however, plenty of ways you can help speed up her recovery, and the staff will guide and encourage you. You'll want to spend as much time at the hospital with your little baby as often as your schedule will allow it.

HOLDING AND TOUCHING
The power of touch is well documented and can greatly enhance your baby's recovery. Even if your baby needs to stay in an incubator for a while, you may be able to hold her for brief periods each day. If this is possible, you will be encouraged to tuck her up against you, known as "kangaroo care," so she can feel your warmth, hear your heartbeat, and smell your scent. Babies held like this have been shown to gain weight more quickly. If it isn't possible to pick up your baby, the sides of the incubator have holes, and you'll probably be allowed to put your hands in to stroke her body for a few minutes at a time.

TALKING AND SINGING
Your baby can recognize your voice from before the birth. Talking and gently singing to her is immensely soothing for her. Keep your voice calm, positive, and reassuring. You could even leave a recording of your voice for her to listen to when you're not around.

FEEDING YOUR BABY
Breast milk is the most important source of nutrition for your baby. If she's too small to hold and feed, the hospital staff will encourage you to express your milk to give her through a syringe, tube, bottle, or cup so she gets antibodies to strengthen her immune system. If you're finding it hard to express enough milk, she may be offered breast milk that has been donated to a hospital milk bank. If it's known that you may deliver early, you could hand express (see p.347) colostrum to store in the freezer for your baby.

PRACTICAL CARE
Becoming involved in your baby's everyday care—changing her diaper and keeping her clean—is reassuring for her, and can make the transition to life at home easier. The nurses can advise you on hygiene and how to handle her, making sure you wash your hands frequently and possibly wear a mask.

TAKING CARE OF YOURSELF
Part of helping your baby involves looking after yourself. Eat healthily and rest when you can, so that you have the energy to focus on and care for your baby. Keeping a diary to record what happens each day can help to clear your mind, and provides an outlet to express your thoughts and feelings. Staying informed will also help to ease your mind: Write lists of questions to ask your baby's doctor, and keep notes of what you're told by the hospital staff to refer back to.

Bonding with a baby in the NICU

Spending time with your baby and helping her to grow familiar with your presence will start the bonding process.

- The staff in the unit will be able to tell you how much time you can spend holding or touching your baby. Listen to their advice and always do as much as you can. Your physical presence is immensely empowering for your baby, so even if it's only talking at this stage, you will be helping her.

- Your touch matters, so stroke your baby, or simply lay your hand on her belly or arm, or hold her tiny fingers.

If you're able to get her out of the incubator, hold her against your skin. Get involved in the rhythm of her day, tuning in to her as much as possible.

- Overcome feelings of helplessness by asking the doctors and nurses how you can be involved in your baby's everyday care. Even in an incubator, she will need cleaning and changing, so ask the nurses if you can help with this. Similarly, try to be involved in her feeding times as much as you can. There are plenty of things you can do to bond with your special-care baby.

Getting to know each other

You've just added a whole new person to your family, with her own personality, likes, dislikes, and sense of humor. You are likely to feel a sense of excitement, curiosity, and wonder as you look forward to your new life together.

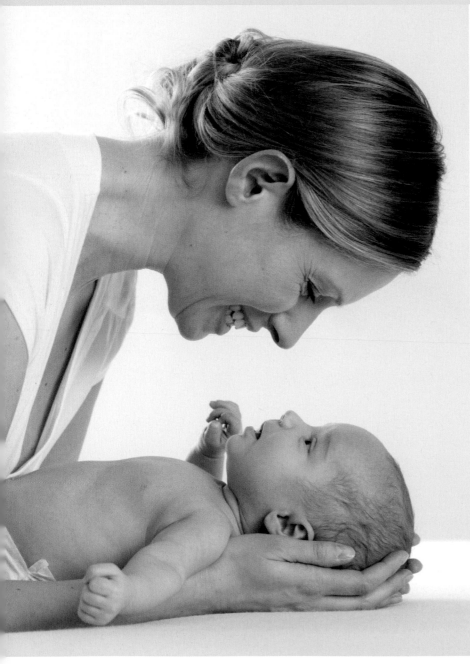

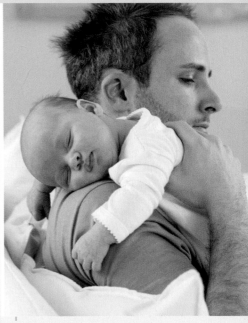

BONDING TIME WITH DAD
The time your partner spends touching, stroking, and kissing your baby will help them to develop their own special bond.

EYE-TO-EYE
One of the best ways to get to know your baby is to spend lots of time making eye contact. Hold her close to your face, chatting and singing to her as you do so. When she makes a sound or facial expression, respond with a noise or a smile. Before long, she will try to copy your movements, poking out her tongue and moving her mouth.

"Within a few weeks—or days—your baby will start to show signs of her budding personality, reminding you of her uniqueness"

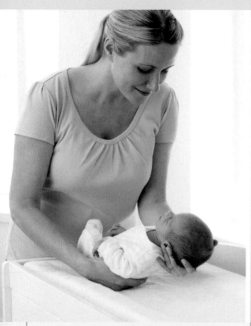

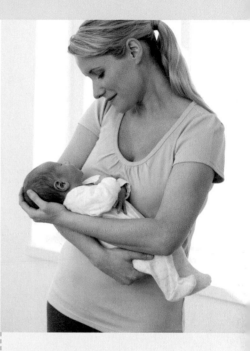

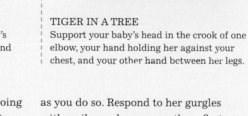

CAREFUL LIFTING
Gently place one hand under your baby's head and neck, then slide your other hand underneath her bottom as you lift her.

TIGER IN A TREE
Support your baby's head in the crook of one elbow, your hand holding her against your chest, and your other hand between her legs.

CRADLING YOUR BABY
Lay your baby across one arm, supporting her bottom with that hand and using the other hand to support her head.

Getting to know your baby is an ongoing process. The time you spend talking to, touching, and holding her increases her trust in you and builds your relationship.

Bonding

Creating strong bonds with your baby in these early weeks helps her to feel secure and gives you confidence in your abilities as a parent. Both you and your partner should chat and sing to your baby as much as possible, making eye contact

as you do so. Respond to her gurgles with smiles and answers—these first "conversations" teach her that when she speaks, someone listens and responds.

Breastfeeding naturally promotes bonding; or if you're expressing or bottle-feeding, dad can get involved, too. Diaper-changing, bathing, and bedtime are all perfect opportunities for you and your partner to interact with your baby.

Try to limit the amount you pass your baby around, so that she gets to know the people closest to her first and becomes secure in your company.

Holding your baby

Babies often have a preference for how they like to be held. Your baby may enjoy being held face down over your arm, or she may find this unsettling and prefer to be cradled so she can see your face. As she grows and gains neck control, she may like to be held over your shoulder so she can see the world go by. Try different holds, always supporting her head, to find positions you both find comfortable.

Our postpartum care

Once you leave the hospital, you're far from alone: Your ob/gyn, your baby's pediatrician, and a lactation consultant, if necessary, will support you during the first few months of life with your new baby.

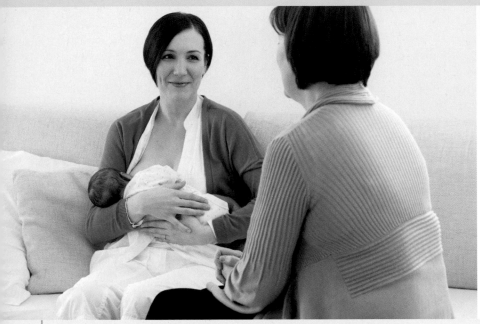

TALKING OPENLY AND HONESTLY
An appointment with the pediatrician is not only an opportunity to check on the health of your baby, but is also a time when you can talk freely about any concerns you may have about your parenting techniques.

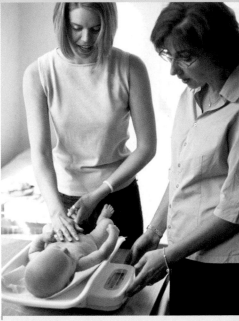

WEIGHING YOUR BABY
Checking that your baby is gaining weight appropriately is an important element of her continued care after the birth.

Taking your baby home can be daunting. It can seem incredible that anyone so unproven in the business of parenting can be set free so soon to care for a precious new life. However, you are more than capable of caring for your baby, and her whole world revolves around you and your partner. In the first days, weeks, and months, you will have a number of routine scheduled appointments with your pediatrician to make sure that everything is as it should be. You will also have a thorough checkup with your ob/gyn six weeks after the birth.

Making sure you're OK

Before you are released from the hospital, your doctor (and nurses) will be sure that you're well on the road to recovery from the birth. If you had a tear or episiotomy (see p.311), or a caesarean, they'll check how you're healing. Your doctor will also feel (palpate) your abdomen to make sure your uterus is shrinking back properly, and she'll check your blood pressure. She'll ask if you're

passing urine and stools normally and whether your bleeding, or lochia (see p.330), is under control.

It's normal to feel emotional and weepy in the week or so after the birth (see p.375), and the pediatrician may check that these feelings aren't cause for concern. She may ask you questions about your emotional welfare, possibly using a questionnaire. If you're finding it hard to cope or feel sad, confiding in your ob/gyn or pediatrician can be very helpful, and they will be able to offer support and practical advice.

Finally, if you're breastfeeding, the pediatrician should ask you if you're happy with how things are going, will give you advice if you need it, and may check your breasts for signs of cracked nipples and mastitis.

YOUR SIX-WEEK CHECKUP

Shortly after the birth, you'll be asked to arrange an appointment at your ob/gyn's office for your six-week postpartum checkup. Your doctor will check your physical health, making sure that any stitches have healed well and your blood pressure is fine; and may also check that your abdominal muscles are returning to normal. You may be asked to provide a urine sample to rule out a urinary tract infection; and she will ask if you've suffered any urinary incontinence. This is common after having a baby, since the pelvic floor muscles are weakened, making it harder to hold on when you need to urinate. If this is a problem, she'll discuss pelvic floor exercises (see p.67) to regain strength in your muscles.

If you are due to have a Pap smear, this will be arranged for three months from now, and you will also be asked about your plans for contraception.

Apart from your physical health, she or he will ask how you're coping and assess your emotional well-being. This is a good moment to discuss any concerns you have about you or your baby.

Making sure your baby is OK

Each time you bring your baby to see her pediatrician, the doctor will weigh your baby and record her weight, length, and head circumference. By plotting these details on the growth chart in her medical records, she can keep an eye on your baby's growth pattern and ensure that she is putting on weight steadily.

If it hasn't already been done at the hospital, your pediatrician will give your baby a blood test, sometimes called a "heel prick test," before she is two weeks old. This involves taking a drop of blood from your baby's heel to test for certain conditions. Although this is thought to give your baby a moment of discomfort, it does help to detect some fairly serious conditions that, if found early on, can often be successfully treated. It tests for the following:
• A deficiency in an enzyme called phenylketonuria (PKU), a rare metabolic condition that can cause mental handicap.
• An underactive thyroid gland (hypothyroidism), which causes your baby to have a slow metabolism, poor growth, and developmental problems.
• Galactosemia, which can cause blindness, developmental delay, and death.

Several provinces test for up to 25 other hereditary conditions, including sickle cell trait, cystic fibrosis, and MCADD. Ask your doctor which tests are done in your area.

YOUR BABY'S FIRST CHECKUP

Your baby will have her first appointment at the pediatrician's office when she is four or five days old. This is an extension of the checks given in the hospital, to confirm that nothing has changed and there is no cause for concern.

Your pediatrician will check her hips, genitals, heart, eyes, spine, and palate. He or she will also check your baby's hearing and movement, and ask about her general behavior, including whether or not she has begun to smile.

REGULAR PEDIATRIC VISITS

You'll be expected to make regular appointments with the pediatrician during your baby's first year to ensure that she's growing properly (and not gaining too much or too little weight). Your baby will also be vaccinated at these checkups. It's important to attend these appointments regularly for your baby's well-being. Some pediatricians have weekend office hours, if it's difficult for you to visit during regular business hours.

You baby's immunization schedule

Your baby's specific immunization schedule will depend on where you live, but here is a typical program:

At 6 to 32 weeks
• Rot, to protect against rotavirus

At 2 months, 4 months, and 6 months
• DtaP-IPV-Hib, to protect against diphtheria, tetanus, pertussis (whooping cough), Haemophilus influenzae, and polio
• Pneu-C-13, to protect against pneumococcal disease

At 6 to 23 months
• Influenza, to protect against the flu

At 12 months
• MMR, to protect against measles, mumps, and rubella

• Men-C, to protect against meningococcal disease

At 15 months
• Varicella, to protect against chicken pox
• Pneu-C-13

At 18 months
• DtaP-IPV-Hib
• MMR

At 4 to 6 years
• DtaP-IPV-Hib

At 12 years
• HB, to protect against hepatitis B (if not given in infancy)

Girls aged 9 to 13 years
• HPV, to protect against human papillomavirus

Breastfeeding my baby

This is not only the most nutritious and rewarding way to feed your baby, but also the simplest and most convenient way. It is recommended that you breastfeed for at least the first six months of your baby's life.

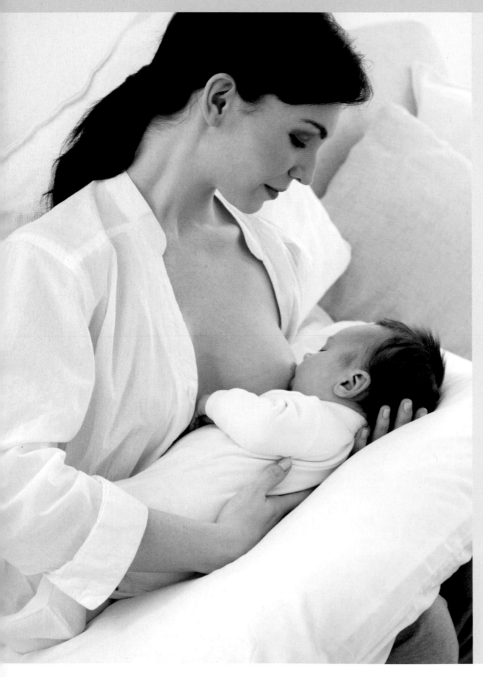

Breastfeeding your baby has scores of benefits for both of you (see p.238–239). The watery pre-milk, colostrum, that your breasts produce in the first few days is the ideal first food for your baby as it is rich in nutrients and antibodies to protect her from infection. Breast milk also has long-term benefits for your baby, reducing her risk of childhood obesity, diabetes, allergic conditions such as eczema, and the risk of heart disease later in life.

There are plenty of bonuses for you, too. Breastfeeding helps you regain your figure more quickly as your body uses more energy to produce milk. It also benefits your health, reducing your risk of developing breast and ovarian cancer.

Your milk supply

Your body produces milk on a supply-and-demand basis. From the moment your baby starts sucking after birth, your body gets the message to start producing milk, and two to five days later your milk "comes in," replacing the colostrum you produced originally. Your breasts will feel heavy and full, so you will need to ensure that your baby empties them at each feed to avoid uncomfortable engorgement. Your milk production continues in this

TUMMY-TO-TUMMY
Your baby needs to face you "tummy-to-tummy" to latch on well and feed properly. Use a pillow to raise her and have supportive cushions for your back and arms to ensure you and your baby are comfortable during feeds.

"As well as providing the best nutrition for your baby, breastfeeding helps you to establish a warm, nurturing relationship"

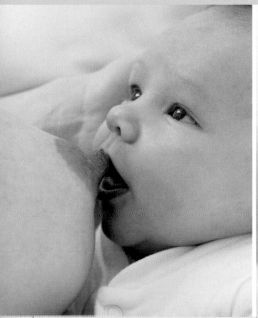 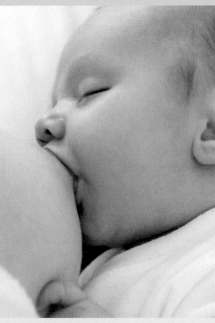 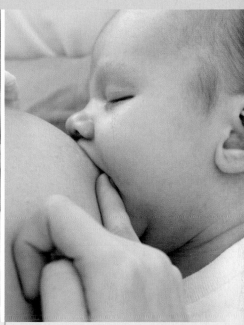

MOUTH OPEN WIDE
Your baby's mouth needs to be gaping for her to latch on well. Once it's open wide, direct your nipple toward the roof of her mouth.

A SUCCESSFUL LATCH
With your areola and nipple in her mouth, your baby's sucking stimulates the milk ducts in the breast tissue to release your milk.

TAKING YOUR BABY OFF THE BREAST
Carefully insert your clean little finger into the corner of your baby's mouth to break her suction before removing her from the breast.

way, with your body producing more or less milk according to your baby's demands. It's also good to know that the composition of breast milk adapts constantly to meet your baby's changing nutritional needs.

It's best to avoid any attempt at a schedule in the first few weeks; instead, feed your baby whenever she is hungry—her tiny stomach can digest only small amounts of milk at a time. There will no doubt be times when she seems dissatisfied after feeds, and you'll worry that you're not producing enough milk. This is common

during growth spurts: Feeding her more will mean your body produces more to catch up with demand, after which the frequency of feeds will settle down.

How to breastfeed

A common misconception is that because breastfeeding is a natural way to feed your baby, it follows that it should be easy, too. While it's definitely true that

some women take to breastfeeding effortlessly, it's more usual for it to take a bit of time and practice to get right. Here are a few pointers.

CHECK YOUR BABY'S POSITION
The first thing to check is that your baby is positioned properly so that she can latch on well. She is correctly positioned if you and she are tummy-to-tummy, her face opposite your breast. You may need to raise her on a pillow; once supported, she'll be able to wrap her lower arm around your side and feed comfortably.

STIMULATE YOUR BABY'S FEEDING REFLEX

Your baby is born with a "rooting" reflex (see p.333), which means that she opens her mouth and turns her head when she feels your skin and senses that food is near. Gently stroking her cheek or corner of her mouth sets off this reflex, and she will open her mouth wide. Once her mouth is as open as it can be, she is ready to latch on to your nipple (see below).

LATCHING ON YOUR BABY

Attaching your baby to your breast correctly, known as latching on, is the key to successful breastfeeding. As your baby opens her mouth wide, her tongue should be down and forward. Aim your nipple toward the roof of her mouth and bring her to your breast, rather than your breast to her. When she is properly latched on, she'll have all of your nipple and some of your areola (the dark area surrounding the nipple) in her mouth. As you watch her nursing, her lower lip should be rolled outward and her chin should rest on your breast. You'll see her lapping at your breast, drawing back

with her jaw—not sucking through her cheeks—and you'll hear only a low-pitched swallowing noise, rather than a smacking sound.

EMPTYING EACH BREAST

Work on the principle that your baby should empty one breast before moving on to the next. This will ensure she gets both the hydrating foremilk (which is thinner and thirst-quenching) and the thicker, nutrient-dense, and sustaining hindmilk. Emptying your breast is important for you, too, because it helps prevent blocked ducts or either breast becoming engorged (see p.346).

TAKING YOUR BABY OFF THE BREAST

Your baby's sucking is immensely strong, so it's very important to unlatch her correctly (even if she's fallen asleep)—otherwise she will pull on your nipple, which is painful and can lead to soreness. Put your clean little finger into the corner of her mouth, and gently "pop" her suction, softly pulling her mouth away from the breast.

Positions for breastfeeding

Whichever position you choose to nurse your baby in, you need to be sure that you will be comfortable for the duration of the feed and will be able to support your baby without straining yourself. Make sure primarily that your back is well supported and that you have arm rests or cushions if you need them.

THE CRADLE HOLD

Many moms find the cradle hold the easiest position for latching on. Your baby's tummy lies across your tummy while you cradle her head in the crook of your arm, and your opposite hand supports her head. A variation is the cross-cradle hold, in which your baby is supported mostly by your opposite hand and arm. A pillow underneath raises her to the right height for your nipple.

THE FOOTBALL HOLD

In this position, your baby's body is tucked under your arm on the side of

CRADLE HOLD
This classic breastfeeding position enables you to support your baby in your arms while you sit in a comfortable upright position.

LYING-DOWN HOLD
If you had a caesarean, you might find lying down for a feed works well, since it avoids putting strain on your abdomen. Prop yourself up on your elbow if it's comfortable to do so.

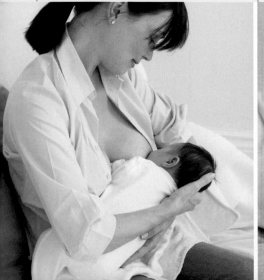

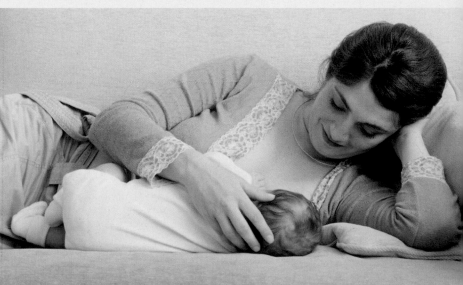

your body that she's feeding on, and her feet point behind you, as if you were holding a football. You can use your hand on the same side to guide and support her head. You may find this position more comfortable after a caesarean, since it takes the pressure off your abdomen.

THE LYING-DOWN HOLD

Mastering the art of breastfeeding lying down is fantastic for feeding at night. Lie your baby alongside you, and use your opposite hand to guide her head, then let the bed do the work of supporting your baby. Take care to make sure that you are "tummy-to-tummy," and that she has latched on properly.

Burping your baby

All babies need to be burped after a feed, and sometimes in the middle of one. Burping stops air from getting trapped in your baby's digestive system, which can make her fussy and uncomfortable.

If you haven't burped your baby and eventually the air bubble does come up, she may bring up some milk, too. (If you're bottle-feeding your baby—see pp.348–349—it's especially important to burp her, as she's more likely to gulp in air as she sucks through the nipple.)

There are several positions for burping your baby. A good position for newborns is to hold her upright with her head supported against your shoulder, then gently rub or pat her back until she burps (sometimes you will be able to feel the air bubble making its way up her body). She is still likely to bring up a little milk as she burps, so it's a good idea to put a burp cloth over your shoulder to protect your clothes.

When her neck muscles are a little stronger, you can try sitting her on your lap, with your forearm supporting her tummy and chest and your hand supporting her chin and head, while you rub her back with your free hand. Or you could try laying her across your legs, facing downward and supporting her in the same way, but keeping her more horizontal.

Safeguarding your milk supply

Just as you did during pregnancy, you should eat healthily while breastfeeding. You need to replenish essential nutrients used in milk production. Be aware that substances in food and drink can pass into breast milk, so you should be sure that whatever you ingest is healthy for your baby, too. Keep caffeine intake low to avoid keeping your baby awake. Also, tiny amounts of alcohol can end up in your milk, so abstain or keep your intake to a minimum—say, no more than one or two drinks, once or twice a week.

Some moms wonder if eating peanuts while breastfeeding will increase the risk of their baby developing a peanut allergy. There is no evidence of this, but talk to your pediatrician if you're worried.

Breastfeeding is dehydrating, so drink plenty of water. Sip a glass of water while you feed your baby so that you can replenish fluids as you go along. Fruit juices and milk are also hydrating, but avoid soda, tea, and coffee.

FEEDING TWINS
Mothers of twins often find the football hold enables them to feed both babies at the same time and keep an eye on what they're doing!

BURPING
Helping your baby to burp during or after a feed will help her to settle more easily. Support her well as you gently rub her back.

DRINK, DRINK, DRINK
Get into the habit of having a glass of water with you as you breastfeed to help prevent you from becoming dehydrated.

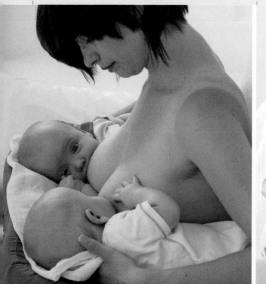

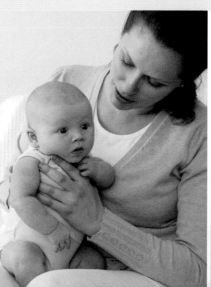

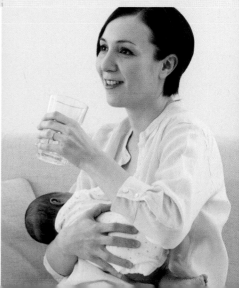

Troubleshooting

Chances are you've never had a hungry little mouth attached to you before, or it's been a few years since you last breastfed, and you will find that it takes a few days for your nipples to get used to this new role. As a result, it's normal for your nipples to feel tender and sore until they grow accustomed to having your baby suck on them for several hours a day. This can make breastfeeding a very stressful experience in the early weeks, and this is the point at which many women give up. However, if you make sure that your baby latches on well, you will soon find your nipples are less sore and that feeding becomes easier. If problems do arise, there are tried and true ways to help ease discomfort and get breastfeeding back on track.

SORE AND CRACKED NIPPLES

While a little bit of discomfort is perfectly normal when you start to breastfeed, sore and cracked nipples are more serious—and painful.

The most likely reason for sore, blistered nipples is that your baby isn't latching on properly. Check your technique and try different positions until you find which works best. Ask your pediatrician, your midwife, or a lactation consultant to watch you latch on your baby so she can offer advice. Remember, too, to break your baby's suction safely (see p.344), without pulling her away from your breast.

To make feeding easier, start your baby on the side that is least sore, saving the sore nipple from her most vigorous sucking. You can apply a purified lanolin ointment to your nipples to encourage healing and provide protection—the ointment doesn't need to be washed off before nursing. If you want to avoid creams, rub a little breastmilk at the end of a feed over your nipple to speed up healing. It's helpful to expose your breasts to the air for brief periods between feeds.

If your nipples continue to be sore and cracked and you're really struggling, talk to your pediatrician, your midwife, or a lactation consultant. She may suggest that you express milk for a while so your

nipples have a chance to heal. Bear in mind, however, that switching to a bottle can put your baby off the breast (although some switch happily between the two), and you'll still need to get your baby to latch on well to prevent soreness when you start breastfeeding again.

Finally, if you use breast pads, change them regularly—damp pads can cause or exacerbate sore nipples—and avoid using plastic-backed pads, which prevent air from getting through.

ENGORGED BREASTS

It can take a while for your body to adjust to the rhythm of feeding, and breasts can become hard, swollen, and lumpy in the first couple of weeks as the milk ducts become clogged. If milk isn't cleared during feeds, your breast can become engorged, which can be very uncomfortable and even raise your temperature. Nursing on demand and letting your baby empty a breast before moving on to the next one will help.

Expressing excess milk (see opposite) can relieve the pressure. This can be

---

REMOVING YOUR BABY WITH CARE
To help prevent sore or cracked nipples, take care when you remove your baby from the breast. Break the suction by using your little finger to gently push her mouth away from your breast.

INSTANT RELIEF
Far from being an old wives' tale, placing cold, bruised cabbage leaves in your bra can help relieve the discomfort of engorgement; the enzymes in the leaves reduce swelling and inflammation.

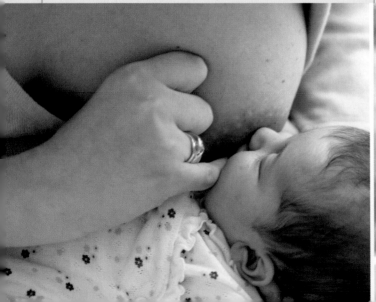

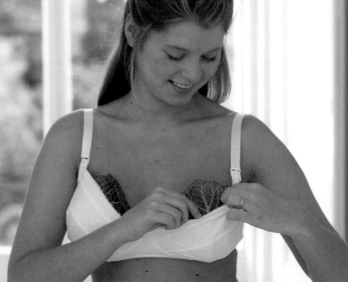

especially helpful when your milk comes in and your breasts feel very full. Express just enough to relieve the pressure, but not so much that your body thinks it has to make yet more milk to replenish the supply.

If your breasts are engorged for longer than a few days, your baby may not be drinking all the milk you're producing, possibly because she isn't latching on well. Check your baby's latch and give her time to take a full feed, making sure a breast feels empty before moving her to the other side. If the problem persists, talk to your pediatrician or consider hiring a lactation consultant for a home visit.

DEALING WITH MASTITIS

If engorgement persists and the milk ducts fail to clear, you can develop a painful infection of the breast tissue called mastitis. The tissue around your duct may have become swollen, causing the duct to close and forcing milk into the breast tissue, which results in a red, sore, lumpy patch on your breast that

feels hot and stings. The breast tissue around the closed duct can become infected, triggering flu-like symptoms.

Let your doctor know if you feel feverish so that any infection can be treated swiftly with antibiotics. The temptation is to stop breastfeeding if it becomes painful. However, it's important to continue feeding through an infection and express excess milk; you need to relieve the engorgement to help clear the milk ducts. Placing warm washcloths or a cold compress over your breast while you're not nursing can relieve the sore, hot feeling, and you should try to get plenty of rest. Also make sure you have a supportive, well-fitting nursing bra; a poorly fitting, tight bra can increase the pressure on your milk ducts, making the symptoms of mastitis worse.

Expressing milk

When breastfeeding is established, you can start to express your milk if you wish. You can freeze your milk so that

your baby has a supply if you're away from her, and your partner can get involved with feeding. It also provides instant relief from engorgement.

You can express milk by hand or with an electric or manual pump. Manual expressing can be efficient, but takes a bit of practice at first, and many women find breast pumps easier. Breast pumps have a suction cup attached to the pump, which extracts your milk and collects it in a bottle.

To express manually, put your fingers underneath your breast and rest your thumbs on top. Lean over a clean bowl and gently squeeze your thumb and forefinger together, without sliding them over your skin, so that you squeeze the tissue behind your nipple. Hold for a few seconds, then release, and repeat this until your milk comes out.

Store your milk in a sterilized container. You can keep it in the fridge (below 39°F/4°C) for up to five days; in the fridge's freezer compartment for up to two weeks; or in a dedicated freezer (below -0.4°F/-18°C) for six months.

EXPRESSING BY HAND
There's an art to expressing manually, but once you perfect your technique, you may find this an efficient way to express milk.

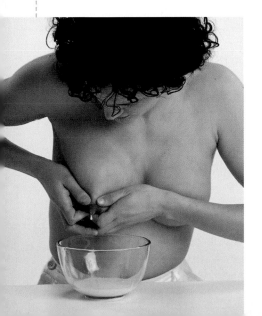

Our breastfeeding experiences

I was determined to breastfeed all three of my babies. The first week or so each time was really painful, but my doctor gave me lots of practical tips for getting through the discomfort, and in the end, for me, each time it became one of the most rewarding experiences of motherhood. CH

Once I got the hang of breastfeeding, I really enjoyed it. I breastfed all three of my babies, and being aware of the pitfalls before encountering them really helped me feel more confident. However, that's not to say that it wasn't challenging when my first baby turned out to be a very slow eater with a weak suck! She fed every one to two hours for weeks and would always fall asleep while eating. My milk

took over five days to come in, and when it did, my body had had so many mixed messages that I leaked badly. It wasn't until my second was born I realized how weak the first's suck had been—number two was the opposite! Now I'm really glad to be able to help other mothers, because if I learned anything, it was that sometimes when you think breastfeeding is going wrong, it's really going just as planned! LJ

Unlike many first-time mothers, I found latching on my babies fairly easy—I was really lucky. However, I did find that I wasn't producing enough milk to satisfy them, so after a few weeks supplemented their daily feeds with formula. TL

Bottle-feeding my baby

If you're not comfortable with breastfeeding or not able to breastfeed, you can still give your baby a good start with formula. In the beginning, your baby will need to feed little and often.

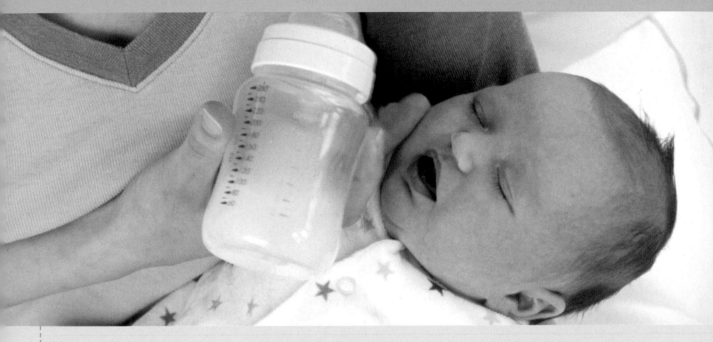

CRADLE YOUR BABY
Hold your baby in a slightly upright position and gently rub her cheek to stimulate her rooting reflex and get her ready for a feed.

Preparing bottles can seem time-consuming at first, but it's easy once you get into a routine. It's important to keep all your feeding equipment scrupulously clean, because formula is a breeding ground for bacteria, which can make your baby very sick. Clean all nipples and bottles carefully in hot, soapy water with a bottle brush.

Making up bottles

Read the manufacturer's instructions carefully before you begin, and mix the formula exactly as they describe, using the scoop supplied to measure the powder. Don't dilute or strengthen the mixture, as either can upset your baby's digestive system.

Use cooled, once-boiled water to make up your baby's feeds. Ideally, the water should still be fairly hot when you add the formula, then left to cool for a while. Avoid bottled water, which has a high concentration of minerals.

Place the bottle on a level surface and crouch down to make sure you've added the right measurement of water before you add the scoops of powder. Fill the scoop and level it with a knife, without patting it down, then tip it into the water. Once you've added the required number of scoops, replace the cap and shake the bottle vigorously until the powder is dissolved.

"If breastfeeding isn't possible for you, it's reassuring to know that you can raise a healthy, happy baby on formula instead"

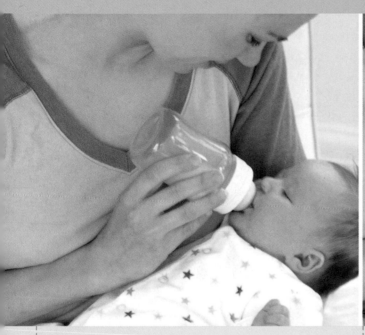

GIVING A BOTTLE
Gently insert the nipple into your baby's mouth. Hold the bottle upright so the milk covers the nipple and your baby isn't swallowing any air.

FINISHING A FEED
As with breastfeeding, gently put your clean little finger into the corner of your baby's mouth to break her suction and remove the bottle.

CAN I STORE BOTTLES?

Unless you need to leave a bottle for someone else to feed to your baby, for example daycare staff or a nanny, it's best to make up bottles as you go to reduce the risk of bacteria breeding. If you do need to make bottles in advance, store them at the back of the fridge below 39°F (4°C) for up to 24 hours.

If you're going out, it's safer to fill bottles with hot water to the right levels and take appropriate quantities of powdered formula in a clean, sealed container to add to the water when you need to feed your baby. Containers are available that are specifically intended for transporting powdered formula in measured batches.

Giving a bottle

First, test the temperature of the milk by pouring a drop onto your wrist: It should be warm, not hot. Hold your baby semi-upright to give her the bottle. As with breastfeeding, make plenty of eye contact. It can help to raise your baby on a pillow, and make sure you're well supported, too. Insert the nipple gently into her mouth and tip the bottle up so the milk covers the nipple and the baby doesn't take in air while feeding. When your baby is finished, remove the bottle carefully and gently burp her (see p.345). If she starts to fuss during a feed, she may need burping before you continue, or she may simply have had enough. Don't encourage your baby to finish the bottle if she seems to have lost interest. Discard any milk that is left over in the bottle and make up a fresh bottle for her next feed.

My baby's diapers

Your baby is going to wear diapers every day for more or less the next two to three years—and probably for even longer at night. You'll soon discover that keeping her bottom dry and clean will help to keep her happy and content.

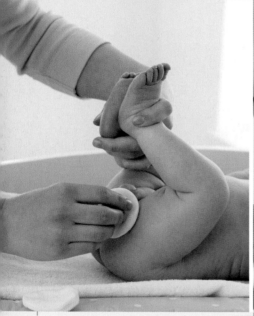

A THOROUGH CLEAN
Use damp cotton pads or a washcloth to clean your baby's bottom. Wipe in his creases to make sure you've cleaned everything.

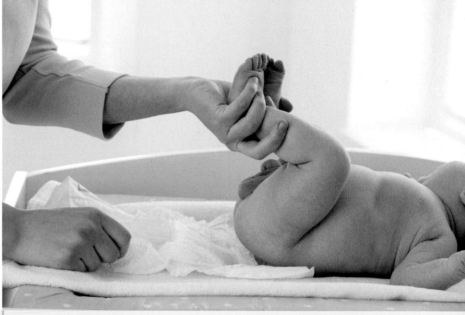

POSITIONING THE DIAPER
With your diaper at the ready, hold your baby's feet in one hand, then gently lift his bottom and slide the clean diaper underneath him, so the tabs are at his waistline.

The first time you change your baby's diaper, you may find yourself unsure of how to handle her, clean her, and get rid of the contents of the old diaper all at the same time. However, with at least six to eight diaper changes a day at first, you will soon have diaper changing down to a fine art! You will also become quickly attuned to when your baby needs a diaper change, which will usually be after a feed, and each time your baby soils her diaper. Making sure she doesn't spend too long with a wet diaper on will help protect her skin from soreness.

Your baby's stools

Initially, you may find the contents of your baby's diapers somewhat alarming. There's a lot of variation in babies' stools, but rest assured that there's usually nothing to worry about.

Your baby's first stools will be dark green and tarry as she passes the meconium that was in her intestines before birth (see p.215). Once breast-feeding is established, her stools will become yellow or yellowy-green and runny, sometimes with curdles of milk.

She doesn't have diarrhea—this is exactly what newborn stools should be like. The stools of formula-fed babies are slightly darker and thicker.

Newborn stools can vary in frequency, too, from after each feed to once every couple of days. Breastfed babies tend to have more frequent stools.

If your newborn's stool is dry, she might be dehydrated, so mention this to your pediatrician, and offer her extra feeds to make sure she is getting enough fluids. Also tell her doctor if you find any blood or mucus in her diaper.

"Make diaper-changing time a sociable one: Smile at your baby and sing and talk as you change her to make the process feel like fun"

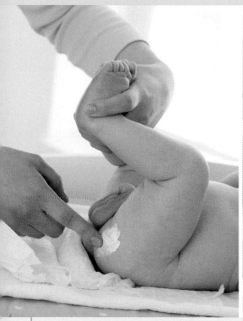

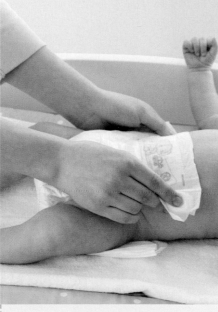

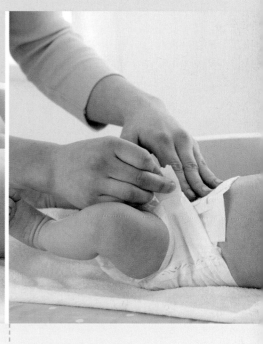

PROTECTING YOUR BABY'S BOTTOM
Continuing to hold your baby's legs, apply a thin coating of barrier cream over his bottom and in his creases.

PULL UP THE DIAPER
Gently bring the diaper up between your baby's legs. If you have a baby boy, make sure his penis is facing downward.

SECURE THE DIAPER
Secure the diaper at the front, making sure that you can put your thumb between it and your baby's tummy.

Changing a disposable diaper

Diaper changing isn't every baby's favorite activity, so being organized so that you can change her speedily and with the minimum of fuss will make this far less stressful. Gather everything you need before you start, or better still, have a designated diaper-changing area where you keep diapers, washcloths and/or cotton pads, a changing mat, barrier cream, and a diaper pail or bags.

Wash your hands, then lie your baby down on her changing mat—you can put a towel on top of the mat for comfort and warmth if you wish. If she has had a bowel movement, use the old diaper to wipe away the poop, then fold the diaper up and dispose of it. If you have a boy, when you undo the old diaper, hold it over his penis for a moment before removing it in case he chooses this moment to urinate.

Clean your baby's bottom with a damp washcloth or damp cotton pads. Her skin is sensitive, so avoid using soap or detergents, which can also wash away the natural oils and make her more prone to diaper rash (see p.353). Wipes are convenient, but many contain chemicals that can be harsh on your baby's skin, so use these sparingly (maybe when you're away from home) and opt for chemical- and fragrance-free ones.

If you have a girl, always wipe from front to back to prevent bacteria from getting into the vagina or bladder and causing an infection. Apply barrier cream if you wish, then put the clean diaper on (see above).

Changing a cloth diaper

There are a number of different types of reusable diapers, but the easiest to manage are those that are self-fastening. You'll need plastic outerpants or wraps (unless your diaper has a built-in waterproof outer layer), a clean, dry diaper, a liner, and, if required, a pad for extra absorbency. Thicker disposable or reusable pads are useful for nighttime to keep your baby drier.

As with disposable diapers, have everything you need to clean and change your baby ready at the start. Lie her on her changing mat. If she has had a bowel movement, you can lift out the diaper liner; most liners are biodegradeable and can be flushed down the toilet with any bowel movements. Remove the soiled and/or wet diaper if necessary and place it in a bucket with a tight-fitting lid for laundering. You can keep a very mild bleach and water solution in the bucket to work on stains and prevent odors.

Prepare your new diaper by laying a clean diaper on a wrap, with a diaper liner on top.

Clean your baby's bottom as usual (see p.351). Slide the new diaper under her bottom, then fasten the diaper (see below). Secure the plastic wrap over the diaper, ensuring that it is firmly fastened. When you've finished, run your fingers around the leg openings to make sure that the outer wrap completely covers the diaper to avoid leaking.

Diapers and skincare

Keeping your baby's bottom clean and rash-free is an essential part of her care. Find a diaper that suits your baby's needs and your lifestyle.

- Until your baby is about four months old, you can expect to go through up to eight disposable diapers each day. Save money by stocking up on additional diapers when they are on sale or buying in bulk.

- If you want to use cloth diapers, experiment until you find a brand you like. Find out about diaper services available locally, and ask for a trial pack to be sure you're happy with a system before investing in it.

- Look into diaper services that launder reusables for you.

- Try doubling up cloth diapers at night or when you go out.

- If you buy diapers in bulk, take care that you don't buy too many in a size that your baby is likely to grow out of soon.

- Massaging your baby with oil every day will help to keep her skin supple. It also adds a protective barrier to prevent it from drying out, which minimizes the risk of diaper rash.

- At first, avoid wipes and diaper creams that may contain harsh chemicals.

ARRANGE YOUR BABY'S DIAPER
Place a clean diaper liner inside the new clean diaper, putting it into position so it is ready to put on your baby.

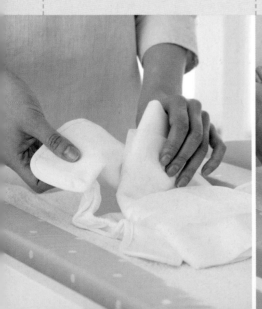

CLEAN YOUR BABY
Use a clean washcloth or a damp cotton pad to clean your baby's bottom, wiping from front to back with a girl.

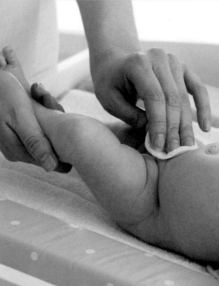

PUTTING ON THE DIAPER
Place the diaper under your baby, then bring the front up between her legs and secure the diaper. Add a waterproof wrap if you wish.

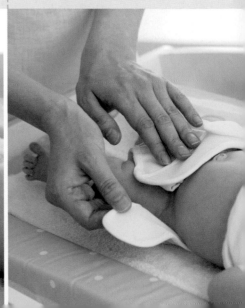

Dealing with diaper rash

At some point, most babies get diaper rash, which is caused by the skin becoming wet. Diaper rash looks red and sore, and may be pimply, sometimes spreading over your baby's buttocks.

The best way to avoid a rash is to give your baby some diaper-free time each day, and change her diaper often. If she develops a rash, zinc-oxide cream helps healing. Different diaper creams and lotions may also help. If a rash is severe or persistent, your doctor may prescribe a mild corticosteroid cream. If there are white patches on her bottom, she may have a yeast infection, and your doctor may prescribe an anti-fungal ointment.

Trying different diapers

As with many aspects of baby care, figuring out what works best for you and your baby comes with trial and error. Over time, you may decide you want to try a different type of diaper, perhaps to save money, or to use a more eco-friendly brand. Or you may decide to combine diapers, maybe using cloth diapers in the day and switching to more absorbent disposables for the night. You may also find disposables more convenient when you're out and about, allowing you to dispose of the soiled diaper, rather than having to carry a dirty cloth diaper around with you.

A TEAM EFFORT
Changing diapers is one aspect of caring for your baby that dads—and other family members or friends—can help with. Helping with your baby's everyday care allows your partner to define his role and feel involved, and, of course, encourages the bonding process.

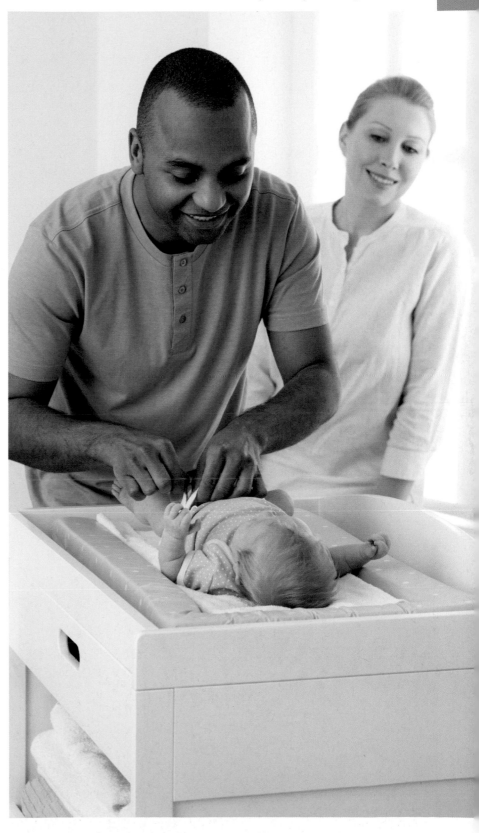

My baby's sleep

Nights of disrupted sleep can come as a shock at first, and you may wonder how you will manage. Don't despair—your baby will eventually learn to keep more civilized hours; in the meantime, you can encourage her toward this.

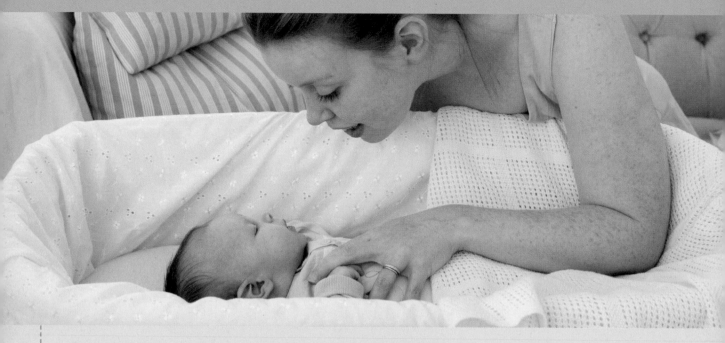

LEARNING TO SETTLE
Avoid the temptation to put your baby into her bassinet if she falls asleep during a feed. Burp her, talk to her gently, and then put her down and encourage her to settle herself.

The amount of time newborns spend sleeping varies from baby to baby, with some needing a great deal of sleep, up to 20 hours a day, while others need very little and may sleep for only around 10 hours. In general, however, a newborn during the first few weeks of life will sleep roughly 15 to 18 hours in a 24-hour period, often in short bursts of two or three hours at a time—even through the night, since she will need to nurse at regular intervals. Take heart: Around six weeks, a pattern will begin to emerge, and your baby should start to sleep for longer stretches at night as her tummy grows and goes for longer between feeds.

Bearing in mind that you are unlikely to enjoy an unbroken night's sleep for a while, aim to build in rest periods during the day for you, too. Many mothers find it hard to follow the principle of sleeping when their baby sleeps—there's always so much to do! However, this isn't a luxury, it's a necessity; you'll be much better equipped to cope with the demands of new parenthood if you are well rested.

If you do feel like catching up on chores when your baby is sleeping, attempt only one or two achievable tasks that make daily life with your baby more organized, such as replenishing your diaper bag, putting laundry into the washing machine, or gathering some snacks and a drink for you to have beside you as you feed her later. You'll feel as though you've gotten something done, but you won't be pushing yourself too hard.

"During the first 48 hours after the birth, your new baby is likely to sleep a great deal—after that, anything goes"

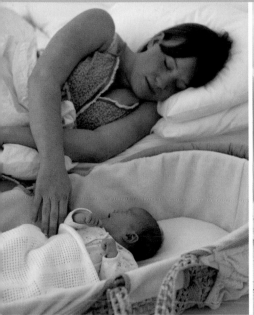

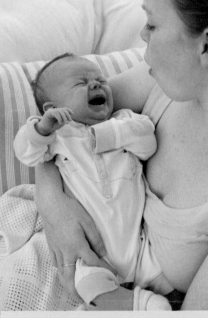

SIDE-BY-SIDE
Safety guidelines recommend that your baby sleep in your room until she's six months old, and you will probably find it reassuring to keep her close by at first.

SOOTHING YOUR BABY
Never put your baby to bed while she's crying. You want her to be calm and content so that bedtime is a positive experience. Soothe her first, then put her in her crib.

Follow your baby's lead

For the first four to six weeks, it will be much less stressful for everyone if you don't try to get your baby into a routine. Your baby's tiny tummy means she needs to feed little and often at first, so let her nurse when she wants to nurse and sleep when she wants to sleep. Then, slowly and gradually, as you get to know her internal clock, you can start to mold the day a little bit so that it begins to suit you, without upsetting her.

Do be aware that if your baby becomes overtired, she'll find it harder to drift off, so napping every few hours is important. Learn the signs that your baby is tired—she may rub her eyes, fuss with her fists up by her ears, cry, or look tired and drawn.

At around six weeks, you may be able to establish a pattern that suits you both, with naps and activities occurring around the same times each day. You'll still need to be flexible, though. All babies have fussy days, and on other days you may have activities and appointments that mean you can't put her in bed at the usual time. Work to a rough pattern rather than a strict schedule; eventually a kind of order should emerge.

Encouraging sleep

You can't control when your baby sleeps or for how long, but there are steps you can take to help her feel as comfortable and settled as possible. When she is around two to four weeks old, you can also very gently encourage her toward either being awake (and active) or asleep (and quiet). Although babies won't begin to separate night and day for at least a couple of months, you can still get her used to the idea. By building up a bedtime routine (see p.356), you can help her slowly to recognize that daytime is bright and stimulating, punctuated by naptimes, whereas nighttime is quiet, punctuated only by feeding and diaper changes.

MAKING YOUR BABY COMFORTABLE
Young babies need to feel secure. At first, many feel more snug in the enclosed space of a Moses basket or bassinet.

Making sure your baby is neither too hot nor too cold is important for her comfort, as well as for her safety (see p.357). A onesie and pajamas are

"When you start a routine, stick to a rough sequence; try not to be too rigid, because there will be times when you need to adapt your routine"

sufficient nightwear, or just a onesie in warmer months, and then add a sleep sack or swaddling product so she is snug, but not too warm. Put your hand on her chest to check how warm she is, and add or remove layers as necessary. If the weather is very hot, resist the urge to dress her in only a diaper.

A feed is usually a prerequisite to sleep for young babies. Burp your baby before you put her down to sleep so she doesn't wake in discomfort.

When you put your baby down, stay close by at first, sing her a lullaby or talk to her reassuringly, and gently stroke her head. If she cries when you walk away, return to comfort her, but resist the urge to pick her up. Eventually, if she is secure in the knowledge that you return to her when she cries, she will feel confident that you are always there for her.

A GENTLE ROUTINE

By six weeks, you can establish a regular bedtime routine to help your baby associate falling asleep with pleasurable things. Try the following to get started:
• Make the last activity of your baby's day something calming, such as singing her a soothing lullaby or looking at a book. Even tiny babies can respond to images put in front of them. Make your voice soft and soothing.
• Turn off the television or radio and your telephone to make this time of day free from noise and distractions.
• Give your baby a bath—the warm water and gentle lapping will have a soporific effect on her.
• Keep the lighting soft and low, especially in your baby's room while you're giving her a bedtime feed.
• Look at her reassuringly during a feed, but don't chat or sing to her—she needs to learn that this is quiet time and the time for fun and interaction has passed.
• Once she has finished eating, burp her, then gently put her in her bed and leave the room. If she cries, go back and gently reassure her—but without speaking. Simply stroke her face or tummy to settle her and leave the room again. You may have to keep going back for a while, but eventually she'll learn that, even though you always come back, there's no real fun to be had at this time of day, and it will become a natural event to fall asleep.

How our babies slept

When my baby first came home from the hospital, his day and night were completely mixed up and he slept when I wanted him to be awake and was awake at night, when I definitely wanted him to sleep! After a few weeks of slow adjustment—playing with him a little more during his daytime periods of wakefulness and not stimulating him when he became alert at night—he gradually began to shift so that night and day were more along my lines. CH

My first baby hated to go to sleep by herself and wanted to be rocked to sleep all the time. It took me a long time to realize that by far the kindest thing for all of us was for me to stop going for the easy option and giving in, and to find the energy and resolve to gently reassure her every time she cried, but then leave her to drop off alone. TL

I knew the advice was to work toward your baby settling herself rather than being fed or rocked to sleep. My baby often feel asleep while nursing. I wondered why parents and experts alike maintained that this could cause sleep problems, but then my three-month-old started waking every two to three hours in the night wanting a feed to get back to sleep. After a couple of sleepless nights, I was determined to separate the last feed of the night from my baby falling asleep. This was difficult, since nursing had become a cue for my baby to fall asleep. Then I figured out the (incredibly useful) routine of feeding followed by bath, pajamas, and a bedtime book. Bathing after nursing meant she was awake, or was woken, after her last evening feed, and no longer needed a feed to settle back down if she woke in the night. LJ

Both my babies slept through the night by 10 weeks; before then, they needed feeds every two to three hours. Going out in the fresh air each day helped them recognize the difference between day and night, and was very good for me! VB

Safe sleeping

Whether your baby is in her own bed or you are co-sleeping (see p.246), you need to ensure that she sleeps safely. Crib death, or Sudden Infant Death Syndrome (SIDS), is the unexplained death of a young baby, usually while sleeping. Thankfully this is rare, but you will want to do all you can to minimize the risks. Some factors you can't control—for example, babies with a low birth weight, premature babies, and baby boys have an increased risk. However, in the past few decades, pre ventable risk factors have been identified, and today there is plenty that you can do to protect your baby.

• Don't smoke during pregnancy and after the birth. Avoid smoky environments while you're pregnant and also once your baby is born, and don't let anyone smoke in the house.

• Experts recommend that you keep your baby with you at all times until she is six months old, including having her sleep in your bedroom during the night. Place her to sleep on her back. If you wish to cover her with a thin blanket, you must place her in the feet-to-foot position, with her feet at the bottom of the crib and the blanket pulled no higher than her chest and tucked tightly under the crib mattress so she can't wriggle under it.

• Aim for a temperature of 64°F (18°C) in her room.

• Never use pillows, comforters, or bumper pads in her bed.

• Never fall asleep with your baby in an armchair or on the sofa.

• Breastfeeding your baby reduces the risk of SIDS.

FEET TO FOOT
It's best to avoid blankets altogether, but if you do use one, use the "feet-to-foot" position: Place your baby with her feet at the end of her crib so that she can't wriggle down under the blanket. Tuck the blanket under the mattress on three sides and place it at chest height.

• If you think your baby is sick or she has a temperature, take her to the doctor.

• Recent research suggests that babies who suck on a pacifier as they sleep have a lower risk of SIDS.

• There are additional safety sleeping guidelines if you decide to co-sleep with your baby. However, many Canadian medical organizations frown upon co-sleeping, so consider the messages from these groups before moving your baby into your bed. If you want to try anyway, your mattress should be firm and your baby shouldn't get too hot: Pajamas and a sleep sack should do. For safety reasons, you should not use pillows, blankets, top sheets, or other loose bedding in your bed if your baby is sleeping with you; they all pose a suffocation risk. You could try using a bed "divider," which keeps your baby safe in her own space. Never co-sleep with your baby if you have been drinking or smoking, are very tired, or have taken medication that could make you unresponsive or drowsy. Don't co-sleep with your baby if she was under 5lb 8oz (2.5kg) at birth, premature, or is under three months old.

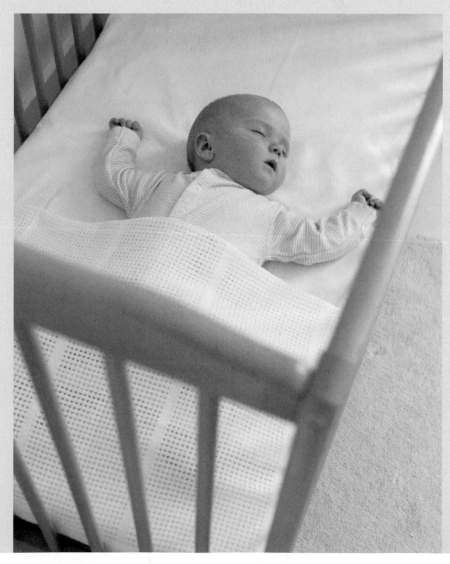

Soothing my baby

Responding to your baby's cries is instinctive, even if at first you're unsure exactly what she needs. While you're getting to know what her different cries mean, it helps to have a few comforting techniques to try out.

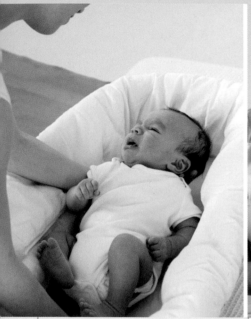

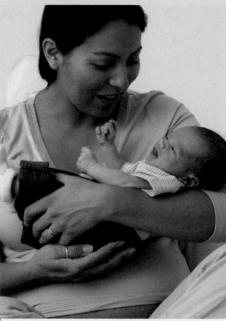

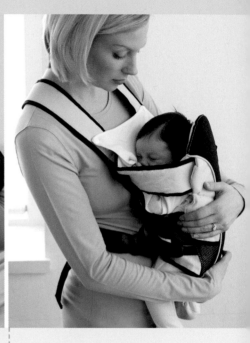

RESPONDING TO YOUR BABY
Don't leave your newborn to cry for long—this will just increase her distress. Young babies often need a comforting cuddle.

ROCK-A-BYE
Rocking and singing to your crying baby will often be all she needs to calm her. Sometimes babies just need to know that you're there.

CLOSE TO YOU
Your baby may feel instantly soothed when held against your chest; she can hear your heartbeat and is rocked by your movements.

All babies cry as a way to communicate their needs. Crying should never be ignored, because it means that your baby is uncomfortable or unhappy—and it's up to you to find out why. This can be tricky at first because your newborn is so new—and if you're a first-time mom, you don't have prior experience to guide you. However, as you get to know your baby, you will learn to interpret her signals and cries and respond to them with ease. Until then, it's helpful to know the common causes of crying and what to do about them.

Causes of crying

There are several reasons why babies cry, most of which aren't nearly as worrying as you might think. Babies cry when they are hungry; have gas; need a diaper change; are overstimulated or tired; are hot or cold; or simply want a cuddle. Your baby might cry, too, if she is bored or fretful, if something startled her, or if she suddenly can't see you. If none of these appears to be the problem, your baby may be suffering with colic (see opposite). If your baby is very distressed

and nothing soothes her, or her crying is out of the ordinary (either in terms of pitch or because it's out of character), call your pediatrician.

Helping your baby settle

If your baby is still upset after you have fed and changed her and she's not too hot or cold, you will need to find other ways to soothe her. Holding her close so

"Crying is your baby's first means of communication; responding to her cries helps her to feel secure and loved"

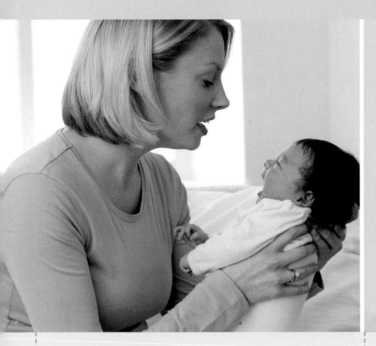

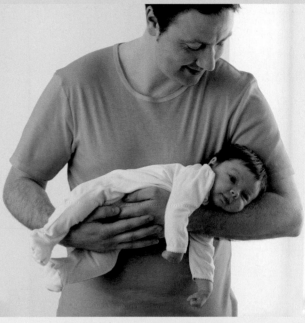

SMILING AND TALKING
Your reassuring voice and smiles will help your baby understand that the world is all right. Try not to show her that you're distressed by her crying, since this will upset her more.

THE TIGER HOLD
Holding your baby face down, securely against your forearm, can soothe a colicky baby, as it allows you to rub her back while rocking her.

she can hear your heartbeat and gently rocking her is instantly reassuring. "White noise," such as the vacuum cleaner or washing machine, can help, too, as it may remind her of being in the womb. A walk in her stroller or a drive in the car are good distractions, but try not to rely on these methods.

Some babies are soothed by being wrapped snugly or swaddled. Try tucking a blanket around her below the level of her head, being sure that she can move a little. If she is soothed by sucking, you could give her a pacifier.

SUFFERING WITH COLIC
If your baby's crying is persistent or frantic, hard to soothe, and occurs at a similar time each day, and if she clenches her fists or brings her knees to her chest, she may have colic. This isn't fully understood, but frequent burping during feeds can help relieve it. If you're breastfeeding, cutting gas-producing foods, such as broccoli and cabbage, from your diet may help. If your baby is bottle-fed, changing her formula might help, but consult your pediatrician first; switching formula can upset the

digestive system. If the colic is severe, your doctor may prescribe an antispasmodic solution.

At home, soothing, rocking, and cuddling your baby through the difficult period can help, as can a warm bath and a gentle massage (see pp.366–367). Share the load with your partner—a colicky baby can be tiring and upsetting for parents, so it's important that you both take a turn and get a break. Reassure yourself that however bad it seems, colic usually disappears by the time babies reach three months of age.

Keeping my baby clean

In the first few weeks of life, your baby doesn't need a daily bath—sponge bathing is all that's required to keep her delicate skin fresh. For babies who don't like being immersed in water, this is definitely the way to go.

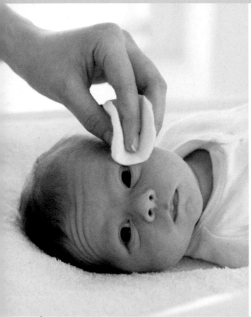

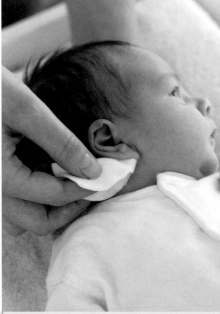

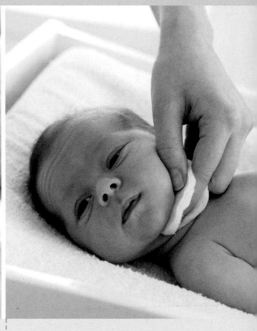

CLEANING YOUR BABY'S EYES
Wipe around the eyes, first under the eye, from the nose outward, then above the eye. Use a separate cotton pad for each eye.

KEEPING YOUR BABY'S EARS CLEAN
Wipe around your baby's ears, but not inside them, beginning at the front and going up and around the back, into the crease.

CLEANING YOUR BABY'S NECK
With a cotton pad or washcloth, work into each of your baby's neck folds, where fluff and milk can accumulate and irritate the skin.

Keeping your baby clean is part of her daily care. She may not get particularly mucky, but giving her a sponge bath daily or every couple of days will prevent milk deposits or grime from accumulating. This is important because if dirt is allowed to build up, it could irritate your baby's delicate skin.

Ensure that the room where you wash your baby is warm and draft-free, and you have everything you need to clean her on hand before you begin (see p.236) so you won't need to leave her unattended and can wash her quickly and efficiently.

Giving a sponge bath

You'll need to clean your baby's face and bottom each day. You can also wipe her hands and feet, and under the armpits. A sponge bath allows you to get your baby clean without dipping her in water. Talk or sing to her throughout to reassure her.

First, lay your baby on her changing mat on a secure surface. You may want to put a towel on top of the mat for comfort and warmth. Fill your bowl or sink with lukewarm water and test the temperature with your elbow to ensure that it is warm, but not hot.
• Start by washing your baby's face. Dip a cotton pad into the water, then gently run it around your baby's eye, smoothing away any goop. Discard the pad and use a clean one for the other eye so you don't pass infection from one eye to the other.
• Use cotton balls or a damp washcloth to wipe around her ears and neck, taking care to concentrate on the creases.
• Now wash the palms of her hands and the skin in between her fingers. Then

"Always wash your hands carefully before cleaning around the umbilical stump, because it can easily become infected"

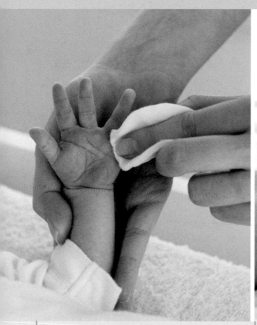

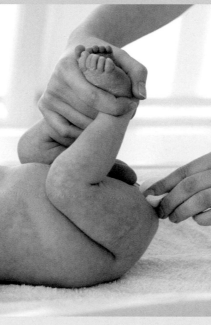

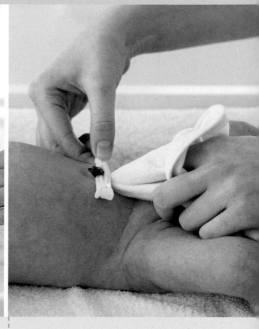

YOUR BABY'S FINGERS AND TOES
Wipe between each finger and each toe, gently drying them with a towel once you're done to keep them from becoming irritated.

CLEANING YOUR BABY'S BOTTOM
Lift up your baby's legs to clean around his bottom. If you wish, use a little pH-neutral baby wash to make sure it's really clean.

AROUND YOUR BABY'S CORD
Use a washcloth, rather than cotton balls, which can get tangled, to wipe around the cord, taking care not to wet the actual wound.

gently lift her arm to clean the creases in her armpits.
• Next, gently wash between each of your baby's toes and down the insides of each leg, wiping into any creases.
• Wash her genital area carefully—a baby's genitals can be swollen after the birth. If you have a boy, don't attempt to pull back on his foreskin, which will still be attached; and if he's circumcised, be very careful around the wound.
• Place your hand on her chest and support her chin, then tip her gently onto her side so that you can wipe her back

and bottom. If you wish, you can use some pH-neutral baby wash on her bottom, then rinse it with clean water.
• Tip her back onto her front, wrap her snugly, and pat her dry.
• Apply diaper cream before you put her diaper on, if necessary, then dress her right away so she doesn't get cold.

CLEANING THE UMBILICAL STUMP
It's important to keep your baby's cord stump clean and dry to prevent an infection. Folding down the top of your

baby's diaper will help to keep urine and feces off the stump and keep it dry.

To keep the area clean, wash your hands, then use a clean, thin washcloth to gently wipe around the area of the stump; if you think the area is particularly dirty, you can use a tiny bit of baby wash. Gently pat around the area with a towel to dry it, and let the air get to it for a few minutes before dressing your baby. It is quite normal for the stump to look a little mucky, but if it appears at all red or swollen, talk to your baby's pediatrician.

Bathing my baby

Giving your baby her first bath can be nerve-wracking: She may object to being undressed and bathed, and you may be anxious about dropping her! Soon you'll both gain confidence, and bathtime will become a special part of the day.

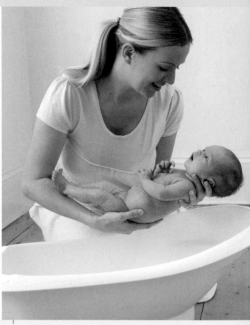

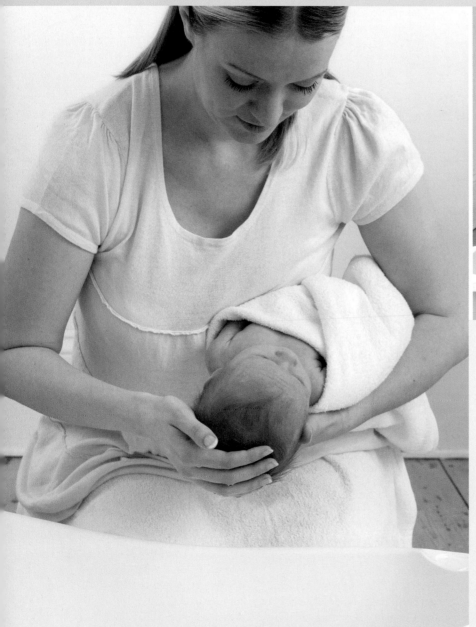

PUTTING YOUR BABY IN THE BATH
Remove your baby's towel, then hold her firmly under her neck and bottom and lower her gently into the water, letting her feet touch the water first. Talk to her constantly to reassure her.

A HAIR WASH
If you're washing your baby's hair, swaddle her in a towel, then hold her under one arm and support her neck while lowering her over the bath. Use your free hand to cup water over her head. You don't necessarily need to use baby wash for her hair at this stage.

"Over time your baby will begin to enjoy the feeling of warm water on her skin and find bathtime a happy and soothing experience"

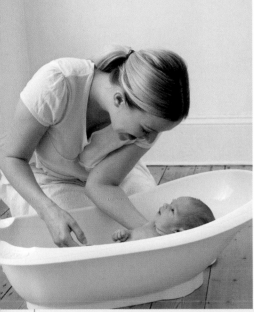

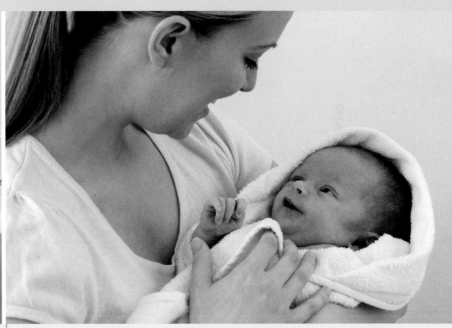

A GENTLE WASH
Support her head and neck with one hand, and use the other hand to wash water over her so she gets used to how it feels.

DRY AND SNUG
As soon as you lift her out of the bath, wrap her snugly in a warm towel and gently dry her all over, including in all her creases to prevent them from rubbing and becoming sore.

It's best to wait until the umbilical stump has dropped off before giving your baby a bath. While sponge baths (see pp.360–361) are fine most days, you might want to bathe her once or twice a week if she enjoys it. Preparation is key to helping bathtime run smoothly: Keep the room warm and draft-free and have all you need at hand (see p.236). You may find a baby bathtub easiest. You can put it on the floor, or a secure, level surface so you don't have to bend over. Or you can use a sink (if the taps aren't in the way) or even the big bath.

• Fill the bath before you undress your baby. The water should be around 95–100°F (35–38°C). You can use a bath thermometer, or test the temperature with your elbow to ensure it's warm, but not hot. You need just enough water to cover her to her middle once she's in. If you wish, you can add a few drops of pH-neutral baby bath, swirling it around before you put her in.
• Hold your baby firmly as you lower her into the bath, supporting her neck all the time. Rest the back of her neck and head on your forearm, using your hand to grip

her gently but firmly around the top of her arm, and leaving your other hand free to wash her. When you wash her back, lean her forward a little, supporting her chest and chin.
• If you're using a big bath, put a non-slip mat down. Never leave your baby unattended in the water—even for a second.
• Dry her as soon as you take her out. If you wish, you can rub a little oil into her skin to stop it from becoming too dry, then cuddle her in a warm, dry towel before dressing her.

Dressing my baby

Your newborn baby's wardrobe may be simple—just onesies and pajamas—but getting her changed can be trickier than you might think. Being methodical and handling her gently but confidently will help make it easier.

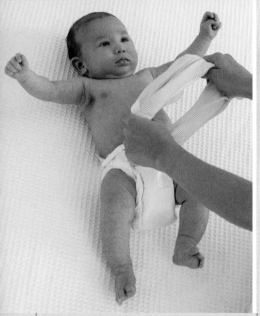

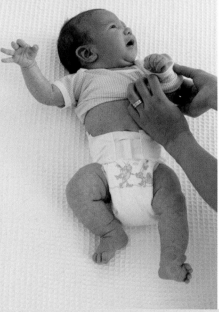

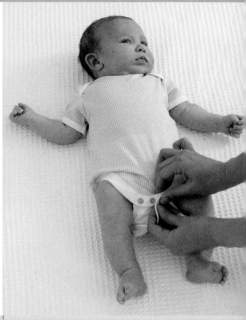

OVER THE HEAD
Pull the neck hole wide, and slip the onesie over the head, gently raising her head and keeping the fabric off her face as you do so.

IN WITH THE ARMS
Gather the material at the arm and poke your baby's hand through, stretching the sleeve wide with your free hand.

FASTEN TOGETHER
Gently tug down the edges of the onesie and fasten the snaps between your baby's legs, over her diaper.

For your baby's first few weeks and even months, choose clothes that have as few fastenings as possible, are made from stretchy material, and allow you to change her diaper without completely undressing her. Onesies and footed pajamas are ideal; your baby can wear them night and day. Save dresses, pants, or items with tricky fastenings for later.

In the daytime, layering items of clothing means that you can remove or add items according to changes in temperature and whether you are indoors or out.

Putting on a onesie

You will need around six onesies to start with. Onesies are essential for babies: In the summer, your baby may need to wear only a short-sleeved onesie (and perhaps

some socks, since her extremities may get cold); and in the winter she'll need a onesie underneath her other clothes to keep her warm. Choose ones with overlapping pieces of fabric on the shoulders, which make them easier to get over your baby's head. Make sure they have snaps in the crotch to stop them from riding up.

As you lower the onesie over her head, talk to your baby and play peekaboo, so that in the brief moment when she can't see you she can still hear you. You may find that she kicks or protests while

"Newborn babies tend to like having clothes on—the fabric offers a reassuring layer of security against the big wide world"

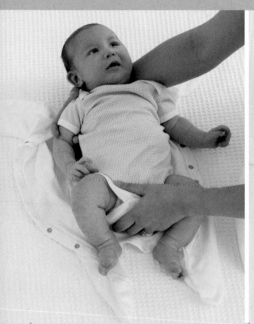 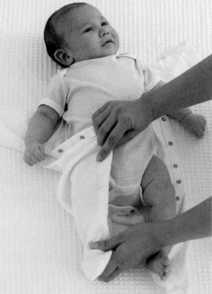 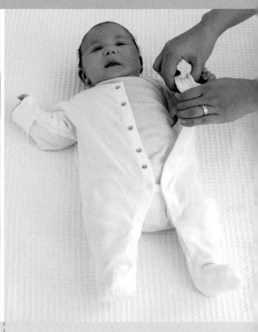

OUTFIT FIRST, THEN BABY
Lay out the open pajamas on a flat surface with the arms splayed and the legs folded down, then place your baby on top.

IN WITH THE LEGS
Gently fold up your baby's legs and tuck them into the feet holes. Once both legs are in, fasten the snaps just to the diaper.

FINISHING OFF
Bunch the sleepsuit's arm, and put your fingers in to guide your baby's hand through. Repeat on the other arm, then fasten all the snaps.

you're doing this—keep reassuring her as you gently pull her hands through the arms of her onesie and pull the onesie down her body (see above, opposite).

Removing a onesie is trickier. Undo the snaps, then roll up the onesie. Pull on the sleeve with one hand, while the other hand reaches inside the onesie to gently pull out her arm. Once both arms are out, put your fingers in the neck hole and gently pull the onesie up and over her face, taking care not to catch her nose. Lift her head gently with one hand while you slide the onesie out from under her.

Putting on pajamas

You will need around six one-piece pajamas, too. These are perfect for your baby: They keep her feet warm, and are front-fastening so you can get her into them (and out of them) quickly. Most have snaps down the legs, so you can untuck her legs from them and pull the bottom half up to change her diaper.

If you're worried about your baby scratching her face, you can buy

sleepsuits that have built-in mittens; make sure they are roomy enough to let your baby stretch her fingers. Remember that babies grow quickly, so if her toes look cramped with her legs at a full stretch, it's time to move up a size.

Again, smile at your baby and reassure her as you maneuver her arms and legs into the pajamas before snapping it up (see above). It's easy to remove pajamas: You simply undo the snaps, gently pull out her legs, then pull on the sleeves so that, as she naturally retracts her arms, they come free.

Massaging my baby

Baby massage is a great way to explore your baby's body and relax her. Massage also helps bonding, improves your baby's sleep, encourages healthy weight gain, and even aids cognitive development. It's time to get started!

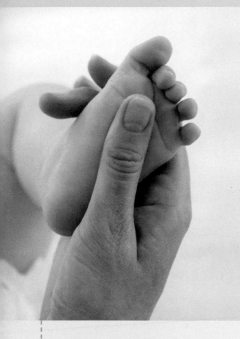

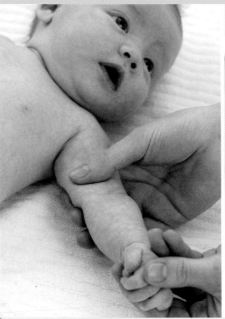

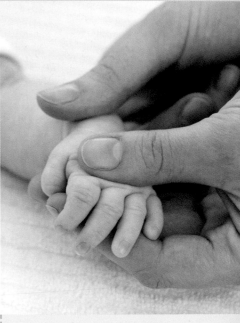

MASSAGING THE FOOT
Hold your baby's foot and use your thumb to stroke down the sole, then gently massage each toe before moving on to the leg.

STROKING YOUR BABY'S ARM
Hold your baby's hand; gently stretch out her arm and use your other hand to stroke down her arm from the armpit to the hand.

MASSAGING YOUR BABY'S HAND
Gently hold your baby's wrist in one hand, and with your other stroke the back and palm of her hand, then each finger in turn.

The power of touch enhances your baby's emotional and physical health. She will feel loved and cared for, and if your baby was premature, massage can help her to thrive. One study even claims that babies who are massaged have fewer colds. There are also benefits for you. When you massage your baby, your body produces the feel-good hormone oxytocin, which can help you overcome baby blues, or simply feel calmer and more connected to your baby. Massage helps dads to bond, too, so this is a great activity for your partner to get involved in.

You don't need to learn special strokes to massage your baby—it's enough simply to run your hands over her body, in rhythmic, slow movements. She'll soon let you know what feels good.

Getting started

Choose a time when your baby is content, well fed, and rested; she will become restless and fractious if she's hungry or tired when you start out. If she cries at any time, stop and give her a

reassuring cuddle and try again another time. Also, don't massage your baby if she has a temperature or you think she might be unwell.

When you're ready, lay out a towel or blanket in a warm, quiet room. Make sure you have enough space to move around her, so that you can sit comfortably at her feet and at her head. Remove her clothes. It might be more restful for you if she keeps her diaper on, but if you aren't worried about accidents, take it off so you can easily get to her tummy.

"Your baby loves to be touched by you and will relish the sensation of your hand massaging her skin—and, of course, your undivided attention"

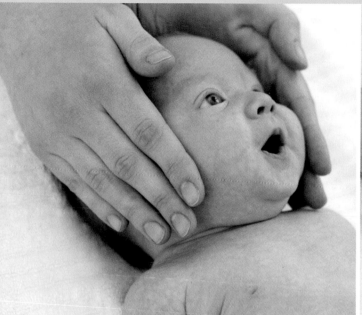

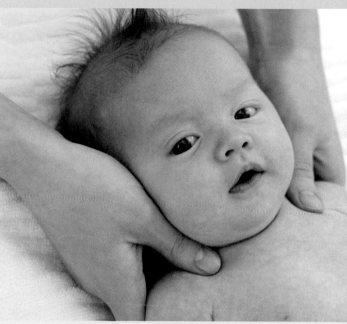

MASSAGING THE HEAD
Talk to your baby in a soothing voice while you sit behind her and lay your hands on either side of her head, then use your thumbs to gently stroke across her brow.

A GENTLE SHOULDER MASSAGE
Place your thumbs at the tops of her shoulders with your fingers behind, then sweep your fingers and thumbs together and very gently squeeze the flesh in her shoulders.

FEET FIRST

Begin with your baby's feet so you can sit in front of her at first. Make plenty of eye contact, talk to her gently, and give reassuring smiles.

• Hold her foot and gently run your fingers over the top of it and softly squeeze each toe. Use your thumb to gently press all over the sole. Hold one leg in your palm, and use the other hand to stroke up and down her leg, front and back. Repeat on the other leg.

• Move up to her tummy. Use lighter pressure here—making gentle strokes over her tummy. Move your hands up and down and in circles, keeping the motion clockwise, so that you are working in the direction her food passes through. Then stroke your hands gently across your baby's chest.

• If she is happy, move on to her arms, massaging from her armpit to her hand. Gently rub each finger and use your thumb to pad all over her palm.

• Reposition yourself at her head, smiling and talking to her the whole time. Gently massage her shoulders and forehead, using light, feathery strokes (see above).

USING OILS

You may be tempted to use essential oils on your baby because the scents seem pleasant to you, but you should avoid placing these potent substances on your baby's sensitive skin without a go-ahead from your pediatrician. Even then, you must exercise caution to keep essential oils away from your baby's genitals, eyes, or mouth. If you'd like to incorporate oils into your massage, it's safer to simply use a bit of olive oil. (All oils—including olive oil—should be kept away from your baby's eyes, mouth, and genitals.)

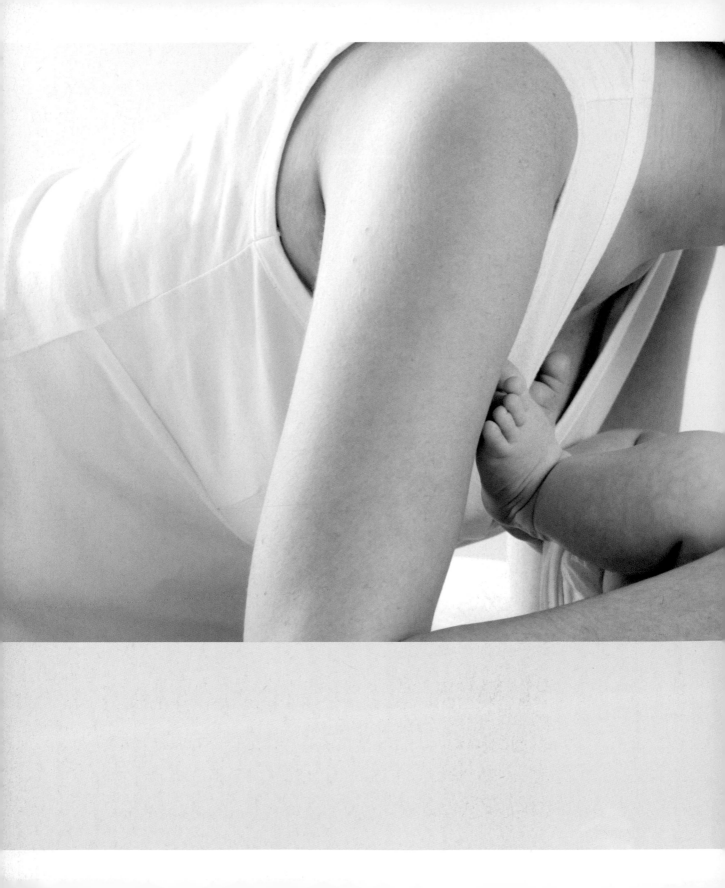

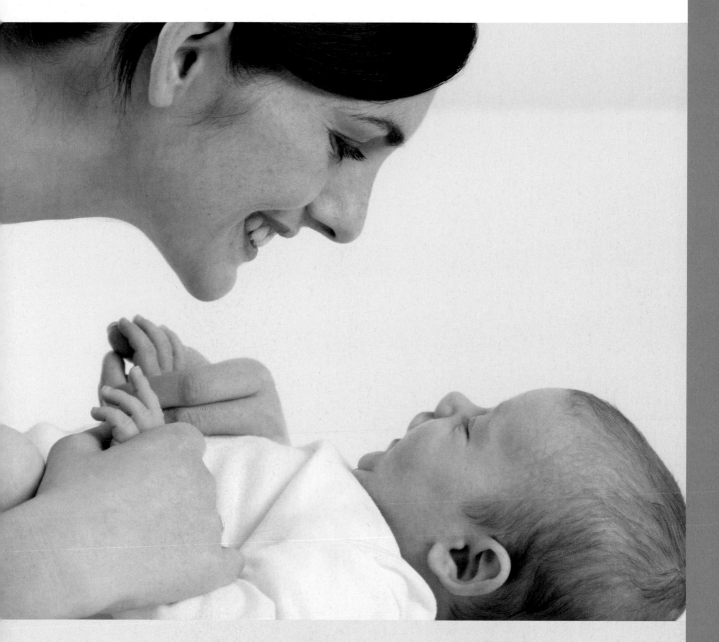

My first weeks as a mom

As your body begins to heal, and you adjust to life with your new baby, it's important to take care of yourself and get the support you need.

Recovering from the birth

Even the most straightforward labor can leave you tired, emotional, and a little uncomfortable. Taking time out for yourself, and using techniques to aid recovery will give you the energy and resources you need to enjoy motherhood.

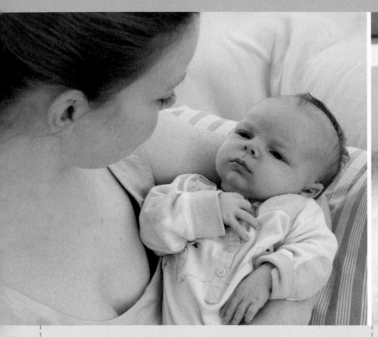

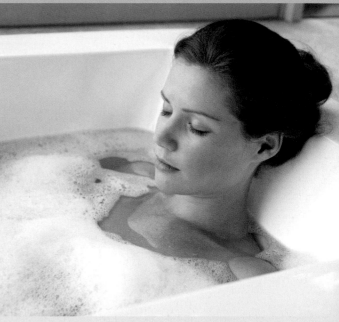

RELAX AND ENJOY
Your priority in the first few weeks of your baby's life is to concentrate on recovering from the birth and getting to know him. Everything else can most definitely wait.

TAKE TIME FOR YOURSELF
It can be difficult to squeeze in some relaxation time, but you'll feel rejuvenated by a little treat, even if it's just a hot bath or five minutes on your own to drink a cup of tea.

Although it can be tempting to rush straight back to your usual routine, it is important to rest and recover after the birth. Most women experience a few uncomfortable side effects, but you'll soon be back on your feet again.

Your new life

You may be experiencing a whirlwind of emotions and activity as you get to know your new baby and start to get a handle on your new life as a family. Sleep may be at a premium, and you may find that you are so busy or tired that you forget to eat. These are two things that simply can't be ignored during the postpartum period. You'll need sleep not only to recover from the birth and encourage your body to heal, but also to provide you with the resources to breastfeed, feel confident in your new role as a mom, and give you enough energy to get through the day. This means sleeping when your baby sleeps—no matter how many dishes are in the sink—and sitting down with your feet up to rest whenever you can.

If you were a busy person before, you may find it a challenge to stop and relax; however, it is essential for your emotional and physical health and well-being.

Similarly, breastfeeding, recovering from the birth, caring for a newborn, and keeping your emotions on an even keel all require plenty of nutrients, not to mention calories. If you can't manage to eat three good-sized meals a day, make sure you are eating plenty of healthy snacks. A healthy sandwich on whole-grain bread or some cheese and fresh salad will supply you with energy and nutrients, as will a bowl of soup and a crusty roll. Ask for help on the cooking front if you don't have time to make nourishing meals; the benefits of a healthy diet during this period cannot be underestimated.

Getting back on your feet

You may be sore after the birth, and experience some postpartum bleeding, pain in the perineum, discomfort when using the bathroom, and even headaches. To speed up your recovery, it helps to know how to deal with common postpartum complaints.

PERINEAL PAIN

Your perineum will have been stretched during labor, and may have been stitched if you experienced tearing and/or an episiotomy. Adding a handful of baking soda and a drop or two of lavender oil to a warm bath can encourage healing and ease any itching. An ice pack, a bag of frozen peas wrapped in a damp dishcloth, or a gel pad designed for the perineal area can ease discomfort and reduce swelling. Keep a bottle of cool water by the toilet, and pour it over your vagina when you urinate, to soothe the area. Pelvic floor exercises can encourage the blood flow to the area, which will facilitate healing.

AFTERPAINS

As your uterus shrinks back to its pre-pregnancy size, you can experience cramping, particularly when you are breastfeeding (which encourages the release of the hormone oxytocin). First-time moms may feel mild contractions, while those who have given birth previously may find that afterpains are very painful, as more forceful

---

How we recovered

Sitting down was very painful after the birth of my 9½-pound (4.3-kg) baby, who was delivered using forceps. I used gel pads, which I had kept in the freezer, to numb the area, which was a massive help. My first baby was delivered by caesarean section, and a week or so after her birth, I started going for short walks. It felt strange and uncomfortable at the beginning, but became easier each day. TL

I found taking the advice of my doctor, accepting practical offers of help from friends, and a mixture of trying to get moving but with plenty of extra rest, worked best. CH

I relied very much on the support of my husband (who helped with everything from cooking and cleaning to 2am diaper changes) to help compensate for the fact that I was essentially breastfeeding around the clock and getting very little sleep. Breastfeeding definitely helped me shed the pregnancy weight I'd gained, and since I was already committed to a healthy diet long before I got pregnant, I simply allowed myself to eat according to hunger. Also, I made a point of taking daily walks with my baby, which was great for exercise and to escape the house! LJ

---

contractions are required to reduce the size of your uterus. Use your breathing exercises when you experience cramping, and try to keep your bladder empty by going to the bathroom every hour or so. A full bladder displaces the uterus, making the contractions less efficient.

Massaging your lower abdomen frequently during the three days after the birth can also help to prevent your uterus from relaxing too much (and therefore prevent the need for it to contract so forcefully). Finally, if all else fails, ask your doctor if you can take an over-the-counter painkiller to ease discomfort.

UNCOMFORTABLE BOWEL MOVEMENTS

You may find that you are nervous about having a bowel movement after all that activity at the site, and actively resist going to the bathroom. Many hospitals will ask you to confirm that you have had one before you can be discharged; however, this is not always the case. There is no doubt that bearing down can be a little uncomfortable, so it is important to keep your bowel

movements loose. This involves eating plenty of fiber-rich foods, such as fresh fruit and vegetables, legumes, whole grains, or even just a bowl of freshly popped popcorn. Along with this, you'll also need to keep well hydrated—drinking between six and eight large glasses of water a day—to encourage movement along your intestines. If you are struggling, your doctor can prescribe a gentle laxative to get things moving. You can also try using your breathing exercises to help you get through the first couple of experiences. The truth is, it is likely to be much easier than you think!

BLEEDING

Bleeding after the birth is known as postpartum bleeding, and this discharge—which is blood and tissue from the lining of the uterus—is known as "lochia." Immediately after the birth it can be quite heavy, and very red. You may find that it comes out in a rush if you've been lying on your back for a while. Over the coming weeks, it will become pinker and lighter until, around 10 days after the birth, there is just a small amount of white or yellowish discharge. Some women bleed for up to four weeks; however, things usually settle down before then. If you do experience very heavy bleeding (particularly with heavy clotting), or if your discharge is smelly, report this immediately to your doctor or midwife, who can rule out any infection, or hemorrhaging (see p.321).

INCONTINENCE
It's not unusual to experience a little bladder incontinence after the birth, particularly when you cough, sneeze, or laugh. Sanitary pads will help to soak up little accidents (change them frequently), and pelvic floor exercises (see p.67), done several times a day, will soon restore your muscle tone to normal.

WEIGHT LOSS
Many moms are aghast to find that they don't look significantly smaller after having given birth. However it can take a while for your body to get back into shape, and if you were a little unfit before the birth, it can take longer.

Breastfeeding is the single best way to lose pregnancy weight, because your body will call upon fat stores to provide energy for producing milk. Sensible eating and some gentle exercise will also help you to lose weight naturally. Don't even think about dieting; breastfeeding requires optimal levels of nutrients from your diet, and as a new mom you'll require plenty of good food to sustain energy levels.

HAIR LOSS
During pregnancy, high levels of the hormone estrogen cause more hair follicles than usual to enter the growth phase. After your baby is born, your hormone levels change dramatically, often causing the hair-growth cycle to become disturbed. This is quickly rectified; however, many hair follicles enter a "resting phase," causing excessive hair loss (molting). This normally takes place between six and thirty weeks after the birth. You may be alarmed by the amount of hair you are losing—which can total about two-fifths of your hair—

but you won't have bald patches. Rather, the hair loss results in overall thinning. Rest assured that once your body has settled down and hormones returned to pre-pregnancy state, the molting will stop, and your hair will begin to regrow.

HEADACHES
Many women become temporarily dehydrated after a long labor and failing to keep up fluid levels when breastfeeding, which can cause headaches. Feeding your baby is thirsty work, so make sure that you keep yourself hydrated throughout the day with plenty of water. If your headaches are caused by tension, a light massage by your partner, focusing on your temples, neck, and shoulders, can help. If all else fails, acetaminophen, in the correct doses, is safe to take while breastfeeding.

STRETCH MARKS
Amazingly enough, your skin will shrink to fit your reduced size after pregnancy, but it may be looser in some areas and is also subject to stretch marks. These

FAMILY LIFE
You'll be astonished by how quickly your baby changes over the first few weeks, so take time to admire and enjoy her.

SOOTHING YOUR BABY TO SLEEP
Wearing your baby in a carrier will free your hands for other activities, while keeping him calm as he hears your heartbeat.

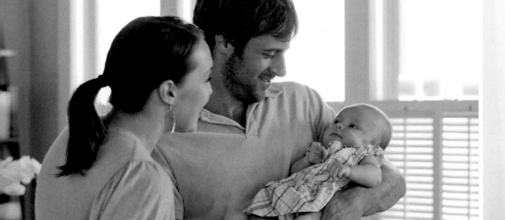

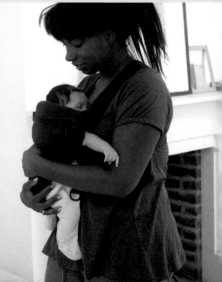

appear first as dark, often raised or even puckered skin, most commonly on your abdomen, breasts, buttocks, and thighs, and occur because the production of collagen in your skin is interrupted when it is rapidly stretched. Once stretched and weakened, the skin can tear, leaving marks that can take some time to fade. A few months after the birth, they will start to look less angry, becoming silvery or white. They are, however, unlikely to disappear completely. You can buy creams and oils to reduce the appearance of stretch marks (see p.196), but their efficacy is questionable. Instead, try massaging a little vitamin E oil into the affected areas, to encourage the growth of healthy collagen.

Recovering from a caesarean

A caesarean section is a major operation, and although you may feel just fine immediately after surgery, it's important to take the time to rest and recover. You will be offered medication to deal with any pain, and this will be carefully monitored and chosen so that you can begin and continue to breastfeed.

It's normal to feel incredibly tired and tearful—particularly if the caesarean was not planned—and you may also feel somewhat shocked. Make sure you take advantage of all the professional support offered in the hospital, and if you need more information to understand why a caesarean was necessary, ask.

You can breastfeed as normal, but you may find it more comfortable to place a pillow across your abdomen, to support the weight of your baby. Lying on your side to breastfeed, with your baby beside you, may be more comfortable because you are not putting weight on your stomach. You can also use a pillow to press down on your abdomen when you laugh, cough, or go to the bathroom, to ease any discomfort. Ask your doctor or nurse to show you how to roll out of bed and get upright so you don't need to use your abdominal muscles, and ask for

your baby to be handed to you, rather than attempting to lift him yourself. You shouldn't lift anything heavier than your baby for the first six weeks, including your toddler, if you have one. It is also recommended that you do not drive for at least six weeks after the birth, which is roughly the time it takes for all of your tissues to heal completely. You should not exercise during this period, either.

It's very common to breathe too shallowly after surgery because you are fearful of any pain; however, you need to breathe deeply to prevent a chest infection. Move your ankles frequently and stay as mobile as you can to prevent clots from forming in the veins in your legs. Wear oversized underwear that won't put any pressure on your scar, and keep the area clean with regular, warm showers.

Most importantly, look after yourself. You and your baby should be your first and only priorities until you feel yourself again, and this can take a few weeks. You'll probably need more rest than moms who delivered vaginally, so get—and accept—as much support as you can.

CATNAPS
Handing over your baby to your partner will give you some much-needed time to rest, and he'll enjoy the opportunity to bond with her and establish his own routines.

SHARING THE LOAD
You may need to alter the division of labor within the household, since most of your time will be spent caring for your new baby.

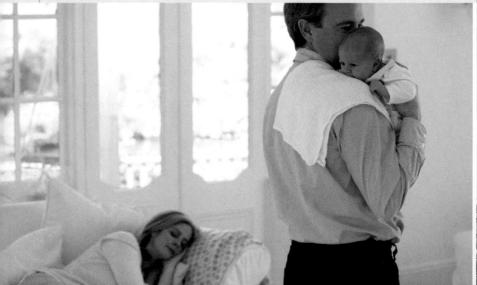

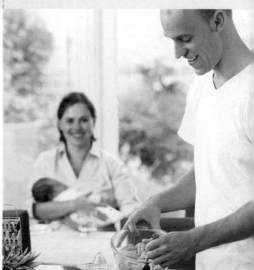

My emotional recovery

Fluctuating hormones, lack of sleep, and natural anxiety about caring for your baby can make you feel a little unsettled. It may take some time to establish an equilibrium, but you'll soon feel yourself again and ready to enjoy parenthood.

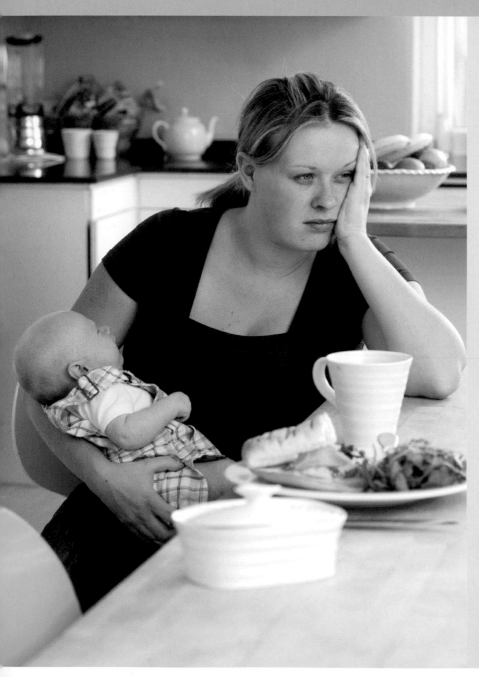

Taking care of yourself can most definitely hasten your emotional recovery from the birth, and help you to achieve more stable moods and a longer fuse! This means eating regular, healthy meals, which keep your blood-sugar levels steady and help you to feel more in control, and ensuring that you get plenty of rest. There is no doubt that sleep deprivation exacerbates feelings of helplessness, tearfulness, and irritation after the birth. Even if it means drafting someone to care for your baby while you get a few hours' sleep, or napping whenever your baby drifts off, you must make an effort to make sleep a priority. This is a time to concentrate on caring for your baby, spending time together as a family, and recovering physically and emotionally from the birth. Try not to worry too much about the rest of the world; batten down the hatches and concentrate on negotiating—and enjoying—this period of adjustment.

Time to adjust

Avoid placing pressure on yourself. There is no reason why a new mom has to be superwoman. Let the housework go for a while, and take advantage of periods when your baby is sleeping to get some

FEELING BLUE
You may feel tired, emotional, irritable and out of sorts for a few days after the birth. If it's all too much, don't hesitate to ask for help.

rest. The current advice is to keep your baby in the same room as you for the first six months, so curl up on your bed and put your feet up. There are very few women who adjust to new motherhood instantly, and it will take some time to establish a routine that works for you and your baby, and to determine the best ways to meet his daily needs. It can be a tiring process, full of trial and error; no new parent is perfect, so lower your expectations, and enjoy the experience.

BABY BLUES

Once the elation of holding your baby in your arms fades, it's normal to feel extremely tired and to experience mild depression, characterized by tearfulness, temporary feelings of inadequacy, exhaustion, and anxiety. Known as "the baby blues," it generally occurs around three days after your baby's birth, and can last a few hours or up to five days.

About 60 to 80 percent of new moms experience this temporary condition, which is believed to be caused by a drop in pregnancy hormones along with a surge in those hormones that are required for breastfeeding. Combined with the usual weariness felt after the birth, the shock of unexpected sleep deprivation, and the natural concerns that new moms have about coping with the needs of their newborns, it's not surprising that you can find yourself in floods of tears or irrationally irritated and frustrated for no apparent reason.

Try to relax, and don't be embarrassed about crying or feeling unusually anxious. Explain to your partner how you are feeling, and take all offers of support and help with housework, other children, and even your new baby. Sleep whenever you can, and keep visitors to a minimum. Now is the time to focus on yourself, your baby, and your new family unit until you are feeling like yourself again.

POSTPARTUM DEPRESSION

More serious than the baby blues, postpartum depression (PPD) affects 10 to 15 percent of all new moms. You're more likely to suffer if you have been depressed before, or had a stressful pregnancy and/or a difficult labor. It is, for example, more common in women who have had emergency caesareans.

Symptoms differ between women, and it's normal to experience at least some of these symptoms after the birth as your hormones begin to settle down and you adjust to your new responsibilities. If, however, you suffer from more than one of the following symptoms regularly, and you aren't feeling any better two weeks after the birth, see your doctor. Professional help is usually required.

- Tearfulness
- Anxiety
- Guilt
- Irritability
- Confusion
- Disturbed sleep
- Excessive exhaustion
- Difficulty in making decisions
- Loss of self-esteem
- Lack of confidence in your ability as a mother
- Loss of libido
- Loss of appetite
- Hostility or indifference to people you normally love
- Difficulty in concentrating
- Shame at being unable to be happy
- Fear of judgment
- Helplessness

If you are concerned that you may harm yourself or your baby, you should seek urgent medical advice.

It is sometimes hard for new moms to recognize that there is a problem, because they are so tied up in the daily care of a newborn. It is important for your doctor and your partner, family or friends to take note of any unusual behavior or symptoms, and to get you the help you need. There is no shame in suffering from postpartum depression, which is not only common but a recognized illness.

Recovering from the baby blues

When I suffered from the baby blues, having someone to listen to my worries, give lots of reassurance, put a strong arm around me, and not tell me I was being silly made it a lot better. CH

Fortunately, I was one of the lucky moms who didn't experience postpartum baby blues, but I do believe it should be taken very seriously. It's very hard for new moms to acknowledge feelings of inadequacy or admit to feeling negative in general. Any time a new parent feels this way, they should be reassured that they are not alone, and given as much support as necessary. LJ

I had a feeling of being housebound after the birth of my second baby, which I found frustrating. There was only a small window of time in which I felt I could leave the house during those first few months, since I was staying in for feeds, meals, and naps for both children. Luckily it didn't last too long. Trying to spend an hour a day on my own really helped to lift my mood, whether it was spent going for a walk, meeting a friend, doing some exercise, or sleeping! TL

Sleep is definitely a factor in the baby blues. Although I didn't experience them, I did have wobbly moments. One day I felt like I had been breastfeeding for 24 hours straight. I expressed some milk, my husband fed the baby, I slept for six hours, and I felt like a new woman. Having a very positive, upbeat husband definitely helped, too. NK

Adapting to life as a mom

You'll soon settle into parenthood and experience the joy of caring for a child. It can take some time to find your feet, so try not to doubt yourself—if there's one thing for certain about life with a new baby, it's the fact that it is unpredictable!

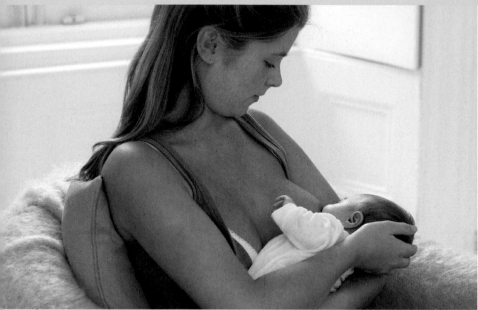

FEEDING ON DEMAND
Don't expect your newborn to feed at set times; in the early days, she will nurse almost constantly as she works to build up your milk supply to meet her needs.

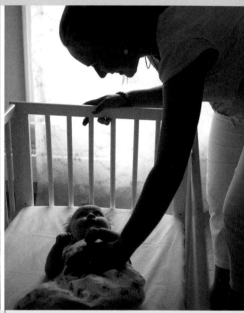

REGULAR NAPS
You will soon begin to recognize when your baby is tired. Try to put her down when she is still awake, so she learns to settle herself.

Many parenting experts would have you believe that you can "train" your baby to sleep, wake up, and feed according to a schedule—usually yours! The truth is that every baby is different, and their sleep and feeding patterns, and even their temperament, will change constantly. While there is no harm in setting up a basic routine that will help to make your baby feel secure, and possibly give you an inkling when you might have a few moments to do something else, it must be flexible, and it should be adjusted to meet your baby's needs.

Natural instincts

The single most important job of any new mother (and father) is to protect and nurture their children, keeping them safe, well nourished, clean, and comfortable. Most parents have a natural instinct, which comes to the fore once the dust settles. It is entirely normal to feel out of your depth when you have a tiny baby in your arms who refuses to settle, appears to cry for no reason, and seems impossibly fragile. It can take a few weeks to understand her cries, and to find the best ways of soothing her.

Bathing, feeding, and settling her down to sleep will soon become second nature, as you grow more confident in your role. Even then, you can expect everything to change—as she needs more frequent feeding during a growth spurt, suddenly decides that nighttime is playtime, or refuses to respond to the tricks you've used to settle her in the past.

ESTABLISHING A ROUTINE
Don't even think about routines for at least the first few weeks. You'll need time to bond and get to know each other, and your baby's own routine will eventually

"There's a big difference between strict scheduling and an elastic routine that can bring a gentle rhythm to your baby's days"

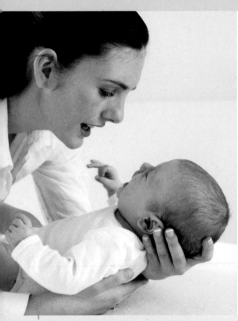

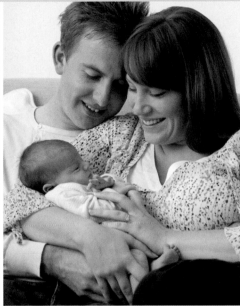

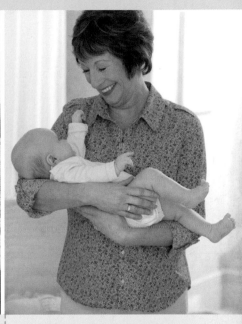

YOUR FASCINATING FACE
Your baby loves listening to you talk and watching your face. Even at this age she'll be learning the basics of communication.

YOUR NEW FAMILY
Although you can take turns caring for your baby in order to get a little rest, it is also important to spend time together as a family.

WELCOMING GRANDPARENTS
Grandparents can offer invaluable help and guidance, and create a bond with your baby that will enhance both of their lives.

begin to assert itself. Once you establish what she likes and when, and how she responds to settling down to sleep, feeding time, bathing, and diaper changes, you can build a routine of your own. Most babies respond well to routines, as they grow to learn exactly what to expect, and when. For example, even young babies get used to the idea that a nice warm bath—with a feed and a lullaby or story—is followed by snuggling down to sleep in her bed.

You'll find it much easier to encourage her to establish healthy sleep habits if you are consistent in your approach.

If you are breastfeeding on demand, there is no question of scheduling her feeds; she will need to nurse as often as possible to stimulate your milk supply and get what she needs; however, you can discourage "snacking" or comfort feeds, and make sure she empties both breasts when you settle down together.

A pattern of feeding will eventually emerge (even though it may be subject to change as she grows and develops), and you will find that her early-morning feed usually keeps her satisfied for a few hours, and that feeding her before you eat your lunch can buy you a little time

to sit down and enjoy it! Settling in a familiar chair, with her usual blanket, can lead her to associate this with feeding, and she will anticipate it and take part. She may be sleepy after a little baby massage or playtime with mom or dad, or regularly close her eyes when she's had a good feed. This in itself is the start of a routine that you can gently adjust and guide as the weeks go by.

Use a schedule as a guideline only, and don't force it. All babies have fussy days, and other days you may have activities or appointments that mean you aren't where you should be come naptime or bath time. Flexibility is fine, as long as you do things in roughly the same order, and lead up to bedtime with much the same series of events. You can start by taking a walk at roughly the same time each day, as well as playtime, reading, or singing to your baby, and her daily bath.

Trial and error

Of course, when you have a fussy baby on your hands even the most successful routine can fly out the window, and it's important to be prepared for this. Babies cry to communicate with you, and it can be difficult to figure out what they are trying to say.

Generally speaking, babies cry when hungry, uncomfortable (perhaps they are cold or too hot, or need a diaper change), tired or overstimulated, and even *under*-stimulated and in need of distraction. They may simply want to be held by mom, rather than dad, or the reverse—or want the comfort of suckling, at your breast or on a pacifier. There's no

doubt that some babies respond well to regular sucking, and will settle immediately.

About a quarter of young babies suffer from colic (see p.359), which is characterized by uncontrollable crying (often around the same time of day or night), and drawing up of their knees in clear discomfort. The cause of colic is unclear, but the good news is that most babies have outgrown it by three months.

Over time, you will begin to recognize your baby's cries—know that she is hungry or lonely, or that it's time for a nap. You'll recognize when she needs a cuddle, or even a little time on her own, to gaze quietly at her new surroundings. She may not enjoy diaper changes or baths, and you'll develop techniques to make these more fun—or get them done quickly!

Parenthood is all about adapting, using a trial-and-error approach to find out what works best for you and your baby, and being prepared for the fact that what works one day will most definitely not work on others.

Taking time out

Although it can be tempting to assume full care of your baby when you are breastfeeding—and probably spending long hours with her—it is important to take a little time off. It can be hard to relinquish control, particularly if you've established a gentle routine that works well and you know exactly how to settle her, but dad will need a chance to develop his parenting skills, too, and will enjoy the opportunity to bond, set up his own routines, and figure out the best way to meet your baby's needs. Try to set up a regular time when he can take over—perhaps taking her for a walk on Saturday mornings, bathing and reading to her in the evenings, giving the occasional bottle of expressed milk, and enjoying a regular playtime together.

Take these opportunities to do something for yourself. Try not to feel guilty about reading a book, catching up with friends, taking a long, warm bubble bath, sleeping, or even just enjoying an uninterrupted cup of coffee. There will

KEEP YOUR BABY CLOSE
Carrying your baby in a carrier means that you can do light housework without leaving him on his own.

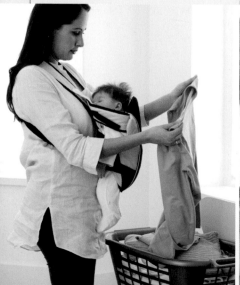

BEING SOCIABLE
Many moms find that sharing time with other new mothers is not only relaxing, but a great opportunity to swap stories and tips.

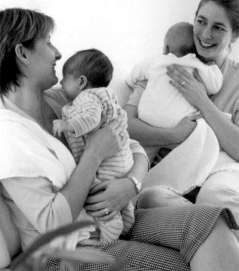

A LITTLE FRESH AIR
All babies require fresh air, and getting into the habit of taking regular walks will lift your mood and help you to regain fitness.

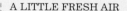
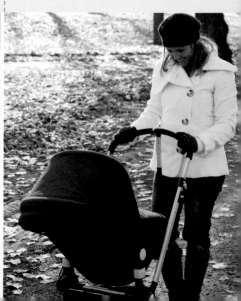

always be lots of things to catch up on around the house, but recharging your batteries is essential for your physical and emotional health, and just an hour or two being yourself again—not just a mom—can make a big difference to your energy levels, your mood, and even your relationship.

GETTING OUT AND ABOUT

It's easy to get into the habit of spending a lot of time on your own in the house, particularly if you know that your baby will sleep between certain hours. When faced with lugging a diaper bag, a stroller, car seat, and a potentially restless baby on an outing, then having to find a quiet place to feed her, it can seem much easier to stay put.

However, fresh air is good for you and your baby (and gives you both a good dose of vitamin D, when you spend some time in the sunlight), and keeping active will help you to recover from the birth much more quickly.

Moreover, spending time with friends—particularly if they have babies of the same age—can be reassuring and rewarding, and renew your sense of fun. While babies are delightful, endlessly entertaining, and completely fascinating to doting moms and dads, there is nothing like a little adult conversation to get your brain working and raise your spirits. Friends in your prenatal group can offer an opportunity to swap tips and experiences, as well as express doubts and concerns. If you haven't got a ready-made network of "baby friends," find a local La Leche League chapter, or seek out a new moms' group at your pediatrician's office or community center.

Don't hesitate to go out on your own, too. An evening with old friends may be just what you need to feel positive again. There is no reason why dad or another capable adult can't feed your baby a bottle of expressed milk, and try settling her down to sleep. This may be tricky in the first few weeks when your milk

supply is still being established, but once you are able to express, and clearly making the quantity of milk your baby needs to put on weight and remain content, you can escape on your own from time to time.

MOM TO ALL

If you have other children, it can be difficult to juggle things in the early days, and you may feel that you are spreading yourself too thin to attend to everyone's needs. Try not to be too hard on yourself. If you can negotiate a little time alone with each child and try to keep up with regular activities, such as reading together or painting, you will discourage any feelings of jealousy and reassure your children that they are very much wanted and loved. Even much older children will require time and reassurance that they are still important. Reading a book or watching a movie with them while you are nursing will be precious time, and little effort for you.

Looking after yourself

Being a new mom is wonderful, but can be exhausting and confusing as well. Don't get too anxious about all the conflicting advice. Try these tips:

• Listen to advice from other moms and helpful relatives, but make your own decisions based on your individual situation, beliefs, and needs. Don't get bullied into doing something that you aren't comfortable with, such as topping up a perfectly healthy breastfed baby with formula, or offering your contented baby a pacifier.

• The more you and your partner share your baby's day-to-day care, the closer you will feel and the more confident you will be to meet his needs. Don't leave sharing to chance; talk through the main

tasks and divide them up as much as you can. Review this division of labor often, to reduce resentment if you feel things are not even.

• Getting sleep is one of the biggest priorities for new parents, so agree to regularly take turns caring for the baby so the other parent can take a nap.

• While visitors are lovely in the early days, they can be exhausting. Try setting up a schedule, where you have one or two guests every couple of days rather than a houseful at one time.

• Visitors can also increase your baby's risk of being exposed to illness. A runny nose or cold in an adult or older child can cause fever, fussiness, and refusal to feed

in a newborn. Ask visitors to come only if they are well, and make sure that everyone who comes into contact with your baby washes their hands.

• There is no "right" way of doing things. If you focus on recommendations for health and safety, and stop worrying so much about getting things "right" in terms of spending a certain number of hours monitoring your baby's development and being a perfect parent, then you are most definitely getting it "right."

• Don't forget the importance of recharging your own batteries. It is essential that you pay attention to your own emotional and physical well-being, or the act of parenting can become a chore rather than a pleasure.

Getting back in shape

As long as your baby was delivered vaginally and you didn't experience any complications, you can begin gentle exercise shortly after the birth. While exercise can help your recovery, take things slowly and don't push yourself.

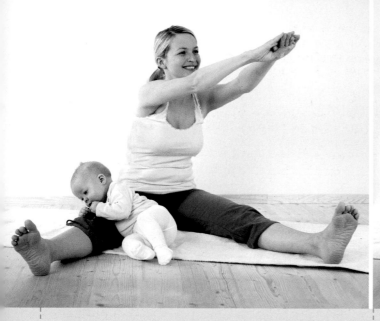

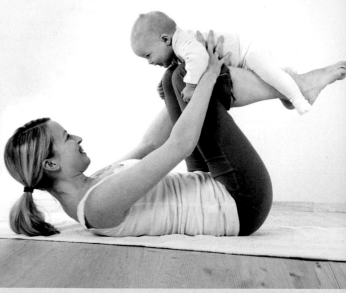

START WITH STRETCHES
Although you may not feel like exercising for at least a few weeks after the birth, some gentle stretching can help to encourage healing.

HELPING MOM EXERCISE
Include your baby in your exercise sessions; she'll think it's playtime, and you'll get a light workout, too!

Even if exercise was not a feature of your pre-pregnancy life, it's a good idea to introduce it now. Not only will you lose those pregnancy pounds more quickly, but it will encourage the release of "feel-good" hormones known as endorphins, which can make you feel more positive throughout the postpartum period and beyond. What's more, you are your baby's primary role model, and will want him to adopt a healthy, active lifestyle once he is a little older. Making exercise a part of your regular routine will create healthy habits that can last a lifetime. Go for a long stroll in the local park, or park your baby's stroller under a tree and do a little stretching. Take him to a mom-and-baby yoga class, or let him visit the gym nursery while you go for a swim or get a workout on a stationary bicycle.

Many women meet regularly in the park to power-walk with their strollers, and you may find this a sociable, fun experience. Getting in shape will help you cope better with the demands of parenthood, and keep up with your active baby when he finds his feet.

Do, however, set realistic goals. In the early weeks, sleep deprivation is likely to put a damper on your best intentions, so don't become frustrated if you find yourself with little or no extra energy. Wait until you are feeling more energetic before stepping up your expectations. There are most certainly days when plopping yourself on the sofa with your baby is all you will be able to manage.

If you had a caesarean section, you should wait until your doctor gives you the all-clear at your six-week checkup before starting to exercise.

My six-week checkup

Between six and eight weeks, your doctor will examine you to ensure that you are recovering well after the birth. This is an opportunity to bring up any concerns about your health, no matter how minor.

YOUR PHYSICAL HEALTH

Your uterus will be palpated to make sure it is firm, and that your bleeding has stopped. In some cases, women continue to experience a little light bleeding for many months; you may also have had your first period. While exclusive breastfeeding does, in many women, prevent ovulation, this is not always the case.

Your perineum or any caesarean scar will be assessed to ensure that it is healing well, and your doctor will check that your bowels and bladder are functioning normally. Your blood pressure will be taken, and if you have experienced any problems with tears or abnormal bleeding—or pain during intercourse—a vaginal examination may be required. If your stitches are still in place (these can take up to three months to dissolve in some women), they will be checked.

If you suffered from anemia during pregnancy, or are more tired than expected and exhibit signs of anemia (see p.384), a blood test may be ordered to check your hemoglobin levels. Your urine may also be tested to make sure your kidneys are working properly, and that there is no infection. Finally, if you are not immune to rubella (German measles) and were not given an immunization before you left the hospital, you will be offered one now.

YOUR EMOTIONAL HEALTH

Your doctor will discuss any concerns you have about your own health, and chat about how you are doing with breastfeeding. She'll be happy to talk through any issues relating to your baby's birth, and also ask you how you are sleeping, eating, and being supported at home. This is an important opportunity for your healthcare team to assess whether you are suffering from any signs of postpartum depression (see p.375). It's important to be honest in response to any questions asked; there is plenty of support available for women who need a little extra help in the months after their babies are born.

YOUR BABY

Your doctor will ask about feeding, and encourage you to continue breastfeeding, while offering suggestions for any problems that you might be experiencing, such as engorgement, sore nipples, or milk-supply issues.

If you have concerns about the baby, you should bring up those questions the next time you visit the pediatrician's office. However, most doctors are happy to see the babies that they delivered during the six-week checkup, so don't feel that you must leave your newborn at home, especially if you don't have a babysitter at the ready.

CONTRACEPTION

Some women become pregnant before their periods return, and a surprising number are already pregnant again by their six-week checkup. Don't leave contraception to chance! Your doctor will discuss the various options, and help you to choose a method that is most appropriate for you and your lifestyle. If you do choose to have an IUD (intra-uterine device), this may be inserted now. At the same time, a Pap smear may be taken.

The postpartum or six-week checkup marks the official end to your regularly scheduled appointments pertaining to your pregnancy—unless you have complications that need further visits. You will still have plenty of support when you need it, but the time has now come to get on with the business of being a mom!

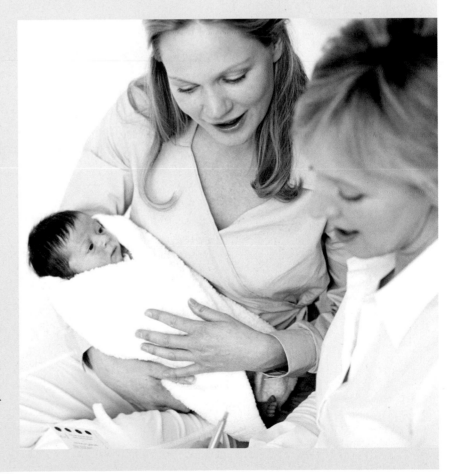

Life as a family

Although the first few weeks of family life will pass in a blur, it won't be long before you can settle into and experience the rewards of parenthood. Set up gentle routines and work on maintaining healthy habits and relationships.

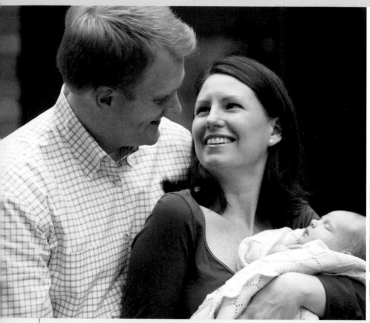

A LITTLE AFFECTION
Although physical intimacy may not interest you at the moment, comforting hugs will reassure both you and your partner how much you mean to each other.

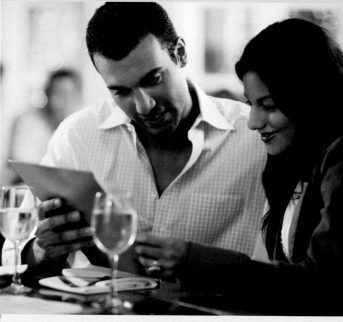

TIME ALONE
Don't underestimate the importance of spending time on your own with your partner. Schedule some regular dates and hire a responsible babysitter to help keep your relationship strong.

Working on keeping your relationship with your partner strong will help ensure that you become the best possible parents. Both of you will need support and reassurance, so try to establish healthy communication now.

Your relationship

Try to remember that your partner may be feeling equally unsettled after the labor and birth, and struggling with the demands of a new baby. Many dads, particularly when their partners are breastfeeding, feel a little left out and sometimes inadequate, when mom has clearly mastered the art of bathing and diaper-changing more quickly. Including your partner, asking his advice, giving him opportunities to be alone with your baby (not just having him thrust at him the moment he puts the key in the door), and enjoying time together as a *family* can reduce tension and resentment, and ensure that he feels involved.

Talk about your expectations and your concerns; take time to reassess your roles to ensure that there is no resentment brewing or hurt feelings. The very best parents are those who work as a team, so establishing and cementing your bond as a couple is a very important part of establishing healthy family life. With the buzz of having a newborn in the house, it can be easy to forget that couples need time alone with one another—and time off from babycare. See if you can find a willing grandparent to give you a break from time to time, to give you some space to go out for a meal or even just a long walk. It's amazing how quickly a change

"Make time for your relationship, and create regular opportunities to sort out issues as they arise, rather than bottling up resentment"

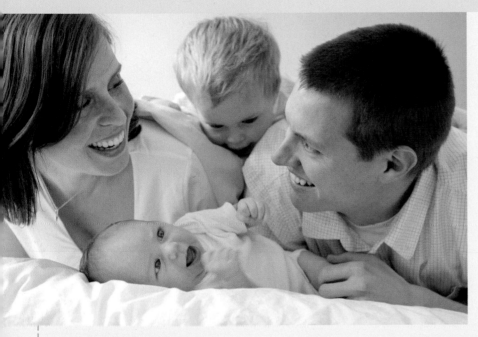

ROOM FOR EVERYBODY
A new baby will bring joy to your family, no matter what its size. Take time to relax and enjoy family life. For parents, memories of this happy time in their lives are very precious.

of scene can reinforce your relationship and help you to value each other again.

You will have many challenges in the years to come, from juggling work, finances, and family life to supporting each other through difficult times and decisions. Raising children is never easy, and you may both have very different ideas of what this entails. Working to get yourself on roughly the same page— or at least respectful of one another's views and values—can help to make the process more successful and reduce any tension.

RESUMING INTIMACY
Sex may be the last thing on your mind if you are feeling battered by the birth, and so tired that you fall asleep the moment your head hits the pillow, but intimacy is important for all relationships, and your partner may need physical reminders that you still care for him. This can take the form of cuddling up together in the evenings, or just remembering that a hug or a kiss can work wonders to reassure you both that you are still attractive, lovable people (as opposed to simply harassed parents).

When you do feel more like intimacy, you may feel a little nervous—particularly if your shape has changed dramatically or you had stitches after the birth. Be open about your feelings; you will probably find that your partner is nervous, too. Take things slowly, making sure you have plenty of foreplay to warm things up. Changing hormones may cause your vagina to become unusually dry, particularly while you are breastfeeding, so you may want to experiment with a gentle lubricant. Most importantly, don't forget about birth control (see p.381).

FAMILY LIFE
A new baby in the house can upset even the most established routines, and make your other children feel left out. Bear in mind that your newborn does have very defined needs, but as long as he's happy, clean, and well-fed, he'll be perfectly content to join in with the family.

You can encourage a healthy relationship between your children—and help your other children feel loved and wanted—by making time for them all. Try to get a little help with your baby from time to time so you can settle down to read or play with your older children, or take them out for a treat.

Try to make sure that their regular activities, such as swimming or toddler gym, continue to take place, so they don't feel disgruntled or let down. Encourage them to play a role in your baby's care, which will help them feel important and involved.

Concerns and complications

The majority of pregnancies are straightforward, with no concerns for mother or baby. For the few who do encounter a problem, expert care provides successful treatment or support to deal with ongoing conditions.

Pregnancy and labor

During pregnancy, a few women experience complications and symptoms that require additional prenatal care. Thankfully, most problems are identified and dealt with successfully.

■ ANEMIA

This occurs when you have low levels of hemoglobin, the protein in your red blood cells containing iron that carries oxygen around your body. If it is left untreated, anemia increases the risk of a premature delivery, low birth weight, and postpartum hemorrhage. Blood tests in pregnancy check your hemoglobin levels so that treatment can be given if they're low. While results may be normal early on, it is not unusual for women to develop anemia in the last two trimesters.

Iron deficiency is the main cause of anemia in pregnancy. During pregnancy, you need extra iron to cope with an increased blood volume and the demands of your growing baby and the placenta. Other less common reasons include a deficiency of folic acid or vitamin B12; inherited blood disorders such as sickle cell disease; severe pregnancy sickness; being pregnant with twins or other multiples; having babies in close succession; or a heavy menstrual flow before pregnancy. Symptoms include feeling tired, weak, and dizzy, and you may be unusually pale. You may also have palpitations, shortness of breath, irritability, and poor concentration. Many of these are common symptoms of a normal pregnancy, but it's important to report symptoms to your doctor or midwife just in case.

Treatment is usually in the form of iron supplements. However, these can cause constipation, which can be relieved by including plenty of fiber and fluid in your diet. If your anemia is mild, you may prefer to increase your iron intake through your diet (see p.49).

■ HYPEREMESIS GRAVIDARUM

While nausea and vomiting are common in pregnancy, particularly in the first 12 weeks, some women experience a severe form of sickness, known as hyperemesis gravidarum, when they are unable to keep down any food or fluid.

This condition usually causes weight loss (often more than 10 percent of body weight), dizziness, exhaustion, nutritional deficiencies (in particular iron deficiency), and dehydration. Unlike pregnancy sickness, hyperemesis gravidarum usually continues well into the second trimester, and occasionally for the entire pregnancy.

Around 2 percent of pregnant women experience this condition. The cause isn't clear, but it's thought that it is the result of hormonal and emotional changes, nutritional deficiencies, and gastrointestinal problems. Women are advised to rest, eat very small quantities of food as frequently as possible, and to keep well hydrated with sips of fluids—if necessary, rehydration fluids—throughout the day. There is good evidence that acupressure bands worn on the wrist, acupuncture treatment, and homeopathic remedies can ease symptoms. If all else fails, your doctor may recommend antinausea medication and possibly fluid replacement by intravenous drip in the hospital.

If you suffer so badly that you are unable to keep water down, you must consult your doctor.

■ CERVICAL WEAKNESS

The cervix should remain closed during pregnancy to protect your baby. However, very occasionally it painlessly shortens and opens, a condition known as a weak or incompetent cervix, or cervical insufficiency. This rare condition is usually diagnosed following one or more late miscarriages, or a stillbirth in the third trimester. The cause is thought to be a congenital weakness in the tissues of the cervix, or damage to the cervix from a previous labor or cervical surgery. When the weight of the baby and uterus presses down on the weakened cervix in the second and third trimesters, the cervix may shorten and dilate without contractions, leading to a second-trimester miscarriage, premature rupture of the membranes, or premature labor.

Risk factors for this condition include repeated terminations in early pregnancy; damage to the cervix during a surgical procedure or a previous birth; having an unusually short cervix; a previous late miscarriage; or your mother taking the drug DES (used to prevent miscarriage) when she was pregnant with you.

If a weak cervix is thought to be the cause of a previous pregnancy loss, you may be offered a cervical stitch. This is usually inserted at around 14 weeks. A stitch is placed around the cervix via the vagina, under a spinal anesthetic, with the aim of holding the cervix closed. The stitch is removed at around 37 weeks, after which you will go into labor naturally—although sometimes not for some weeks.

Some women may be offered an abdominal stitch, usually if a previous cervical stitch has been unsuccessful. This can be inserted before pregnancy or in early pregnancy. It is not usually removed, and a caesarean section is required to deliver the baby.

You may be admitted to the hospital if your cervix is found to be dilated prematurely. Your doctor may diagnose this following vaginal bleeding or excessive discharge. If you are less than 24 weeks pregnant, you may either be offered a cervical stitch, or simply recommended to rest in bed until the cervix returns to normal.

Penetrative sex should be avoided if you have a cervical stitch in place, or if your cervix is dilated.

■ OBSTETRIC CHOLESTASIS
This liver disorder affects around 1 in 140 pregnant women, and occurs when the normal flow of bile from the liver is reduced. The main symptom is severe itching all over the body in the last trimester (although it can occur sooner), which is often worse at night and particularly uncomfortable on the palms of the hands and soles of the feet. There isn't usually a rash, although scratching can cause skin inflammation. Some women also develop jaundice, recognized by yellowing of the skin and eyes, which causes you to feel unwell and affects the ability of the blood to clot.

The condition usually disappears soon after the birth, and doesn't seem to cause long-term health problems. However, it can cause complications that may affect the baby's health. These include an increased risk of premature delivery and fetal distress, as well as stillbirth. Obstetric cholestasis runs in families, and is more common in women of Scandinavian, Indian-Asian, Pakistani, or South American descent. If you've had it, there's a 60 to 90 percent chance of experiencing it in a subsequent pregnancy.

If the condition is diagnosed, usually by blood tests, you will be monitored for the remainder of your pregnancy, with more prenatal visits, ultrasounds to check your baby's growth and well-being, blood tests, and regular checks on your baby's heart rate and movements. You will be offered ointments to soothe the itching, and drugs may be prescribed to ease the itching and help your liver to work properly. You will be advised to avoid alcohol and limit fatty foods, which put pressure on the liver.

If both you and your baby are well, your pregnancy can continue to progress as normal; however, some obstetricians prefer to deliver babies early (around 37 or 38 weeks) to reduce the possibility of stillbirth. Rest is beneficial; breathing exercises can help with discomfort, and cool baths soothe itching.

■ GESTATIONAL DIABETES
Insulin is a hormone that allows your body to break down sugar in your blood to be used as energy. During pregnancy, other hormones block the usual action of insulin. As a result, your body needs to produce more insulin to cope with these changes. Gestational diabetes, which usually occurs in the second half of pregnancy, results when your body can't meet these demands. It normally disappears after the birth. If gestational diabetes isn't managed, it leads to a higher risk of preeclampsia (see p.386) and premature labor, and can result in too much amniotic fluid. You are also more likely to develop type 2 diabetes later in life. Your baby may be very large, which can lead to problems with the birth (including shoulder dystocia; see p.319), and suffer from low blood sugar (hypoglycemia) after the birth.

You are more likely to develop the condition if you have a family history of gestational diabetes; if you developed the condition in a previous pregnancy; if you have previously delivered a large baby (over 9lb/4.5kg); if you are overweight or obese; or if you have polycystic ovary syndrome (PCOS).

There are rarely any symptoms, so your urine will be checked for sugar content at each prenatal appointment. If you are considered to be high risk, a glucose tolerance test (GTT) will be arranged. This involves drinking a glucose solution, and then having the sugar levels in your blood measured at intervals to see how your body deals with it. In some practices, all pregnant women are given a precautionary GTT.

If you develop gestational diabetes, you will be advised to eat more slow-release carbohydrates, plenty of fruit, vegetables, and lean protein, and reduced levels of refined or sugary foods. Exercise is also recommended to help reduce blood-sugar levels. Some women require insulin injections or tablets.

It is recommended that you breastfeed your baby within 30 minutes of the birth to keep his blood-sugar levels stable, or he may require a glucose solution by intravenous drip. He is also at a higher risk of jaundice (see p.389), respiratory distress syndrome, and birth defects.

For this reason, it is important that gestational diabetes is diagnosed and treated properly—in which case the outlook for you and your baby is good.

■ PLACENTAL INSUFFICIENCY

In some cases, the placenta does not implant deeply enough into the uterus to provide the baby with sufficient oxygen and nutrients. This is more likely if you suffer from diabetes, kidney problems, blood-clotting disorders, or high blood pressure; if you smoke, drink too much alcohol, or take drugs; or if you are poorly nourished.

Placental insufficiency affects 3–5 percent of pregnancies, and is usually spotted if the uterus seems smaller than expected or the baby's movements become less frequent.

If placental insufficiency is suspected, an ultrasound will be arranged to measure the baby's growth, with a Doppler scan to assess the blood flow to the baby. The management of placental insufficiency depends on the severity and the gestation of the pregnancy. A balance needs to be struck between the risks of premature birth and the risks if the pregnancy continues.

If delivery is not required immediately, regular ultrasounds and sometimes electronic fetal monitoring will be arranged, in an attempt to establish the best time for your baby to be delivered. If this is calculated to be before 34 weeks, you will be given steroid injections to help your baby's lungs to mature before the delivery.

■ BLEEDING IN LATE PREGNANCY

This is a symptom that cannot be ignored, especially in the latter stages of pregnancy. It may be caused by something harmless, such as changes in the cervix, which won't affect your pregnancy or your baby; it may indicate a potential problem requiring urgent medical assistance; or it can be one of the signs that labor is imminent—particularly if there is mucus in the blood, known as a "bloody show" (see p.277). Bleeding may be caused if the placenta separates from the uterus. This is known as "abruption," and usually causes bleeding associated with pain, which may be very severe. An abruption can risk the life of the mother and her baby, so urgent delivery is needed. This is often done by caesarean section, but a vaginal delivery may be possible.

Bleeding due to placenta previa, or low-lying placenta (see below), is usually painless but, like abruption, placenta previa can require immediate delivery by caesarean section. However, if mother and baby appear to be well following a bleed associated with placenta previa, bed rest and close monitoring will be recommended instead.

If you experience bleeding during pregnancy, you will probably be advised to stay in the hospital for at least 24 hours. It is common for the bleeding to stop without any cause being identified.

■ PLACENTA PREVIA

In early pregnancy, the placenta usually lies low in the uterus; as your uterus grows, the placenta is usually pulled upward, and away from the cervix. In some cases, however, it does not move up, and fully or partially covers the cervix. This is known as placenta previa, a condition which occurs in about 1 in 200 full-term pregnancies.

Placenta previa is more common in women who have an abnormally shaped uterus or placenta (including a large placenta); women who've had several previous pregnancies; in multiple pregnancies; or if there is scarring on the wall of the uterus. It also appears to be more common in women who smoke or have their first babies after the age of 35.

Most cases are picked up during routine ultrasounds, and if there is concern that your placenta is low-lying, you may have more ultrasounds than usual. Symptoms include sudden, painless bleeding in the second or third trimester, with or without cramping. If there is a great deal of bleeding, you may be admitted to the hospital for monitoring, and blood transfusions may be necessary. If bleeding is not profuse, you will need to remain in bed and reduce all activities until your baby is born. A caesarean will be recommended at around 39 weeks if even part of the cervix is covered by the placenta. If there is heavy bleeding, an emergency caesarean may be necessary.

There is no way to prevent placenta previa, but you can reduce the risks by reporting any bleeding quickly.

■ PREECLAMPSIA

Between 2 and 8 percent of all pregnant women develop preeclampsia, which is a potentially life-threatening condition occurring only in pregnancy, and usually after the 20th week. It causes high blood pressure, and results in protein leaking from your kidneys into your urine. The condition can cause growth problems in your unborn baby (intra-uterine growth restriction; see p.388) and put your own health at risk if left unmanaged.

Preeclampsia is associated with eclampsia, a serious illness affecting the membranes of your brain, leading to seizures and convulsions. It can also cause liver and kidney disorders, and fluid in the lungs (pulmonary edema).

Apart from raised blood pressure and protein in your urine, symptoms can include sudden, severe swelling of your face, hands, or feet; severe headaches; problems with vision (including blurring or flashing before your eyes); severe pain below the ribs; and general malaise.

You will be monitored with regular blood-pressure and urine checks, and ultrasounds to measure the growth of your baby and the flow of blood from your placenta to the baby. If all is well, the pregnancy can proceed as normal, although you will need more frequent prenatal checkups. Rest is recommended, and medication may be offered to bring down your blood pressure. If your preeclampsia is severe, you will have to stay in the hospital until the end of your pregnancy, and both you and your baby will have regular monitoring to ensure that your blood pressure is under control and you do not develop complications. The only "cure" for preeclampsia is delivering the baby, so this may be recommended even if your baby is premature. You may be given magnesium sulphate to prevent eclampsia.

■ SYMPHYSIS PUBIS DYSFUNCTION (SPD)

Pain in the pelvic joints is thought to be caused by a slight misalignment of the joints and is also referred to as pelvic girdle pain (PGP). It affects about 1 in 4 pregnant women to varying degrees, with 7 percent of sufferers continuing to experience symptoms after the birth.

SPD normally occurs from the second trimester of pregnancy, but can happen at any stage. Symptoms include pain in the pubic area, groin, the inside of your thighs, and sometimes in your lower back and hips. You may hear a clicking sound when you walk, and feel as though your bones are grinding together. It can be hard to open your legs, which is why it's important to be diagnosed before labor, when the pubic bones will be under extra strain. Treatment involves wearing a pelvic support garment—like a girdle that fits under your bump—and using crutches if walking is difficult. You may be referred to a physiotherapist, who can give you gentle exercises to help strengthen the muscles around the joint, and offer advice about posture and

activities. Anti-inflammatory medication isn't recommended in pregnancy, which can make the condition difficult to manage. However, acetaminophen can ease the pain, and chiropractic and osteopathy can be helpful. It normally takes between three and six months to recover fully after the birth; however, if the problem continues, you may need to consider corrective surgery.

Rest as often as you can, and avoid lifting and carrying, walking long distances, and even climbing stairs. Inform your doctor, so that she can refer you for treatment, and measure how far you can comfortably open your legs in labor so that she can record this in your file. A caesarean may be recommended.

After the birth

■ MASTITIS

This is an inflammation of the breast tissue, normally caused by an infection, or by blocked ducts and engorgement. If an infection is the cause, your breast may become red, hot, swollen, and release pus from the nipple. You may also experience a fever, shivering, muscular aches and pains, and nausea and vomiting. In the case of engorgement, your breasts may become red, swollen, lumpy, and very sore, with ducts full of milk appearing as hard threads along the surface. Blocked ducts result in tender, hard lumps where milk has not emptied from the breast.

It is safe to breastfeed your baby, even if you have an infection. In fact, regular feeding will encourage the flow of milk and reduce swelling. If you do have an infection, antibiotics will be prescribed. Expressing a little milk, while pressing on areas that are sore and hard, can bring relief. Alternate cool and hot compresses on the affected area to reduce inflammation and pain, and to promote milk flow. Placing cold cabbage

leaves in your bra can be soothing. You can help prevent mastitis by ensuring that your baby feeds from both breasts and empties them fully, and that she is correctly latched on (see p.344).

■ BLADDER PROBLEMS

Some temporary incontinence (leaking of urine) is normal after the birth. Not only are your pelvic floor muscles weakened by pregnancy and birth, but the weight of your baby pressing down on the bladder and urethra (which carries urine from your bladder out of your body) may have caused minor damage to the nerves that affect bladder control.

If you had an episiotomy or a difficult birth (for example, with forceps), the area may be bruised and/or swollen, making urination uncomfortable.

The good news is that problems are almost always resolved within six weeks. The best thing you can do is drink plenty of water, and practice your pelvic floor exercises (see p.67) to regain strength and control. In the short term, wearing sanitary napkins can help you feel less self-conscious. If things don't improve after six weeks, talk to your doctor, who can refer you to a specialist.

■ PUERPERAL PSYCHOSIS

This is a very severe form of postpartum depression, also known as postpartum psychosis, which occurs in about 1 in 1,000 women. It is a severe disorder in which sufferers lose touch with reality, experiencing delusions, hallucinations, confusion, and, sometimes, rigidity or extreme flexibility of the limbs.

The cause is largely unknown, but it is more common in women who have had a depressive illness in the past, including postpartum depression. It is usually partners, family, or friends who seek help, because sufferers lose a sense of what is real. Treatment is essential to prevent harm to mother and baby, and may involve a stay in the hospital and antipsychotic medication. In most cases, the condition improves within weeks, but counseling may be required for several months to resolve any issues and monitor the mother's emotional health.

■ PERINEAL PROBLEMS

The perineum is the area between your vagina and anus, which is stretched—and sometimes torn or cut—during the birth of your baby. If you had a vaginal birth, you are likely to experience some discomfort and swelling afterward, even if there are no visible signs of damage. The discomfort is usually worst two days after the birth, then in most cases it becomes gradually less painful, and by ten days, you should feel back to normal. However, it can take up to six months if you have had severe tearing or an episiotomy (see p.311). After the birth, your doctor will check the area to see how it is healing. If pain worsens, or there is any foul-smelling discharge, swelling, or tenderness in the area, or you feel unwell, call your doctor. If an infection is diagnosed, you will be prescribed antibiotics, and will need to take special care to keep the area clean.

If the area is not infected, use a cold gel pack (or ice pack), to relieve pain and reduce swelling. Change pads frequently to keep the area dry, and rinse it often with cooled boiled water, patting it dry with a soft towel.

Problems in babies

Some conditions affecting your baby's health can be identified—and even treated—in pregnancy. In other cases, a problem may be discovered after the birth, and your baby will be referred to a pediatrician for diagnosis and treatment.

■ INTRA-UTERINE GROWTH RESTRICTION (IUGR)

This refers to the poor growth of your baby in the uterus. Causes include placental problems, preeclampsia, infections (such as rubella), high blood pressure, and heart disease. Your baby's size will be monitored during pregnancy to assess whether IUGR is likely to cause complications during or after the birth.

■ DOWN SYNDROME

This is a chromosomal abnormality that affects around 1 in every 1,000 babies. Babies born with this syndrome have one more chromosome than normal (47 instead of 46), which produces some characteristic features, including floppy muscle tone at birth, upward-slanting eyes, a single skin crease running across the palms, and a flatter back of the head. Babies with Down syndrome are more likely to have developmental delays, learning disorders, and heart problems.

Down syndrome is more common in babies born to older moms. Prenatal screening identifies your risk (see pp.116–117), and some women choose to terminate the pregnancy if a diagnostic test indicates that their baby is affected.

If you have given birth to a baby with Down syndrome, you will be given support from the hospital team and advice on how to stay on top of potential health problems, breastfeed successfully, and understand the care that may be required over the coming years. The level of developmental and learning problems varies from child to child, and some require special education. Babies with Down syndrome need regular checkups to watch for common complications. These can include thyroid disorders; sleep apnea; eye, heart, and hearing problems; and gastrointestinal blockages.

■ TALIPES

This is a deformity of the foot in which one or both feet are twisted out of shape or into the wrong position. There are two types: *talipes equinovarus*, also called club foot, where the foot turns inward; and *talipes calcaneovalgus*, where the foot is turned outward. In about half of all cases, only one foot is affected. The condition usually results from the foot being compressed in the uterus, often because of the baby's position. It is also associated with a shortage of amniotic fluid around the baby—known as oligohydramnios—possibly because of increased pressure on the foot.

About 1 in 1,000 babies is born with talipes. It is twice as common in boys and appears to run in families. It is often picked up at the 20-week ultrasound (see p.120), but many cases are not recognized until after the birth, and X-rays are required to confirm the condition.

In mild cases, no treatment may be needed, although exercises may be recommended to help the foot realign. This is usually the case if the condition was caused by the baby's position in the uterus. If talipes is caused by a more complex structural problem, prompt treatment is necessary to manipulate the foot while the tissues are still soft. Braces, manipulation, strapping, and casts may be used over several months. Sometimes babies also need splints to hold their feet in place at night. If manipulation isn't effective, surgery may be required at around six months of age. The prognosis, however, is very good.

■ CLEFT LIP AND PALATE

A cleft is a split in the upper lip (cleft lip) and/or palate (cleft palate), which occurs when the face does not join together properly during pregnancy. Some babies are born with one cleft, while others have both. One in every 700 babies is born with a cleft, which may be caused by genetic or environmental factors, such as smoking, alcohol, obesity, poor diet, and taking certain medications during pregnancy.

You may need some help getting breastfeeding established. Breastfeeding may be challenging, but it can be done, and it is highly recommended. A special feeding plate can be inserted into the roof of your baby's mouth to encourage successful nursing.

The clefts can be repaired using surgery when your baby is a little older— usually after weaning onto solid foods. Until that time, a special orthopedic plate may be used to apply pressure to close and align the cleft before the operation.

■ CONGENITAL HEART DISEASE

This is a general term that is used to refer to birth defects that affect your baby's heart. Congenital heart disease is the most common type of birth defect, affecting 6 out of every 1,000 babies. There are over 30 different types of defect, and they are broken into two main types: cyanotic heart disease, where problems with the heart mean that there is not enough oxygen present in the blood; and acyanotic heart disease, where the blood contains enough oxygen, but there are problems with the way it is pumped around the body.

Congenital heart disease sometimes develops as the result of a genetic condition, such as Down syndrome, or an infection, such as rubella; sometimes there is no clear cause. Some cases are picked up at the 20-week ultrasound; others are not evident until after the birth. For example, babies born with cyanotic heart disease usually have bluish extremities caused by a lack of oxygen. Babies born with acyanotic heart disease don't always have such obvious symptoms, but may have high blood pressure, which weakens the heart muscle, and may experience breathing problems over time.

In most cases, the outlook for babies with congenital heart disease is good, and because heart surgery is now so advanced, at least 85 percent of children will live well into adulthood.

■ UNDESCENDED TESTES

Normally, the testes (testicles) develop inside your baby's abdomen, dropping into his scrotum during the second half of pregnancy. If the testicles haven't descended by the time your baby is born, he is probably suffering from undescended testes (where they stay in the groin), retractile testes (where they move back and forth between the scrotum and the groin), or ascended testes (where previously descended testicles migrate back to the groin).

Testicles sometimes descend naturally in the first 12 months after the birth. It's important to monitor the condition, because testicles that remain in the groin lose their ability to produce sperm, and have an increased risk of developing cancer. If testicles fail to descend, your baby will need an operation, usually carried out before the age of two. This involves making a small incision in the groin, under local anesthetic, and carefully freeing the testicle from the surrounding tissues. The testicle is repositioned via a second incision. There are few complications, and the operation is usually successful.

■ SPOTS AND RASHES

Many newborns develop tiny white spots across the nose, cheeks, chin, forehead, and around the eyes, known as "milia," or milk spots. These appear because the oil glands on the face are still developing, and usually clear up within six weeks. Little red spots and mild rashes are also common in babies, and are normally the result of your hormones still circulating in your baby's body. If the spots appear to cause discomfort, see your doctor to

eliminate the slim chance that he has infant eczema. This can be related to foods in your diet if he's breastfed, his formula if he is bottle-fed, or something environmental, such as laundry detergent. Any rash accompanied by a fever should be assessed by a doctor immediately.

■ SLOW WEIGHT GAIN

There are a few reasons why your pediatrician may be concerned about your baby's weight gain. These include: if your baby does not gain at least .5oz (15g) per day from five days after his birth; he does not regain his birth weight by two or three weeks after the birth; he does not gain at least 1lb (450g) a month for the first four months; or there is a dramatic drop in his rate of growth, as shown on his growth chart.

Most babies lose weight in the first few days after the birth, so try not to panic. Some babies are also slow-gainers, who continue to gain weight steadily, but a little more slowly than other babies. If there are any concerns, your pediatrician will check that your baby is thriving—in other words, that he has plenty of wet and soiled diapers each day, is a good color, is alert when he is awake, and is sleeping well.

■ JAUNDICE

This is caused by a build-up of a pigment known as "bilirubin" in your baby's blood. Bilirubin is a natural by-product of red blood cells, and is usually recycled and cleaned from the blood by the liver. Jaundice results in the skin and the whites of the eyes taking on a yellow hue. About 65 percent of newborns suffer from jaundice, usually because their livers are immature and can't cope with the demands placed on them. This type of neonatal jaundice normally settles as the liver kicks into action, and often disappears by about 10 days after birth.

Other, less common causes of jaundice include: infections, illness, problems with the blood or the thyroid hormones, and genetic conditions.

If bilirubin levels remain high, treatment involves placing your baby under a special blue light, or wrapping him in a light-emitting blanket for a few days, known as phototherapy, to help break down the excess bilirubin. Most babies also need to increase their fluid intake, which can mean plenty of suckling at the breast, and sometimes being given sterilized water to prevent dehydration. Fluids encourage the action of the liver and help to ensure the excretion of bilirubin. Making sure your baby gets plenty of natural light can also help. Sometimes babies will not respond as expected, and then other causes for jaundice will be examined, but this is far from the norm. Rarely, if the levels of bilirubin are very high, your baby may need to have an "exchange" transfusion, which involves taking away some of his blood and replacing it with a blood transfusion.

The condition is usually easily treated or resolves itself naturally, and your baby should be better within a few days. It is important, however, that you agree to treatment if it's suggested, since high levels of bilirubin remaining in the blood can cause brain damage. Treatment will not hurt or distress your baby; because jaundiced babies tend to be sleepier than normal—one reason why it is important to rectify the condition at a time when feeding patterns are being established— he probably won't even notice.

ACID REFLUX

All babies spit up a little milk after a feed. However, some babies have a more severe condition known as acid reflux or gastroesophageal reflux disease (GERD). This is usually the result of a weak or immature lower esophageal sphincter— the valve between the esophagus (the tube leading from the throat to the stomach) and the stomach. This valve stops food from being regurgitated; however, in babies, particularly between one and four months, milk easily bypasses this valve, particularly when your baby is lying down. In almost all cases it resolves itself by 18 months and doesn't harm your baby. However, if your baby brings up a large percentage of his milk, is not putting on weight, seems listless and tired, and is distressed by the vomiting, talk to his pediatrician.

In its more severe form, reflux can be painful, like adult heartburn, as stomach acids leak up to your baby's esophagus and cause inflammation. This can be difficult to diagnose, because babies don't always regurgitate the milk; the milk or stomach acid moves only as far as the esophagus or throat. Your baby may cry during or after a feed, pull away from the breast or bottle, and arch his back and become rigid. If your baby seems to be experiencing pain after or during his feeds, see your doctor. And if vomiting is excessive and causing distress, this should be investigated.

If you are bottle-feeding, there are special formulas designed to stay down. There are also substances that can be added to your baby's regular formula to thicken the milk, which makes it less likely to be regurgitated.

If reflux causes pain, an antacid may be offered to ease the inflammation and reduce stomach acid. If the reflux continues once you have weaned your baby, take care to avoid foods that are acidic, such as citrus fruit and tomatoes.

Your baby may feel better if he is on his tummy, supervised, during the day. Holding him across your forearm so that there is pressure on his tummy can also ease the discomfort. However you choose to ease the condition, your baby should see a doctor to be properly treated.

PYLORIC STENOSIS

This is another feeding problem that also involves vomiting after feeds. It occurs in about 3 out of every 1,000 babies, affecting boys more often than girls.

Pyloric stenosis literally means a narrowed outlet of the stomach, where it meets the small intestine. When your baby feeds, his milk passes through his esophagus then into his stomach, where it is mixed with acid and partially digested. From here, it travels to the small intestine to be fully digested and absorbed by his body. When the pylorus (the stomach outlet) is narrowed, this process cannot be completed efficiently, and milk stays in his stomach longer, becoming more acidic and causing pain. This in turn means that your baby will not get adequate nutrients from his feeds, because the milk is not absorbed properly. If left untreated, pyloric stenosis can be serious.

Symptoms normally begin between two and four weeks, although they can appear after two months. Vomiting after a feed is the main symptom, which may be just a dribble at first—or more forceful, known as "projectile" vomiting—and the milk may appear curdled. Your baby may feed well but continue to be hungry, since he loses most of his feeds through vomiting.

The pylorus tends to become narrower over time, which means that little or no food reaches the bowels, and bowel movements gradually reduce. Affected babies do not gain weight and are in danger of quickly becoming dehydrated.

The condition is treated with a small operation, known as a "pyloromyotomy," for which your baby will need a general anesthetic. Surgery is normally undertaken by keyhole, which involves making only a tiny incision. In almost all cases, the operation is successful, and babies usually recover very quickly and experience no further problems.

Resources

Whether you are seeking information about your maternity rights, or have a specific concern about yourself or your baby, there are plenty of organizations and helplines designed to answer your queries and offer support and advice.

FERTILITY

Assisted Human Reproduction Canada
Information about assisted reproduction.
www.ahrc-pac.gc.ca
(866) 467-1853

Canadian Federation for Sexual Health
Information about sexual and reproductive health.
www.cfsh.ca
(613) 241-4474

Infertility Awareness Association of Canada
Information, support, and assistance for people experiencing infertility issues.
www.iaac.ca
(800) 263-2929

My Fertility
Information about fertility, testing and diagnosis, and therapy options.
www.myfertility.ca
(514) 426-7300

PREGNANCY

Babycenter Canada
Information on conception, pregnancy, and birth; free e-newsletters and forums.
www.babycenter.ca

Canada Prenatal Nutrition Program
Promoting the health and well-being of pregnant women, new mothers, and babies facing challenging life circumstances.
www.phac-aspc.gc.ca/hp-ps/dca-dea/
    prog-ini/cpnp-pcnp/index-eng.php

The Childbirth Experience
Services and resources for families involved in higher-risk pregnancies.
www.childbirthexperience.ca

Healthy Pregnancy
Downloadable guide to making healthy choices during pregnancy.
http://www.healthycanadians.gc.ca/init/
    kids-enfants/pregnancy-grossesse/
    index-eng.php

Motherisk
Information on the safety of medications, infections, chemicals, personal products and everyday exposures during pregnancy and breastfeeding.
www.motherisk.org
(416) 813-6780

Preeclampsia Foundation
Information and support on preeclampsia.
www.preeclampsia.org
(321) 421-6957

Prenatal Nutrition—Health Canada
Guide to healthy eating during pregnancy.
www.hc-sc.gc.ca/fn-an/nutrition/
    prenatal/index-eng.php

Society of Obstetricians and Gynaecologists of Canada
Information on women's health and pregnancy.
www.sogc.org
(613) 730-4192 / (800) 561-2416

Women's Health Matters
Information on women's health issues.
www.womenshealthmatters.ca

LABOR AND BIRTH

Canadian Association of Midwives
Help with finding a midwife in your area.
www.canadianmidwives.org
(514) 807-3668

Childbirth and Postpartum Professional Association
Find childbirth educators, lactation consultants, and doulas in your area.
www.cappacanada.ca
(866) 236-2478

Doulas of North America
Find a doula in your area.
www.dona.org
(888) 788-3662

Lamaze International
Information about the Lamaze approach to pregnancy and birth.
www.lamaze.org
(202) 367-1128

Mama Goddess Birth Shop
Supplies for home or water births.
www.mamagoddessbirthshop.ca
(604) 340-2452

Multiple Births Canada
Support for parents who are expecting multiples.
www.multiplebirthscanada.org
(866) 228-8824

BREASTFEEDING

International Lactation Consultant Association
Find a lactation consultant in your area.
www.ilca.org
(919) 861-5577

La Leche League Canada
Support for breastfeeding moms.
www.lllc.ca
(613) 774-4900

SUPPORT GROUPS

Allergy Asthma Information Association
www.aaia.ca
(416) 621-4571 / (800) 611-7011

Autism Society Canada
www.autismsocietycanada.ca
(613) 789-8943 / (866) 476-8440

Canadian Cystic Fibrosis Foundation
www.cysticfibrosis.ca
(416) 485-9149 / (800) 378-2233

Canadian Diabetes Association
www.diabetes.ca
(416) 363-3373 / (800) 226-8464

Canadian Down Syndrome Society
www.cdss.ca
(800) 883-5608

Canadian Foundation for the Study of Sudden Infant Death
www.sidscanada.org
(905) 688-8884 / (800) 363-7437

Canadian Mental Health Association
Information on postpartum depression.
www.cmha.ca/bins/content_page.
asp?cid=3-86-87-88

Compassionate Friends of Canada
Support for bereaved parents.
tcfcanada.net
(866) 823-0141

Spina Bifida and Hydrocephalus Association of Canada
www.sbhac.ca
(204) 925-3650 / (800) 565-9488

RIGHTS AND BENEFITS

Canada Child Tax Benefit
www.servicecanada.gc.ca/eng/goc/cctb.
shtml

Child Disability Benefit
www.servicecanada.gc.ca/eng/goc/cdb.
shtml

Employment Insurance Family Supplement
www.servicecanada.gc.ca/eng/sc/ei/
family/familysupplement.shtml

Employment Insurance—Maternity and Parental Benefits
www.servicecanada.gc.ca/eng/sc/ei/
benefits/maternityparental.shtml

Quebec Parental Insurance Plan
www.rqap.gouv.qc.ca/index_en.asp

Registered Education Savings Plan
www.servicecanada.gc.ca/eng/goc/resp.
shtml

Universal Child Care Benefit
www.servicecanada.gc.ca/eng/goc/
universal_child_care.shtml

PARENTING

Canadian Association of Family Resource Programs
Provides resources for families and others who care for children.
www.frp.ca
(613) 237-7667 / (866) 637-7226

Invest In Kids
Resources for parents on healthy child development.
fnih.investinkids.ca
(416) 977-1222 / (877) 583-5437

SAFETY

Canadian Red Cross
Health, safety, and first aid information.
www.redcross.ca

Safe Kids Canada
Information and resources about child safety at home and elsewhere.
www.safekidscanada.ca
(888) 723-3847

Workplace Health and Safety for Pregnancy
www.hc-sc.gc.ca/ewh-semt/occup-
travail/whmis-simdut/reproductive-
reproduction-eng.php

GENERAL

AboutKidsHealth
Trusted answers from The Hospital for Sick Children
www.aboutkidshealth.ca

Caring for Kids
Children's health information from the Canadian Paediatric Society
www.caringforkids.cps.ca
(613) 526-9397

College of Family Physicians of Canada
Resources to find a family doctor.
www.cfpc.ca
(905) 629-0900 / (800) 387-6197

Index

Acknowledgments

Contributors' acknowledgments

General Editor: Dr. Virginia Beckett
I would like to thank Peggy Vance at Dorling Kindersley for inviting me to contribute to this project. Her team has been a pleasure to work with. Special thanks to Emma Maule for her gentle encouragement with deadlines!

It is a huge privilege to work in my specialty, caring for women and their families at such pivotal times in their lives. I owe a huge debt of gratitude to my colleagues and my patients who have taught me so much. I continue to learn every day. My parents have encouraged me since I announced my intention to become a doctor at the age of nine. Without their continued support, I would not be able to combine my busy working and home lives. I really do try not to "do too much," Mom!

Finally, "Team Beckett"—Conrad, Rowan, and Lydia. You are my sunshine.

Dr. Moneli Golara
I would like to thank my husband Carlo and my children Emilio and Arianna for their patience during many hours of writing. A special thanks to Karen Sullivan, Emma Maule, Mandy Lebentz, and everyone else at Dorling Kindersley.

Dr. Claire Halsey
I would like to acknowledge the loving support of my family, especially my husband Michael and my three boys, Rupert, Toby, and Dominic. Thanks also to Vicki McIvor and, as ever, it has been a pleasure to work closely with Karen Sullivan and all at DK.

Tara Lee
I would like to thank my husband for his continued support and encouragement through all my work, and to my children for being a constant source of inspiration. They continually teach me new ways of seeing, being, and loving.

I would also like to thank all my teachers and students for guiding me along this path. Thanks also to Kerry who modeled for the yoga pictures in this book, pregnant with her fourth child, and who has taken my yoga classes through each pregnancy since the first one and recently become a pregnancy yoga teacher herself.

Nikki Khan
I would like to thank DK for giving me the opportunity to contribute to this book, but most of all would like to thank my wonderful husband, Haroon, and my daughter, Nadia, for their patience and support during the long hours of writing and for keeping me going as deadlines have approached! I would also like to give a special "thank you" to Karen Sullivan for all her awesome encouragement and guidance! Thanks must also go to my own midwife, Elaine Bowden, who brought Nadia safely into this world and whom I shall never forget! On a final note I would like to thank my late mother (also a midwife!) who gave me the insight to take my chosen career path and the belief to reach for your dreams.

Publisher's acknowledgments:

Indexer Susan Bosanko
Proofreader Angela Baynham
Editorial assistance Andrea Bagg, Judy Barratt, Susannah Marriott
Illustration assistance Debbie and Phil Maizels
Design assistance Charlotte Johnson
Hair and make-up stylist for photography Victoria Barnes
Photographer's assistants Issy Oakes, Sophie Gordon
House location agency for photography 1st Option
Picture research Liz Moore

The publisher would like thank: Jo Godfrey Wood for her assistance at photo shoots; Beautiful Bumps model agency for all their help on this book; midwife Lorraine Gallagher for attending photo shoots and advising so efficiently and enthusiastically, and the following models: Alex and Vivienne Baye; Ila and Blake Beaumont; Kerri Beaumont; Karen Billington and Tim and Finley Barton-Knott; Elena and Luca Bishton; Carly and Finley Blaszczyk; Sebastian Blaza; Nadia Bonomally; Alice Bowden; Chloe Bromley; Lucie Brow; Joannes and Louise Buckens; Mia Carvana; Gill Clarke; Helen, Terry, and Amber Crabb; Smita Crow; Fiona and Quincy Forson; Jimmy Froud and Gemma Sampson; Lorraine Gallagher; Adam Gardner; Susie and Poppy Howe; Cameron and Lanalily Leigh; Bea and Alex Lemos; Juliette Livesey and Rafael Livesey-Howe; Max Mawby; Sanyogita Mayer; Natalia Mikhaylova; Antonia and Troy Miller; Louise Morris and Emily Chapman; Poppy Newdick; Amie Niland; Emily, Matt, and Fraser Norris; Suzy Richards and Maximilian Snead; Katie Roberts; Randa Shebly; Mark Sophoeleous and Chloe Webb; Eve Spaughton; Chloe Stickland; Ashley and Poppy Dainty Streeter; Danielle and Montague Threadgold; Jenny Tollady; Monica Tong; Ben Tully.

Picture credits:

The publisher would like to thank the following for their kind permission to reproduce their photographs:

(Key: a-above; b-below/bottom; c-center; f-far; l-left; r-right; t-top)

18 Getty Images: Jamie Grill / Iconica (l). 21 Photolibrary: age fotostock. 22 Alamy Images: Pilchards (c). Getty Images: Blend Images (l). 23 Getty Images: Science Pictures Ltd (br). 24 Alamy Images: Peter Widmann (r). Corbis: Bob Thomas (l). 26 Science Photo Library: Steve Gschmeissner (l); Professors P.M. Motta & J. Van Blerkom (r). 28 Getty Images: Juan Silva (l). 30 Corbis: Clouds Hill Imaging Ltd (l). Science Photo Library: Eye of Science (r); D. Phillips (c). 31 Science Photo Library: Hybrid Medical Animation (r); Dr. Yorgos Nikas (l, c). 36 Alamy Images: Cultura . 38 Getty Images: Mike Harrington (l); Tetra Images (r). 40 Science Photo Library: Colin Cuthbert (l); John Mclean (l); Mauro Fermariello (c). 41 Science Photo Library: Mauro Fermariello. 44 Science Photo Library: Brian Evans (l). 49 Getty Images: Blend Images. 51 Getty Images: Leigh Beisch (c). 52 Alamy Images: WoodyStock (l). Getty Images: Brian Hagiwara (c). 54 Getty Images: Brian Leatart (r); UpperCut Images (l). 59 Mother & Baby Picture Library: Dave J. Anthony. 60 Getty Images: Stuart O'Sullivan (l). 62 Getty Images: Tracy Frankel. 63 Corbis: Mango Productions (l). 68 Alamy Images: Stock Connection Distribution (c). 69 Getty Images: Bambu Productions (r). 80 Getty Images: Stockbyte / George Doyle (r). 81 Getty Images: Jerome Tisne (r). 82 Alamy Images: Agencja FREE (l). 84 Getty Images: LWA / Larry Williams (l); Smith Collection (r). 88 Getty Images: Superstudio (r). Masterfile: Jerzyworks (l). 89 Getty Images: John Kelly. 90 Getty Images: Sam Edwards (r); Jamie Grill / Iconica (l). 92 Getty Images: Jutta Klee (l). Mother & Baby Picture Library: Ian Hooton (r). 94 Photolibrary: Steve Hix. 100 Getty Images: Dylan Ellis (l). 102-103 Photolibrary: Stockbroker. 104 Getty Images: Ian Hooton / Science Photo Library (r). Science Photo Library: Ian Hooton (c). 106 Corbis: Michael Keller (r). Getty Images: Image Source (l). 110 Getty Images: Ian Hooton / Science Photo Library (r). Science Photo Library: Ian Hooton (l). 112 Getty Images: Ian Hooton / Science Photo Library. 113 LOGIQlibrary: (r). Science Photo Library: P. Saada / Eurelios (l). 114 Dr Pranav P Pandya: (l, r). 115 Mother & Baby Picture Library: Ian Hooton. 116 Science Photo Library: BSIP, ASTIER (l). 118 Alamy Images: Craig Holmes Premium. 119 Science Photo Library: GE Medical Systems. 120 Science Photo Library: Living Art Enterprises, LCC (l, r). 121 Science Photo Library: Dr. Najeeb Layyous (r); Living Art Enterprises, LCC (l, c). 122 Getty Images: Steve Allen (l). Science Photo Library: Dr. Najeeb Layyous (r). 124 Photolibrary: Stockbroker (l). 126 Science Photo Library: Ian Hooton. 128 Mother & Baby Picture Library: Ian Hooton (r). Science Photo Library: B. Boissonnet (l). 132 Getty Images: Alterndo Images (l). 134 Mother & Baby Picture Library: Ruth Jenkinson. 135 Mother & Baby Picture Library: Ian Hooton. 136 Getty Images: Jose Luis Paleaz (l). Mother & Baby Picture Library: Helen McCardle (c). 145 Getty Images: B2M Productions (l). Prof. J.E. Jirásek MD, DSc.: (c). 146 Alamy Images: Chris Rout. 147 Alamy Images: PHOTOTAKE Inc. 149 Prof. J.E. Jirásek MD, DSc.. 150 Getty Images: B2M Productions. 151 Science Photo Library: Anatomical Travelogue. 153 Babybond® www.babybond.com. 155 Lennart Nilsson Image Bank. 156 Getty Images: PhotoConcepts . 157 Prof. J.E. Jirásek MD, DSc.. 159 Science Photo Library: Edelmann. 161 Science Photo Library: Anatomical Travelogue. 162 Getty Images: Katrina Wittkamp. 163 Science Photo Library: P. Saada / Eurelios. 165 Science Photo Library: Dopamine. 167 Science Photo Library: Anatomical Travelogue. 169 Babybond® www.babybond.com: (c). Getty Images: Adam Gault / SPL (r). 171 Science Photo Library: Edelmann. 173 Science Photo Library: Dopamine. 174 Alamy Images: Chris Rout. 175 Wellcome Images. 177 Science Photo Library: Dr. Najeeb Layyous. 179 Dreamstime.com. 180 Getty Images: Simon Stanmore. 181 Science Photo Library: BSIP, Marigaux. 182 Getty Images: Adam Gault / SPL. 183 Alamy Images: Nic Cleave. 185 Science Photo Library: Steve Allen. 187 Alamy Images: Paula Showen (b). Science Photo Library: Dr. Najeeb Layyous. 189 Babybond® www.babybond.com. 191 Photolibrary: Neil Bromhall. 192 Getty Images: JGI. 197 Babybond® www.babybond.com. 199 Science Photo Library: Dr. Najeeb Layyous (c). 201 Babybond® www.babybond.com. 203 Babybond® www.babybond.com. 205 Babybond® www.babybond. com. 207 Photolibrary: Scott Camazine. 209 Science Photo Library: Zephyr. 212 Getty Images: Tom Grill. 213 Science Photo Library: Anatomical Travelogue. 214 Photolibrary: BSIP Medical / Chassenet. 215 Science Photo Library: Dr. Najeeb Layyous. 217 PhototakeUSA.com: LookatSciences. 219 Getty Images: MedicalRF. com (b). Science Photo Library: Dr. Najeeb Layyous (t). 220 Getty Images: Jamie Grill . 221 Science Photo Library: Du Cane Medical Imaging Ltd. 223 Science Photo Library: Dr. Najeeb Layyous. 225 Science Photo Library: Medi-mation. 226 Mother & Baby Picture Library: Ian Hooton. 232 Corbis: Jerry Tobias. 251 Photolibrary: Graham Monro (r). 254 Getty Images: LWA (l). Mother & Baby Picture Library: Paul Mitchell (r). 258 Getty Images: LWA (r). 264 Mother & Baby Picture Library: Ian Hooton (r). 268 Science Photo Library: Simon Fraser (l). 272 Getty Images: Reggie Casagrande (l). Mother & Baby Picture Library: James Thomson (c). 276 Science Photo Library: Anatomical Travelogue. 278 Mother & Baby Picture Library: Ian Hooton. 283 SuperStock: Cultura Limited (l). 286 Getty Images: National Geographic (r). Mother & Baby Picture Library: Ruth Jenkinson (l). 288 Science Photo Library: Astier (l). 290 Getty Images: Science Photo Library (l). Science Photo Library: BSIP, Laurent (r). 302 Getty Images: Roderick Chen (r). Mother & Baby Picture Library: Ruth Jenkinson (l). 304 Corbis: Ocean. 306 Getty Images: ERproductions Ltd . 310 Science Photo Library: BSIP, ASTIER. 312 Science Photo Library: Joseph Nettis (l). 314 Science Photo Library: Tracy Dominey (r); Antonia Reeve (l). 318 Getty Images: National Geographic (l). Science Photo Library: B. Boissonnet (r). 324 Getty Images: Frank Herholdt. 326 Getty Images: Ryo Ohwada (c). iStockphoto.com: Gianlucabartoli (l). 327 Science Photo Library: Dr. P. Marazzi. 328 Alamy Images: Janine Wiedel Photolibrary (l). Mother & Baby Picture Library: Ian Hooton (r). 334 Alamy Images: Alena Sudová (l). 335 Alamy Images: Peter Usbeck. 336 Science Photo Library: Samuel Ashfield. 340 Mother & Baby Picture Library: Ian Hooton (r). 370 Getty Images: Fuse (r). 372 Getty Images: Blend Images / Inti St Clair (l). 378 Getty Images: Plattform (r). 380 Alamy Images: WoodyStock (l, r). 381 Getty Images: Ian Hooton / SPL. 382 Corbis: Tim Pannell (r). Getty Images: Fuse (l). 383 Getty Images: Robert Houser

Jacket images: Front: Jose Luis Pelaez Inc./GetStock.com br Back: Getty Images: Ian Hooton / SPL bl

All other images © Dorling Kindersley
For further information see: www.dkimages.com